WHEATER'S
BASIC
HISTOPATHOLOGY

Commissioning Editor: Timothy Horne
Project Development Manager: Jim Killgore
Project Manager: Nancy Arnott
Designer: Erik Bigland
Indexer: Laurence Errington

WHEATER'S
BASIC
HISTOPATHOLOGY

A COLOUR ATLAS AND TEXT

FOURTH EDITION BY

ALAN STEVENS
MBBS, FRCPath
Consultant Histopathologist to Queen's Medical Centre University Hospital NHS Trust,
Nottingham, UK

JAMES S. LOWE
BMedSci, BMBS, DM, FRCPath
Professor of Neuropathology, University of Nottingham Medical School
Honorary Consultant Histopathologist to Queen's Medical Centre University Hospital NHS Trust,
Nottingham, UK

BARBARA YOUNG
BSc Med Sci (Hons), PhD, MB BChir, MRCP, FRCPA
Senior Staff Specialist in Anatomical Pathology, PaLMS, Royal North Shore Hospital
Clinical Associate Professor, University of Sydney, Sydney, Australia

---

THIRD EDITION BY

H. GEORGE BURKITT
ALAN STEVENS
JAMES LOWE
BARBARA YOUNG

DRAWINGS BY

PHILIP J. DEAKIN
BSc Hons (Sheffield), MB ChB (Sheffield)
General Medical Practitioner, Sheffield, UK

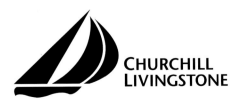

CHURCHILL
LIVINGSTONE

EDINBURGH LONDON NEW YORK OXFORD PHILADELPHIA ST LOUIS SYDNEY TORONTO 2002

CHURCHILL LIVINGSTONE

An imprint of Elsevier Limited

First edition 1985
Second edition 1991
Third edition 1996
Fourth edition 2002

ISBN 0 443 07001 6
Reprinted 2003, 2005

International Edition ISBN 0 443 07002 4
Reprinted 2003, 2005, 2006

British Library Cataloguing in Publication Data
A catalogue record for this book is available from the British Library

Library of Congress Cataloguing in Publication Data
A catalogue record for this book is available from the Library of Congress

Note
Medical knowledge is constantly changing. As new information becomes available, changes in treatment, procedures, equipment and the use of drugs become necessary. The authors and the publishers have taken care to ensure that the information given in this text is accurate and up to date. However, readers are strongly advised to confirm that the information, especially with regard to drug usage, complies with the latest legislation and standards of practice.

ELSEVIER your source for books, journals and multimedia in the health sciences

www.elsevierhealth.com

Working together to grow
libraries in developing countries

www.elsevier.com | www.bookaid.org | www.sabre.org

ELSEVIER **BOOK AID International** **Sabre Foundation**

The publisher's policy is to use **paper manufactured from sustainable forests**

Printed in China

Preface to the Fourth Edition

In the fourth edition of *Basic Histopathology*, we have maintained the format of previous editions, with the teaching text in the form of expanded captions related to high quality labelled photomicrographs illustrating the essential features of the pathology. Each chapter opens with an introductory overview to set the scene, and simple flow charts, line diagrams and revision lists are included where relevant. The text has been updated where necessary, and some sections have been comprehensively rewritten to clarify and emphasise current understanding of the topic. However, the major change in this edition has been the introduction of new photomicrographs and the improvement of many of the previously used pictures using computer manipulation of digitised images. Many of the new photomicrographs have also been generated using a digital camera. We have increased the size of some of the photomicrographs wherever clear layout and pagination permitted it.

This fourth edition still contains some of the original photomicrographs used in the first edition 17 years ago. It is gratifying that no amount of computer jiggery-pokery has been able to improve these original photographs taken by our dear friend and original co-author, the late Paul Wheater.

Alan Stevens, James Lowe, Barbara Young
Nottingham and Sydney, 2002

Preface to the First Edition

Histopathology is an essential component of pathology teaching in all medical and dental courses, nevertheless the scope, content and emphasis on microscopy vary considerably between different centres. Adding to this diversity are the different stages in the preclinical and/or clinical years when the subject matter is presented. This book has been designed to meet as closely as possible the requirements of these many differing courses. We believe that practical microscopy is an important part of pathology teaching, and therefore we have chosen to centre our discussion around appropriate colour photomicrographs as might be done in the lecture room or microscope laboratory. The text has been designed as a series of amplified captions explaining not only the features visible in the labelled colour plates, but also providing some background text in order to relate the subject matter to the theoretical and clinical implications of the pathological processes. Consequently this book should not be regarded as a copiously illustrated introductory textbook of pathology, but rather it is intended as a histopathology companion to any of the many excellent standard pathology textbooks; the text, though more than normally found in an atlas, is thus by no means comprehensive.

The subject matter has been divided into two sections, the first covering basic pathological processes and the second encompassing the common diseases encountered in systems pathology. In general, our material has been taken from both surgical and necropsy specimens of common clinical conditions. Uncommon conditions have been included only where they illustrate important pathological principles. The haematoxylin and eosin staining method has mainly been employed as is standard practice in pathology laboratories, but special staining methods have been occasionally used where appropriate. Rather than specifying numerical magnification factors, each micrograph has been designated as low power, medium power or high power by the abbreviations LP, MP and HP respectively as this is probably more relevant to student needs.

It is our hope that this book will be useful both as a guide in formal practical classes, as well as assisting the student in private study. Although the book is primarily aimed at preclinical and clinical medical and dental students, it would also prove useful for other groups such as veterinary science students, medical laboratory scientists specialising in histopathology, and candidates for post-graduate examinations in surgery and pathology.

Nottingham, 1985

P.R.W.
H.G.B.
A.S.
J.L.

Acknowledgements to Fourth Edition

In a book such as this, the photomicrographs which finally appear represent only a minute proportion of the vast number of microscope slides prepared for review and selection prior to photomicrography.

A great debt of gratitude is therefore owed to the BMS staff in the Departments of Histopathology at QMC, Nottingham and at the Department of Anatomical Pathology, Pacific Laboratory Medicine Services (PaLMS), Royal North Shore Hospital, particularly Janet Palmer, Anne and Ian Wilson, Carol Dunn and Liz Bakowski in Nottingham, and Adele Clarkson, Rob Stewart, Dianne Reader and Liam O'Donnell in Sydney. We are also very grateful to all Staff Specialists and Registrars in Anatomical Pathology at PaLMS who generously provided cases. Particular thanks go to Associate Professor R.P. Eckstein, who provided the photograph for Figure 15.4b. The electron micrographs and acrylic resin sections were prepared by Trevor Gray, Stan Terras, Neil Hand and Jane Watson at Nottingham.

For this fourth edition, our main acknowledgment must be to Anne Kane, of the Department of Histopathology, Queen's Medical Centre, Nottingham who has been responsible for skilfully and patiently improving many of the pictures from previous editions of the book, as well as generating high quality digital images for the new photomicrographs. The authors are extremely grateful for her efforts. We are grateful to Isabella Streeter, Linda Dewdney and Irene Smith in Nottingham for secretarial assistance.

The authors wish to thank the staff of Elsevier Science, particularly Jim Killgore who steered us through the majority of this edition, and Timothy Horne who kept an eye on it throughout.

Contents

BASIC PATHOLOGICAL PROCESSES

PART ONE

1. Cellular responses to injury

Introduction

The constantly changing environment demands a considerable degree of cellular adaptability. Most of these adaptations are at a biochemical level and represent fine regulation of metabolic function. However, many adaptations are also accompanied by structural changes which are visible microscopically. Many such structural changes fall within the normal pattern of growth of a tissue; for example, the thyroid gland enlarges in pregnancy owing to the action of increased thyroid-stimulating hormone on thyroid epithelial cells. This is an example of physiological cellular adaptation to a stimulus within the normal range. In contrast, certain environmental changes lie outside the normal physiological range and result in cell damage and/or failure of the cells to function adequately: these stimuli are termed ***pathological***.

Cells respond to changes in their environment as summarised in Figure 1.1. If a cell makes a successful adaptation to an environmental change, then it will either return to normal or it may make an adaptive change. Such adaptive changes are presented in Chapter 6. If a cell is unable to respond successfully to an environmental change, then the cell may die. This chapter will consider the morphological changes that occur when cells respond to environmental change and what happens when they fail, leading to cell death. There is a further consequence of unsuccessful adaptation to an environmental change, the development of neoplasia, which will be discussed in Chapter 7.

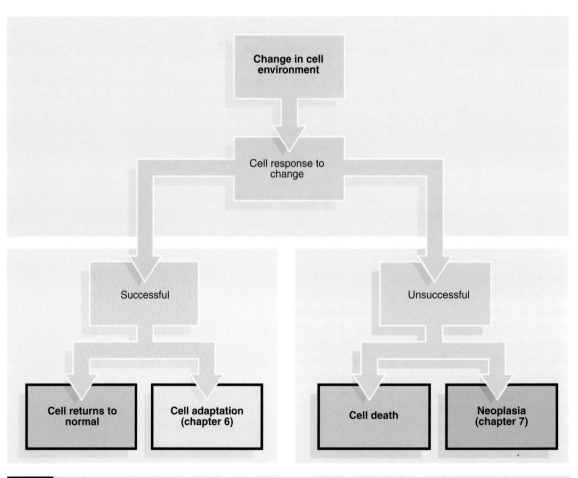

Fig. 1.1 Cellular adaptation

The fate of a cell which is exposed to a harmful stimulus depends in part on the magnitude of the injury, and in part on how vulnerable the cell is to the injury. For example, a cerebral neurone is much more vulnerable to damage following hypoxia than a fibroblast.

When a cell is exposed to a harmful stimulus, before structural changes can be detected, a cell stress response takes place. In this response, the cell turns off most genes and activates a set of genes coding for cell stress proteins, which have cytoprotective effects. While this response has no routine morphological changes, cell stress proteins can be detected using immunochemistry. The common routes and endpoints following cell injury are summarised in Figure 1.2.

Response of cells to injury (see Fig. 1.2)

The ultimate fate of a cell, once exposed to a harmful stimulus, depends on whether the damage affects selected sub-cellular systems, or the cell as a whole. It is still uncertain why a cell decides to undergo apoptosis rather than necrosis – but insights into cell biology are starting to give the answers. If there is mild damage to cell components, including the energy supply, then a cell may develop morphological changes termed cellular degeneration. The commonest structural changes are *cloudy swelling*, *hydropic degeneration*, and *fatty change* (see Figs 1.4 and 1.5). Importantly, such morphological changes are reversible if the causative environmental change is removed or abates. Under such circumstances, a cell may return to normal after removal of damaged organelles through autophagy and the synthesis of new proteins. However, the outcome is not always successful and the damaged cell may still die (see later).

If a cell develops non-selective, irreversible damage to many cell components then it is unable to respond and dies. Following cell death, a series of morphological changes take place termed *necrosis* (Figs 1.6 and 1.7). Necrosis may also take place if, following development of the changes of cell degeneration, the harmful stimulus does not abate.

Selective damage to certain key cellular components may trigger a process of programmed cell death, termed *apoptosis*. This is a highly organised process where intracellular signalling systems bring about destruction of the cell. Damage to DNA, cell surface membrane, or mitochondria are potent stimuli for apoptosis. Additionally, some cells that have initially responded by showing signs of cell degeneration (sublethal cell injury) may enter programmed cell death and die through apoptosis.

Although discussed later in Chapter 7, it is important to note here that some harmful stimuli to cells can cause non-lethal DNA damage that leads to mutations and development of *dysplasia* and *neoplasia*.

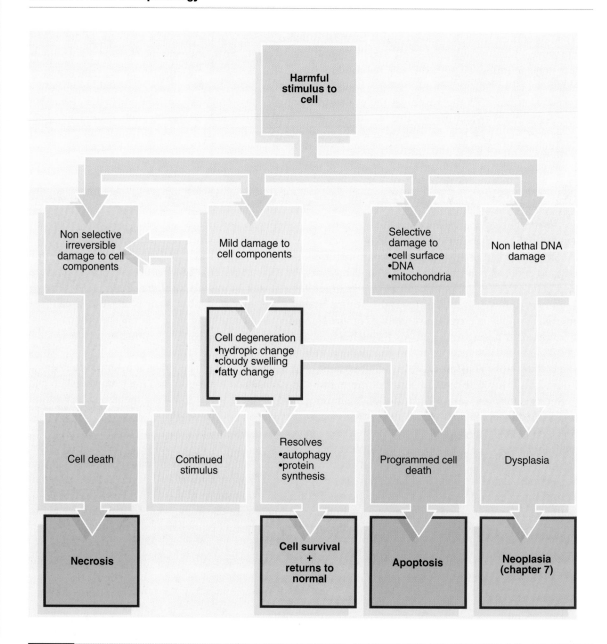

Fig. 1.2 Response of cells to injury

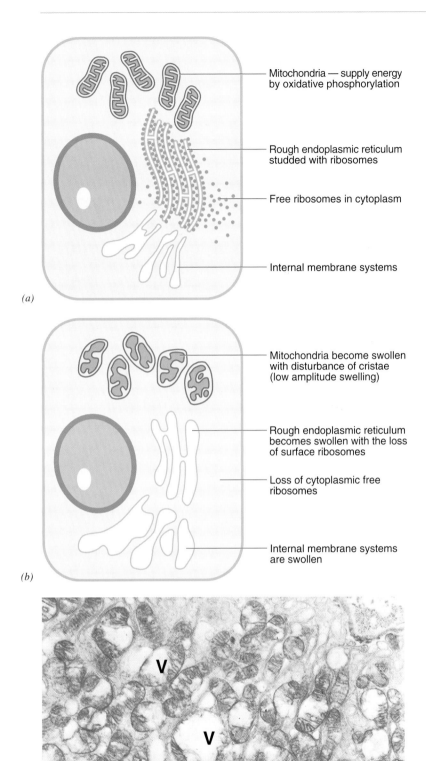

Mitochondria — supply energy by oxidative phosphorylation

Rough endoplasmic reticulum studded with ribosomes

Free ribosomes in cytoplasm

Internal membrane systems

(a)

Mitochondria become swollen with disturbance of cristae (low amplitude swelling)

Rough endoplasmic reticulum becomes swollen with the loss of surface ribosomes

Loss of cytoplasmic free ribosomes

Internal membrane systems are swollen

(b)

(c)

Fig. 1.3 **Early cellular responses to injury**

(a) Normal cell
(b) Reversible cell damage
(c) EM

The first ultrastructural evidence of sub-lethal cell damage is swelling of membrane-bound organelles, particularly endoplasmic reticulum and mitochondria.

In micrograph (c), an electron micrograph of a renal tubular epithelial cell damaged by hypoxia, most of the mitochondria are swollen. Instead of regular stacks of cristae (inner mitochondrial membrane), several of the mitochondria now contain spaces or vacuoles **V** pushing the cristae apart. This is probably a result of accumulation of electrolytes and water owing to early damage to the enzymes of the membrane sodium pump. This change is potentially reversible if the noxious stimulus is insufficient to cause cell death. Further insult leads to destruction of the cristae, more severe swelling of the mitochondria and formation of electron-dense bodies. At this stage, the changes are probably not reversible and cell death occurs when ATP production is insufficient to maintain other cellular functions.

Another manifestation of early cell injury is loss of ribosomes from both cytosol and the surface of the rough endoplasmic reticulum. Inner cell membrane systems, particularly the endoplasmic reticulum, become dilated and swollen. Later, the swelling leads to vacuolation which is visible by light microscopy (see Fig. 1.4). Lethal injury is marked by progressive disintegration of other organelles, particularly lysosomes which release hydrolytic enzymes causing auto-digestion of the cell (*autolysis*).

The mitochondrion is the probable 'transducer' for cell death:

● If there is selective damage to a few mitochondria, intracellular signals promote apoptotic cell death.
● If there is overwhelming damage to most mitochondria, a cell dies and goes through necrosis.

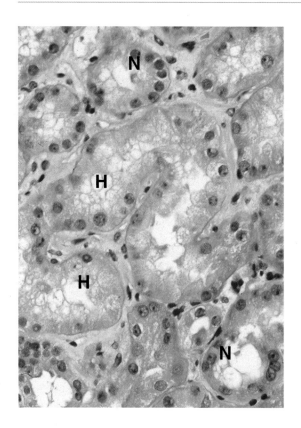

Fig. 1.4 Hydropic degeneration: kidney (HP)

The earliest light microscopic evidence of cellular injury is loss of normal staining intensity of the cytoplasm owing to swelling of membrane-bound organelles. Normal cytoplasm stained with haematoxylin and eosin is light pink with a faint tint of blue; the blue tint (basophilia) is mainly due to the presence of ribosomal RNA. With sub-lethal cellular damage, ribosomes are reduced in number and the normal blue cytoplasmic tint is lost. Swelling of endoplasmic reticulum and mitochondria contribute to further cytoplasmic pallor. This is described as *cloudy swelling* and may be subtle and difficult to identify. With further swelling of organelles, the cell becomes waterlogged and true vacuoles appear in the cytoplasm, which now stains faintly with total loss of basophilia. At this stage, cells are said to exhibit *hydropic degeneration*.

This micrograph shows a section of kidney deprived of blood flow owing to severe hypotension. Undamaged tubules are seen lined by normal staining epithelial cells **N**. Some of the tubules are damaged, the cells being pale and vacuolated and exhibiting hydropic degeneration **H**. Such damage to the renal tubules may lead to acute renal failure.

Cloudy swelling and hydropic change reflect failure of membrane ion pumps, because of lack of cellular ATP, allowing the cell to accumulate fluid.

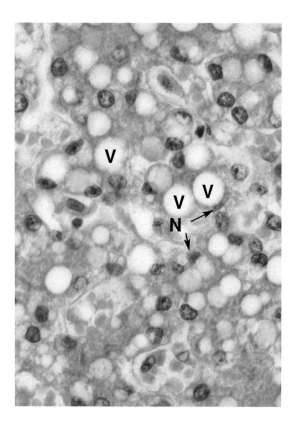

Fig. 1.5 Fatty change: liver (HP)

Fatty change is another manifestation of sub-lethal metabolic derangement seen in certain cell types with high energy demand. It is most common in the liver, as in this example, but also occurs in the myocardium and kidney. The common causes of fatty change are toxins (particularly alcohol and halogenated hydrocarbons such as chloroform), chronic hypoxia, diabetes mellitus and obesity. Impaired metabolism of fatty acids leads to accumulation of triglycerides (fat) that form non-membrane-bound vacuoles in cells, which may displace the nucleus from its usual location.

This example of liver from an alcoholic shows large vacuoles **V** in the hepatocytes with displacement of the nucleus **N**. In conventionally processed tissue, organic solvents used in preparation dissolve out the fat to leave empty, non-staining spaces. Frozen sections can, however, be prepared to preserve the fat, which can then be specifically stained.

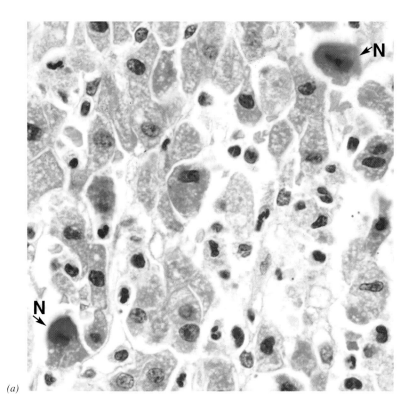

(a)

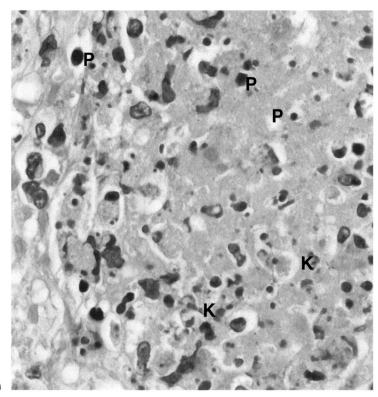

(b)

Fig. 1.6 Cell necrosis
(a) Liver (HP)
(b) Renal cortex (HP)

When a cell has sustained irreversible damage, a succession of histological changes occur which are grouped under the term *necrosis*.

Micrograph (a) is a section of liver from a person poisoned by paracetamol, an hepatic toxin. Many of the hepatocytes are pale-stained and a few exhibit early cytoplasmic vacuolation, indicating sub-lethal injury. Several cells also show histological features of necrosis **N**. The dead cells stain a bright pink (eosinophilia) and stand out from the other cells; this is due to degeneration of structural proteins which form a compact homogeneous mass. Compared to living cells, the nucleus of each necrotic cell is smaller, condensed and intensely stained with haematoxylin (basophilia). This nuclear condensation is termed *pyknosis* and is due to progressive chromatin clumping, possibly as a result of reduced pH resulting from terminal anaerobic metabolism.

Further nuclear changes are seen in micrograph (b), which is a portion of necrotic kidney. Pyknotic nuclei **P** stand out as intensely basophilic, round bodies. Note that the nuclear changes are accompanied by cytoplasmic changes. The cytoplasm has lost definition and the cell margins (plasma membranes) are indistinct.

With further degeneration, the pyknotic nuclei become fragmented into several particles which represent pieces of degenerate nuclear material, a change termed *karyorrhexis* **K**.

Complete breakdown of nuclear material then takes place by release of cellular hydrolytic enzymes, leading to loss of the groups which bind haematoxylin. This process is termed *karyolysis* and, when complete, leaves the dead cell as an anucleate, homogeneous, eosinophilic mass.

Many of the structural changes seen in necrosis are mediated through the action of lysosomal enzymes, liberated through breakdown of internal cell membranes.

BASIC PATHOLOGICAL PROCESSES

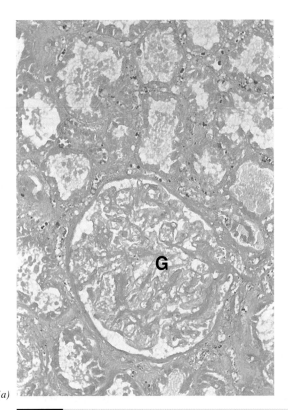

(a)

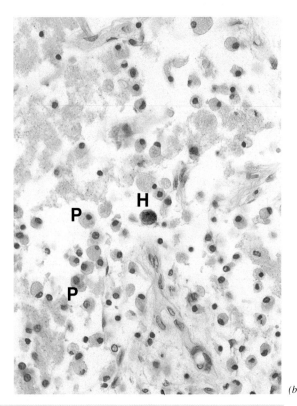

(b)

Fig. 1.7 **Patterns of tissue necrosis**
(a) Coagulative necrosis: kidney (MP)   (b) Colliquative necrosis: brain (HP)

Traditionally, three main patterns of tissue necrosis are described: *coagulative*, *colliquative* and *caseous*. Each term describes the macroscopic appearance of necrotic tissue. In coagulative necrosis, the tissue appears firm as if cooked. In colliquative necrosis, the dead tissue appears semi-liquid, while in caseous necrosis, the dead tissue has a soft consistency reminiscent of cream cheese. These gross patterns correlate closely with histological appearances.

In areas of coagulative necrosis, much of the cellular outline and tissue architecture can be discerned histologically even though the cells are dead. The commonest cause of this pattern of necrosis is ischaemia owing to loss of arterial oxygenated blood.

In areas of caseous necrosis, cells die and form an amorphous proteinaceous mass in which no semblance of original architecture can be discerned. Caseous necrosis is typically seen in tuberculosis, several examples of which are shown in Chapter 4.

The term colliquative necrosis was originally used to describe the macroscopic appearance of necrosis in the brain as a result of arterial occlusion (cerebral infarction), at a stage when the necrotic area was occupied by semi-liquid material. This appearance, however, is not a specific form of necrosis but results from dissolution of tissue after an initial coagulative phase, which is common to all tissues immediately following cell death.

The subsequent liquefaction of dead tissue reflects both tissue composition and the cause of necrosis. In brain, the relative lack of extracellular structural proteins (reticulin and collagen) leads to rapid loss of tissue architecture as autolysis occurs, resulting in the early formation of a semi-liquid mass of dead cells. Otherwise, liquefaction of dead tissues is virtually confined to cases of necrosis associated with pyogenic (pus-producing) bacteria such as in an abscess (Fig. 2.13).

Micrograph (a) is an example of coagulative necrosis in an area of kidney subject to infarction. Note that the architecture of a glomerulus **G** and surrounding tubules is still recognisable despite the dissolution of nuclear material except for a few pyknotic and karyorrhectic remnants.

Micrograph (b) illustrates the liquefaction phase in a cerebral infarct where no residual tissue architecture is preserved; the earlier phase of coagulative necrosis in brain can be seen in Figure 23.2. The necrotic brain is now largely replaced by wisps of pink-staining cellular debris, with phagocytic cells **P** engulfing degenerate material. Some of these contain haemosiderin pigment **H** which is a breakdown product of haemoglobin and is indicative of haemorrhage into the tissue.

A fourth type of necrosis, known as *fibrinoid necrosis*, is principally seen in the walls of blood vessels and is discussed in Chapter 11.

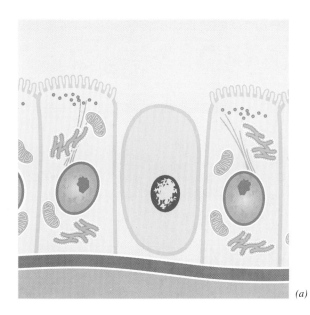

(a)

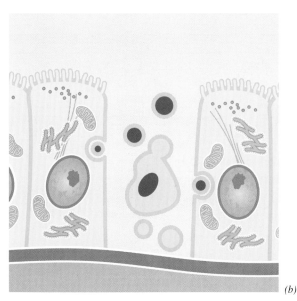

(b)

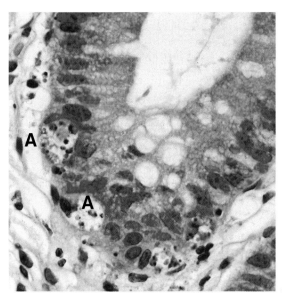

(c)

Fig. 1.8 Apoptosis
(a) Early stage
(b) Later stage
(c) Apoptosis in colonic glands (HP)

Certain stimuli to cells lead to their controlled elimination by programmed cell death in a process called *apoptosis*. While apoptosis is a normal physiological process, for example in development and cell turnover, it is also an important way for elimination of damaged or diseased cells. Normal cells switch off their house-keeping genes and express genes that bring about cell death. When apoptosis is triggered, cells undergo a distinct set of structural changes.

Diagram (a) illustrates how the cell loses specialised surface features and attachments to other cells and structures, becoming 'rounded up'. At this stage proteases, termed caspases, cleave cellular proteins, while endonucleases break down chromatin. The nucleus becomes shrunken with dense condensation of chromatin beneath the nuclear membrane.

Diagram (b) illustrates the rapid fragmentation of the cell into multiple small *apoptotic bodies*, each one being membrane-bound and many containing nuclear remnants. Each fragment is still a vital entity. The surface membranes express factors that facilitate phagocytosis by adjacent cells.

Many stimuli can activate apoptosis. Cell membrane damage, damage to mitochondria, damage to DNA, viral infection, and immune-mediated attack are all common triggers. The benefit of eliminating cells by apoptosis is that individual cells can be eliminated in a way that does not stimulate a tissue response to cell death in terms of an inflammatory response.

Micrograph (c) shows apoptosis in colonic glands in a patient who had a bone marrow graft and is suffering from graft-versus-host disease in which donor immune cells attack host tissues, in this case the colonic epithelial cells.

At least three late apoptotic cells **A** represented by multiple dot-like *apoptotic bodies* are seen.

In tumour pathology, apoptosis is a major factor that limits the growth of a neoplasm. The production by tumour cells of factors that prevent apoptosis is an important mechanism in development of uncontrolled growth.

BASIC PATHOLOGICAL PROCESSES

2. Acute inflammation, healing and repair

Introduction

Inflammation is an almost universal response to tissue damage by a wide range of harmful stimuli including mechanical trauma, tissue necrosis and infection. The purpose of inflammation is to destroy (or contain) the damaging agent, initiate repair processes and return the damaged tissue to useful function. Inflammation is somewhat arbitrarily divided into ***acute*** and ***chronic inflammation*** but in reality the two often form a continuum. Many causes of tissue damage provoke an acute inflammatory response but some types of insult may bring about a typical chronic inflammatory reaction from the outset (e.g. viral infections, foreign body reactions and fungal infections). Acute inflammation may ***resolve*** or ***heal by scarring*** but may also progress to chronic inflammation and it is common for a mixed acute and chronic response to coexist. This chapter describes acute inflammation and its sequelae, while chronic inflammation is discussed in Chapter 3. Many examples of acute and chronic inflammation are illustrated in Chapter 4.

There are three major and interrelated components of acute inflammation:

- **Vascular dilatation**
  - relaxation of vascular smooth muscle leading to engorgement of tissue with blood (***hyperaemia***).
- **Endothelial activation**
  - increased endothelial permeability allows plasma proteins to pass into tissues
  - expression of adhesion molecules on the endothelial surface mediates neutrophil adherence
  - production of factors which cause vascular dilatation.
- **Neutrophil activation**
  - expression of adhesion molecules causes neutrophils to adhere to endothelium
  - increased motility allows emigration from vessels into surrounding tissues
  - increased capacity for bacterial killing.

Fig. 2.1 Mechanism of early acute inflammation (*illustration opposite*)

Acute inflammation may develop over minutes or hours depending on the type and severity of the tissue damage and generally lasts hours to days. Vascular dilatation, increased vascular permeability and neutrophil activation and migration are interdependent processes and all three are required for the full response. Immediately after the tissue damage has occurred, there may be a brief phase of constriction of arterioles but this is followed within seconds by arteriolar dilatation, which leads to increased blood flow to the area. At much the same time, gaps form between endothelial cells of the capillaries allowing protein-rich plasma to leak into the tissue. The dilated capillaries become engorged with red cells and blood flow slows and then stops. The slowing of blood flow brings neutrophils into contact with the endothelial cells, which have been busy inserting adhesion molecules into their plasma membranes. As the neutrophils come into contact with the endothelium, ***adhesion molecules*** on the neutrophil plasma membrane bind to their complementary receptors on the endothelial cells and become stuck. Activation of the neutrophils plays a role here so that activated neutrophils are more likely to stick. Meanwhile in the tissues, the plasma-derived proteins undergo various changes. The ***complement cascade*** is initiated (alternative pathway) forming components with a wide range of

activities. ***Immunoglobulins*** bind to any causative organisms immobilising them, and forming immune complexes that further activate complement (classical pathway). ***Fibrinogen*** is cleaved to form monomers which then polymerise to form a network of ***fibrin*** that impedes the movement of any pathogenic organisms present, and also provides a framework for the movement of neutrophils. The increased fluid in the tissue causes an increased flow of lymph to carry immune complexes and antigenic material to the lymph nodes where a specific immune response is initiated over a matter of days. The neutrophils pass through the basement membrane of the endothelium and move along a concentration gradient of ***chemotactic factors***. When they arrive at the site of injury, the activated neutrophils phagocytose necrotic tissue debris and any pathogenic organisms. The activation of the neutrophils makes them more efficient at phagocytosis and bacterial killing. Opsonisation of bacteria by complement and immunoglobulins renders them more readily phagocytosed.

This entire process is orchestrated by a plethora of chemical mediators derived from injured tissues, bacteria, plasma proteins and leucocytes. The most important of these mediators are indicated at their sites of action. Note that some mediators have multiple actions.

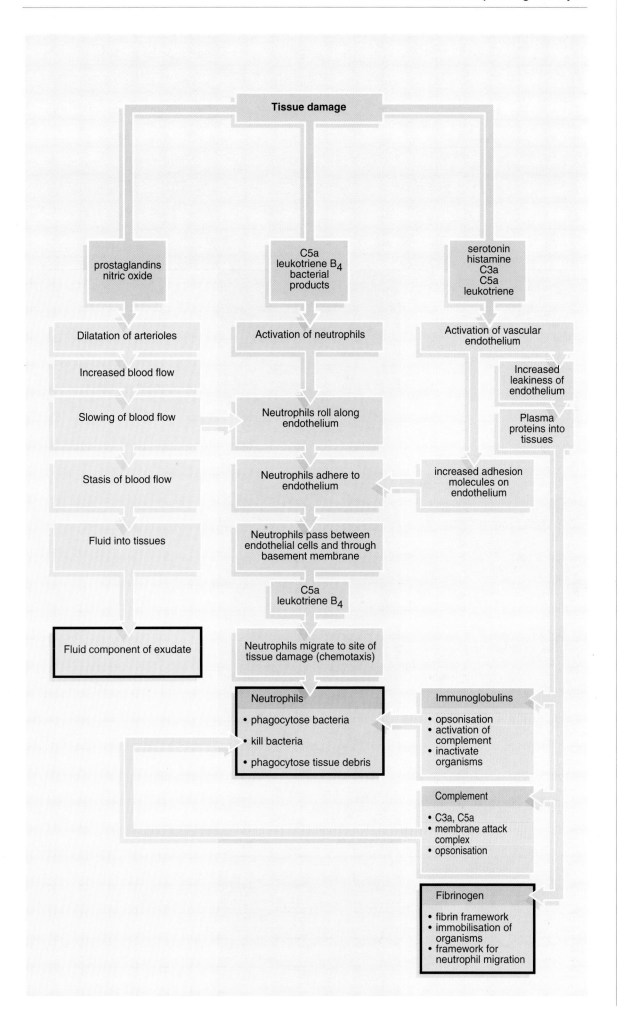

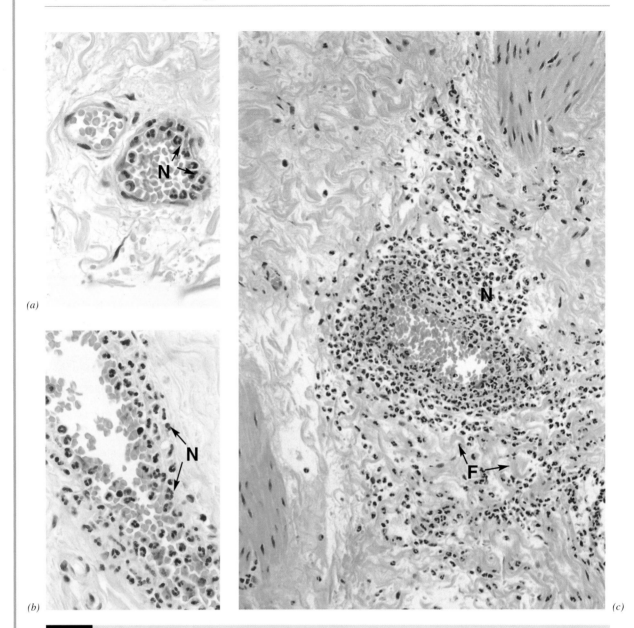

(a)

(b)

(c)

Fig. 2.2 Formation of the acute inflammatory exudate
(a) Early vascular changes (HP) (b) Migration of neutrophils (HP) (c) Early formation of exudate (LP)

This set of micrographs illustrates the sequence of events during the initial phases of the acute inflammatory response described in Figure 2.1. In micrograph (a), two small capillaries are shown. Both vessels are dilated and in the larger, neutrophils **N** line up around the periphery of the vessel, a process termed *pavementation*. These neutrophils are adherent to the endothelium. The surrounding fibrous connective tissue contains clear spaces owing to the accumulation of fluid (*oedema*) between the collagen bundles. Plasma proteins, although not visible, are also found free within the tissue. These include the blood coagulation protein *fibrinogen* which is converted to insoluble *fibrin*, which will later form a meshwork within the tissue.

The neutrophils pass through the vessel wall by extending their pseudopodia between adjacent endothelial cells. The neutrophils then penetrate the endothelial basement membrane and move into the perivascular connective tissue as shown in micrograph (b). Once in the extravascular tissues **N**, the neutrophils are attracted to the site of tissue damage by chemotactic

agents such as the complement component *C5a* and migrate actively towards higher concentrations of these agents (*chemotaxis*); this is shown in micrograph (c). At the site of tissue damage, neutrophils play an important role in destruction of microorganisms. Phagocytosis of organisms is promoted by a coating of immunoglobulin and complement (*opsonisation*) and activated neutrophils are more effective at killing pathogens. These three components, namely water, proteins (including fibrin **F**) and neutrophils **N**, form the typical *acute inflammatory exudate*.

Chemical mediators, although not visible, control this process. Vasodilatation is mediated by *prostaglandins* and *nitric oxide*. Increased vascular permeability is controlled by substances such as the vasoactive amines, serotonin and histamine, complement components *C5a* and *C3a, leukotrienes C_4, D_4* and *E_4, platelet activating factor (PAF)* and *substance P*. Leucocyte activation and chemotaxis are influenced by *C5a, leukotriene B_4*, various *chemokines* and bacterial products.

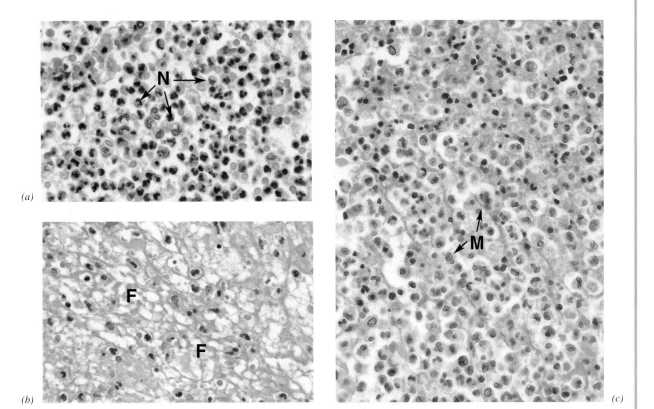

Fig. 2.3 Acute inflammatory exudate
(a) Neutrophilic exudate (HP) (b) Highly fibrinous exudate (HP) (c) Mixed neutrophil–fibrin exudate (MP)

The quality of an acute inflammatory exudate varies depending on the state and nature of the injured tissue and the type of noxious agent involved. These micrographs show established acute inflammatory exudates differing from one another in the number of neutrophils **N** and amount of fibrin **F** present; fibrin strands stain bright pink with H&E staining.

Micrograph (a) shows an acute inflammatory exudate in which neutrophils are the main component, usually the case when the damaging stimulus is a bacterial infection; this neutrophil-rich exudate is commonly called *'pus'*, and this pattern is therefore often called *acute purulent inflammation*.

Micrograph (b) shows an acute inflammatory exudate in which fibrin is the main component (*fibrinous exudate*); this occurs most commonly on serosal surfaces (see Fig. 2.6b).

Micrograph (c) shows a mixed neutrophilic/fibrinous exudate at a late stage, with some macrophages entering the picture.

Once in the extravascular tissues, neutrophils engulf necrotic fragments of damaged tissue, breaking them down with their lysosomal enzymes. When tissue damage has been caused by bacteria, as in lobar pneumonia (Fig. 2.4), neutrophils phagocytose and kill the causative organisms. The activity of neutrophils is limited by their inability to regenerate lysosomal enzymes and, after a *respiratory burst* which generates the hydrogen peroxide used to kill bacteria, the neutrophils degenerate. Mature neutrophils only survive for 3 days but their numbers are

maintained in acute inflammation by new arrivals from the circulation; the systemic response to acute inflammation is release of neutrophils from bone marrow into the blood, resulting in a *neutrophil leukocytosis*. Degenerate neutrophils can be recognised by condensation (pyknosis) and fragmentation (karyorrhexis) of the nuclei and, eventually, cytoplasmic disintegration; this is best seen in micrograph (b).

Although the dominant cell type in the early phases of acute inflammation is the neutrophil, within 24 hours macrophages also begin to migrate into the damaged tissue and by 48–72 hours are the predominant cell type. The macrophages are derived from circulating blood monocytes. Macrophages **M**, a few of which can be seen in micrograph (c), continue the phagocytic work begun by neutrophils and ultimately mop up the degenerate neutrophils and fibrin strands. Unlike neutrophils, macrophages can regenerate their lysosomal enzymes and are capable of sustained activity. The monocytes may also act as antigen-presenting cells to initiate specific immunological responses.

The fate of the acute inflammatory exudate depends on a variety of factors including the nature and destructibility of the injurious agent, the extent of tissue damage and the properties of the tissue in which the damage has occurred.

The process of acute inflammation terminates by one of four main processes: *resolution*, *organisation and repair*, *abscess formation* or *chronic inflammation*.

BASIC PATHOLOGICAL PROCESSES

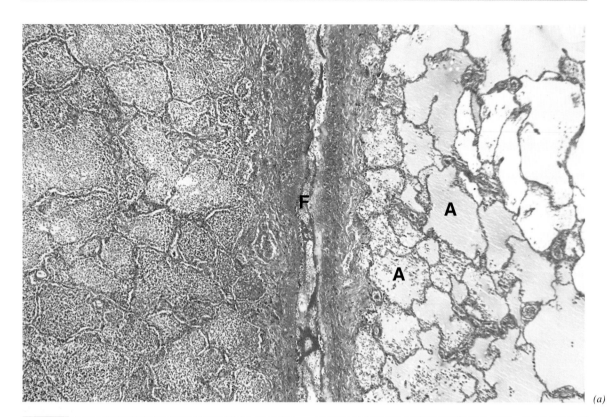

(a)

Fig. 2.4 Acute inflammation of lung: lobar pneumonia (a) LP (b) MP

An important cause of acute inflammation in the lung parenchyma is bacterial infection causing lobar pneumonia. However, the most common type of pneumonia is bronchopneumonia (Fig. 12.5) where infection spreads from the bronchi into adjacent lung tissue. In lobar pneumonia, which is less common now than previously, a whole lobe becomes solidified as a result of a massive outpouring of fluid, fibrin and neutrophils into the alveolar spaces. This pattern of pneumonia is most commonly caused by pneumococcus (*Streptococcus pneumoniae*).

In micrograph (a), a portion of lung is shown with an interlobar fissure **F** running vertically. The lung tissue on the left shows obliteration of alveolar spaces by purple-staining masses of inflammatory cells (mainly neutrophils) with associated fibrin; this is termed *consolidation*. Alveolar walls can still be discerned. The dense inflammatory exudate is sharply limited by the interlobar fissure. The lung on the right of the fissure shows the earliest changes of acute inflammation, with faint pink-staining serous exudate in alveoli **A** and early neutrophil emigration giving rise to a few scattered cells within the alveolar spaces.

At higher magnification in micrograph (b), alveolar wall capillaries **C** are seen engorged with blood. The alveolar spaces are obliterated by an acute inflammatory exudate rich in neutrophils and lesser amounts of wispy pink-stained fibrin. Occasional large, rounded mononuclear cells, macrophages **M**, can also be seen, but these are few in the acute phase of the disease.

If untreated, there are three possible outcomes to lobar pneumonia: death may occur (as in this patient), there may be complete resolution (Fig. 2.8), or, rarely, the exudate may become organised with consequent permanent fibrosis of the lung tissue.

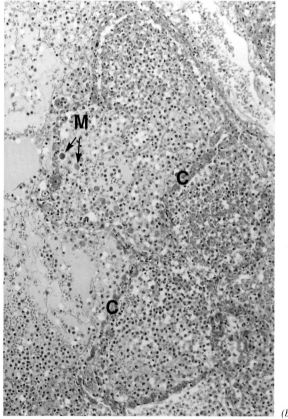

(b)

Clinical features and nomenclature of acute inflammatory processes

The vascular and exudative phenomena of acute inflammation are responsible for the clinical features and were described by Celsus in the first century AD. The *cardinal signs of Celsus* are:

- *redness* (*rubor*) caused by hyperaemia
- *swelling* (*tumor*) caused by fluid exudation and hyperaemia
- *heat* (*calor*) caused by hyperaemia
- *pain* (*dolor*) resulting from release of bradykinin and PGE_2

Galen later added:

- *loss of function* (*functio laesa*) caused by the combined effects of the above.

Clinically, patients who have significant acute inflammation feel unwell and have a fever. This is mediated by cytokines released into the blood (*interleukins 1 & 6, tumour necrosis factor (TNF)* and *prostaglandins*), acting on the hypothalamus. Laboratory investigations commonly reveal a raised neutrophil count in the blood.

The nomenclature used to describe inflammation in different tissues employs the tissue name (or its Greek or Latin equivalent) and the suffix '*-itis*'. For example, inflammation of the appendix is referred to as *appendicitis*, inflammation of the Fallopian tube is termed *salpingitis*, and inflammation of the pericardium is termed *pericarditis*. While this holds true for most tissues and organs, there are notable exceptions in traditional clinical usage. For example, inflammation of the pleura is usually termed *pleurisy*, while inflammation of subcutaneous tissues as a result of infection is usually termed acute *cellulitis*. Many examples of acute inflammatory diseases are presented in the systems pathology chapters, which form the second half of this book. In addition, the nomenclature applied to common forms of acute inflammation is presented in Figure 2.5; the causes given in this table illustrate the most common factors initiating each type of inflammatory response.

Fig. 2.5 Nomenclature and aetiology of common types of inflammation

Tissue	Acute inflammation	Typical causes
Meninges	Meningitis	Bacterial and viral infections
Brain	Encephalitis	Viral infections
Lung	Pneumonia	Bacterial infections
Pleura	Pleurisy	Bacterial and viral infections
Pericardium	Pericarditis	Bacterial and viral infections, myocardial infarction
Oesophagus	Oesophagitis	Gastric acid reflux, fungal infections
Stomach	Gastritis	Alcohol abuse, *Helicobacter pylori* infection
Colon	Colitis	Bacterial infections, ulcerative colitis
Rectum	Proctitis	Ulcerative colitis
Appendix	Appendicitis	Faecal obstruction
Liver	Hepatitis	Alcohol abuse, viral infections
Gallbladder	Cholecystitis	Bacterial infections, chemical irritation
Pancreas	Pancreatitis	Pancreatic enzyme release
Urinary bladder	Cystitis	Bacterial infections
Bone	Osteomyelitis	Bacterial infections
Subcutaneous tissues	Cellulitis	Bacterial infections
Joints	Arthritis	Bacterial and viral infections, immune complex deposition
Arteries	Arteritis	Immune complex deposition

BASIC PATHOLOGICAL PROCESSES

Morphological types of acute inflammation

While the basic process of acute inflammation is the same in all tissues, there are frequently qualitative differences in the inflammatory response seen under different circumstances. Terms describing these variations are widely used in clinical practice and are summarised below:

- *Suppurative inflammation (purulent inflammation)* refers to acute inflammation in which the acute inflammatory exudate is particularly rich in neutrophil leucocytes. Suppurative inflammation is most commonly seen as a result of infection by bacteria where the mixture of neutrophils (viable and dead), necrotic tissue, and tissue fluid in the acute inflammatory exudate form a semi-liquid material referred to as *pus*; hence the term *purulent inflammation*. This is illustrated in Fig. 2.6a. Within tissues, a circumscribed collection of semi-liquid pus is termed an *abscess* (Fig. 2.13). The destruction of tissue may be due as much to release of neutrophil lysosomal enzymes as to tissue destruction by bacteria. Bacteria which produce purulent inflammation are described as *pyogenic bacteria*. They initiate massive neutrophilic infiltration with subsequent destruction of infected tissues. Pyogenic bacteria include *Staphylococci*, some *Streptococci* (*S. pyogenes*, *S. pneumoniae*), *Escherichia coli* and the *Neisseriae* (meningococci and gonococci).

- *Fibrinous inflammation* refers to a pattern of acute inflammation where the acute inflammatory exudate has a high plasma protein content. Fibrinogen derived from plasma is converted to fibrin, which is deposited in tissues. This pattern is particularly associated with membrane-lined cavities such as the pleura, pericardium and peritoneum, where the fibrin strands form a mat-like sheet causing adhesion between adjacent surfaces. This is illustrated in Fig. 2.6b.

- *Serous inflammation* describes a pattern of acute inflammation where the main tissue response is an accumulation of fluid with a low plasma protein and cell content. This is often called a *transudate*, which by definition has a specific gravity of <1.012 in contrast to an *exudate* with a specific gravity >1.020. This pattern of response is most commonly seen in the skin in response to a burn.

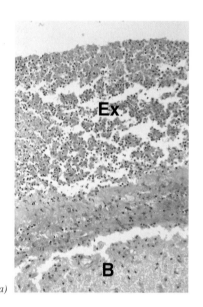

(a)

(b)

Fig. 2.6 Purulent and fibrinous inflammation
(a) Purulent inflammation: acute meningitis (LP) (b) Fibrinous inflammation: acute pericarditis (LP)

These micrographs contrast examples of purulent and fibrinous inflammation. Acute inflammation in the meninges (a) surrounding the brain illustrates an example of an exudate in which very little fibrin is formed. In acute meningitis, the exudate is almost entirely composed of oedema fluid and neutrophils.

Acute meningitis may be caused by bacterial infection (e.g. *Neisseria meningitidis* or *Streptococcus pneumoniae*). Viral and mycobacterial (tuberculous) meningitis are characterised by a chronic inflammatory reaction from the outset and this is reflected clinically by a much more subtle presentation. The presence of pathogenic bacteria in the meninges excites an acute inflammatory exudate in the subarachnoid space in which neutrophils predominate. Macroscopically, this appears as a creamy thick fluid, and the term *acute purulent inflammation* is often used to describe such a reaction. In the micrograph, note the densely cellular exudate **Ex** lying on the surface of the brain **B** in the subarachnoid space.

When an acute inflammatory exudate forms on a serosal surface, the exudate is usually dominated by the presence of large amounts of fibrin. Macroscopically, a shaggy layer of fibrin coats the formerly smooth surface. This is seen in acute pericarditis (b) and also in acute pleurisy and acute peritonitis. In this low magnification photomicrograph, the exudate **Ex** is well established on the epicardial aspect of the pericardium **P**. No myocardium is seen in this micrograph, but epicardial fat **F** is readily identifiable. Acute pericarditis most commonly occurs secondary to death of underlying cardiac muscle (*myocardial infarction*). The acute inflammatory exudate is made up of dense masses of pink-staining fibrin with comparatively few neutrophils.

The usual fate of serosal exudates is organisation via ingrowth of granulation tissue, and eventual formation of collagenous scar tissue binding adjacent serosal surfaces together. If this process occurs in the peritoneal cavity, then bowel loops can be obstructed by these fibrous adhesions.

Outcomes of acute inflammation

The process of acute inflammation is designed to neutralise injurious agents and to restore the tissue to useful function. There are four main outcomes of acute inflammation if the patient survives: *resolution, healing by fibrosis, abscess formation,* and *progression to chronic inflammation.* Three factors determine which of these outcomes occurs:

- the severity of tissue damage
- the capacity of specialised cells within the damaged tissue to divide and replace themselves, a process termed *regeneration*
- the type of agent which has caused the tissue damage.

Resolution involves complete restitution of normal architecture and function. This can only occur if the connective tissue framework of the tissue is intact and the tissue involved has the capacity to replace any specialised cells that have been lost (regeneration). Examples of resolution are recovery from sunburn (acute inflammatory response in the skin as a result of UV radiation exposure) and the restitution of normal lung structure and function following lobar pneumonia (see Fig. 2.8). Regeneration of tissues can play an important part in resolution, for example regrowth of alveolar lining cells following pneumonia. Another example of regeneration is seen in the peripheral nervous system where axonal processes can regrow following damage. This function depends on viability of the cell body of the neurone and is an example of regeneration of one part of a cell, not the formation of new cells.

Healing by fibrosis (scar formation) occurs when there is substantial damage to the connective tissue framework and/or the tissue lacks the ability to regenerate specialised cells. In these instances, dead tissues and acute inflammatory exudate are first removed from the damaged area by macrophages (see Fig. 2.7), and the defect becomes filled by ingrowth of a specialised vascular connective tissue called *granulation tissue* (see Fig. 2.9). This is termed *organisation*. The granulation tissue gradually produces collagen to form a *fibrous (collagenous) scar* constituting the process of *repair* (see Figs 2.10 and 2.11). Despite the loss of some specialised cells and some architectural distortion by fibrous scar, structural integrity is re-established. Any impairment of function is dependent on the extent of loss of specialised cells. Modified forms of fibrous repair occur in bone after a fracture when new bone is created (Fig. 2.12), and in brain with the formation of an astrocytic scar (Fig. 23.2).

Abscess formation takes place when the acute inflammatory reaction fails to destroy/remove the cause of tissue damage and continues, with a component of chronic inflammation. This is most common in the case of infection by pyogenic bacteria. As the acute inflammation progresses, there is liquefaction of the tissue to form *pus.* At the periphery of this area, a chronic inflammatory component surrounds the area and fibrous tissue is laid down, walling off the suppuration (see Fig. 2.13).

Chronic inflammation may result following acute inflammation when an injurious agent persists over a prolonged period, causing concomitant tissue destruction, inflammation, organisation and repair. Some injurious agents elicit a chronic inflammatory type of response from the outset. Chronic inflammation is discussed fully in Chapter 3.

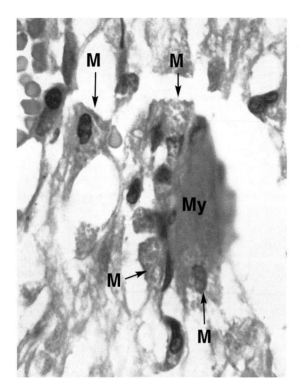

Fig. 2.7 Early outcome of acute inflammation: macrophage accumulation (HP)

As early as the second or third day of the acute inflammatory response, macrophages accumulate in increasing numbers. These enter the tissue in a similar fashion to neutrophils under the influence of chemotactic factors. Macrophages phagocytose cell debris, dead neutrophils, and fibrin. At the same time, lymphocytes begin to enter the damaged area, reflecting an immune response to any introduced antigens.

This micrograph shows an area of cardiac muscle, which has undergone necrosis following blockage of its arterial supply (*myocardial infarction*). The acute inflammatory response has almost run its course, and the neutrophils and fibrin predominant in the earlier stages have been removed by macrophages. All that remains is a soft, loose tissue containing a few necrotic myocardial remnants **My**, one of which is shown here being engulfed by macrophages **M**. The macrophages can be identified under these circumstances by the foamy appearance of their cytoplasm, which also often contains brownish pigment granules. These brown granules are iron-containing pigments (*haemosiderin*) derived from haemoglobin. Further details of the events following myocardial infarction are shown in Figure 10.2.

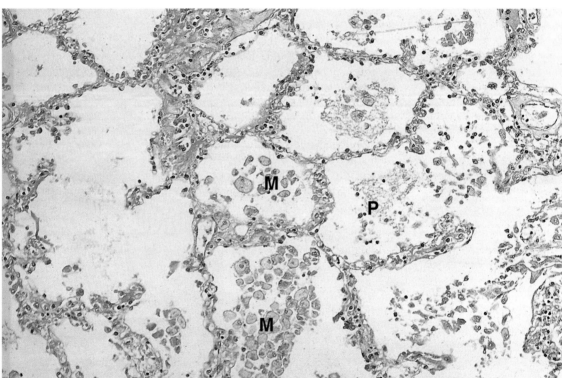

Fig. 2.8 Resolution of acute inflammation: lobar pneumonia (HP)

Occasionally, a damaging stimulus may excite a strong acute inflammatory response with minimal tissue damage. In such circumstances, resolution of the exudate may occur without any need for organisation and repair, thereby leaving no residual tissue scarring.

This phenomenon occurs in lobar pneumonia in which the acute inflammatory response is due to infection by a bacterium, commonly the pneumococcus (see Fig. 2.4). The alveoli of one or more lobes of the lung are filled with acute inflammatory exudate and the loss of respiratory function may be so great as to cause fatal *hypoxia*. This was a common cause of death in previously fit young people in the pre-antibiotic era.

Bacteria are engulfed by neutrophils, and fibrin strands are broken down by *fibrinolysins* derived from plasma and neutrophil lysosomes. Macrophages **M** are recruited and phagocytose necrotic neutrophils, extravasated red cells and other cell debris. Fluid and degraded proteinaceous material **P**, together with the macrophages are then resorbed into the circulation via alveolar wall vessels and interstitial lymphatics, or may be coughed up as brown-coloured sputum. Alveolar spaces are thus cleared of exudate and can participate in gaseous exchange. Regeneration of alveolar lining cells completes the return to normal structure and function.

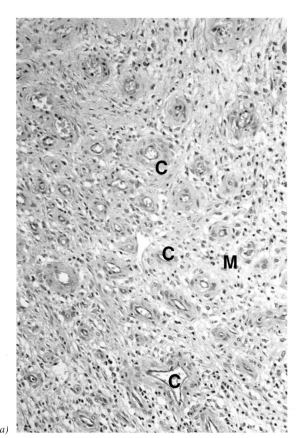

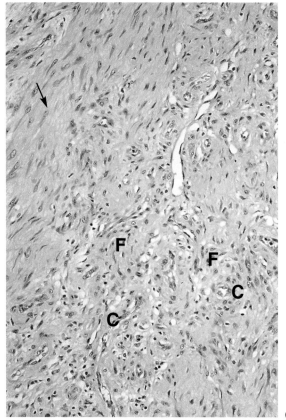

(a)   *(b)*

Fig. 2.9 Granulation tissue

(a) Vascular granulation tissue (HP) (b) Fibrous granulation tissue (HP)

Where there is significant damage to the connective tissue framework, the former site of active tissue damage and acute inflammation becomes occupied by a mixture of proliferating capillaries, fibroblasts, macrophages, lymphocytes and plasma cells, termed ***granulation tissue***.

Capillaries **C** are derived by budding from vessels at the periphery of the damaged area (***angiogenesis***) and form an interconnected network shown in micrograph (a). In this early form, termed ***vascular granulation tissue***, spaces between the capillaries are occupied by macrophages **M**, lymphocytes, proliferating fibroblasts and a loose connective tissue matrix. At the earliest stages, the capillaries are thin-walled and relatively leaky, leading to extravasation of erythrocytes and fluid into the tissue.

With time, most of the vessels regress, collagen is laid down, and the inflammatory cells return to the circulation. The effect of this progression is seen in micrograph (b), where numerous plump activated

fibroblasts **F** can be seen with a few residual lymphocytes and relatively inconspicuous capillaries **C**. This is now termed ***fibrous granulation tissue*** in recognition of the presence of mature collagenous fibrous tissue. Collagen, laid down by the fibroblasts, becomes remodelled in an orderly pattern (arrow) and the fibrous granulation tissue takes on the characteristics of an early ***fibrous scar*** as seen in Figure 2.11.

Granulation tissue is also involved in healing of wounds whatever the cause and site of the tissue defect. In the case of a simple skin incision, where the wound edges are in close apposition and the actual defect is minimal, healing occurs quickly with a small amount of granulation tissue and is termed ***healing by primary intention***. In other situations, the tissue defect will be large and filled with blood clot and a variable amount of tissue debris. In this case, described as ***healing by secondary intention***, organisation and filling of the defect by granulation tissue take considerably longer (see Fig. 2.10).

BASIC PATHOLOGICAL PROCESSES

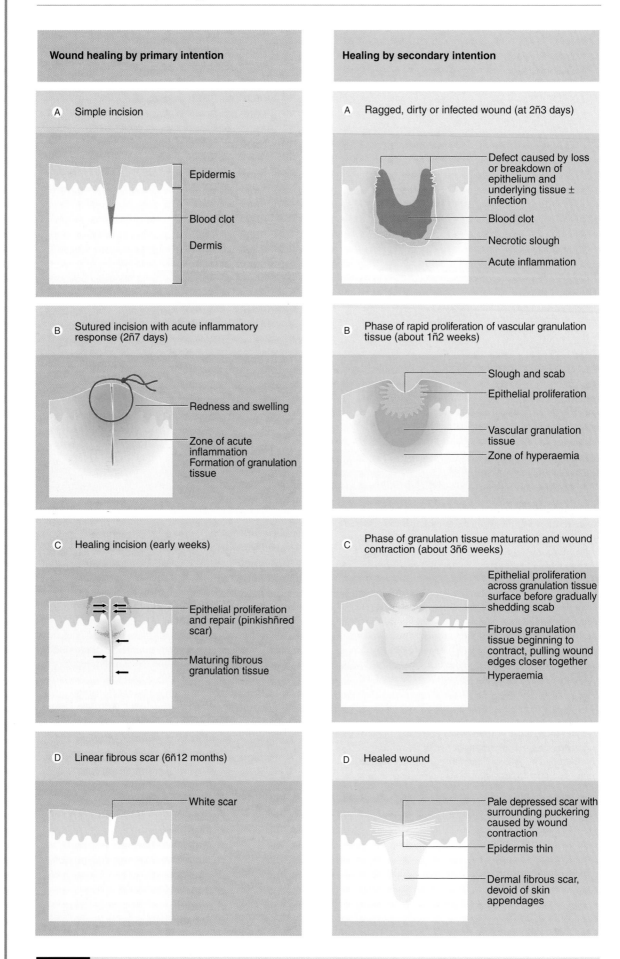

Wound healing by primary intention

A   Simple incision

Epidermis

Blood clot

Dermis

B   Sutured incision with acute inflammatory response (2ñ7 days)

Redness and swelling

Zone of acute inflammation Formation of granulation tissue

C   Healing incision (early weeks)

Epithelial proliferation and repair (pinkishñred scar)

Maturing fibrous granulation tissue

D   Linear fibrous scar (6ñ12 months)

White scar

Healing by secondary intention

A   Ragged, dirty or infected wound (at 2ñ3 days)

Defect caused by loss or breakdown of epithelium and underlying tissue ± infection

Blood clot

Necrotic slough

Acute inflammation

B   Phase of rapid proliferation of vascular granulation tissue (about 1ñ2 weeks)

Slough and scab

Epithelial proliferation

Vascular granulation tissue

Zone of hyperaemia

C   Phase of granulation tissue maturation and wound contraction (about 3ñ6 weeks)

Epithelial proliferation across granulation tissue surface before gradually shedding scab

Fibrous granulation tissue beginning to contract, pulling wound edges closer together

Hyperaemia

D   Healed wound

Pale depressed scar with surrounding puckering caused by wound contraction

Epidermis thin

Dermal fibrous scar, devoid of skin appendages

Fig. 2.10 Wound healing by primary and secondary intention

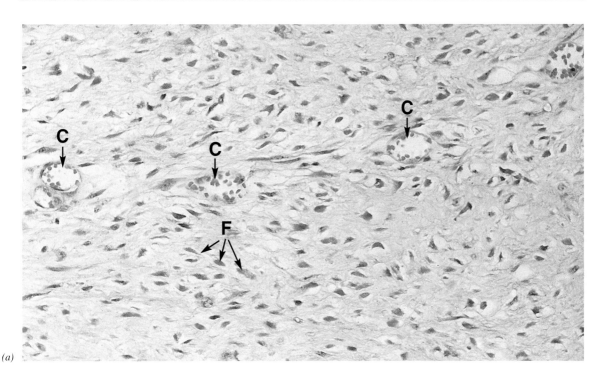

(a)

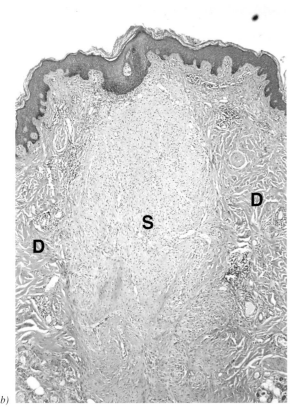

(b)

Fig. 2.11 Fibrous scar
(a) Fibrous scar tissue (HP) (b) Skin scar (LP)

The deposition of collagen within fibrous granulation tissue occurs over a period of many weeks. Collagen is remodelled in an appropriate orientation to withstand the tensile stresses placed on the area of repair. With time, the previously plump and metabolically active fibroblasts regress and become relatively inconspicuous, as shown in micrograph (a) of a typical area of early fibrous scar. Note the condensed nuclei of inactive fibroblasts **F**. Some capillaries **C** persist, accounting for the red appearance of recent scars.

Micrograph (b) illustrates, at low magnification, a recent area of scarring in the skin after healing of a simple incision for biopsy of a skin tumour. Immature collagenous tissue forms a pale scar **S**, which interrupts the normal pink collagen of the dermis **D** on either side. There are no skin appendages in a skin scar. During the ensuing months and years, the cellularity of the scar diminishes, there is progressive loss of capillary vessels and the scar contracts so that after many years a skin scar may be virtually undetectable macroscopically. Note that healing of skin or mucous membrane involves epithelialisation of the surface by proliferation of epithelium at the edges of the defect (i.e. *epithelial regeneration*).

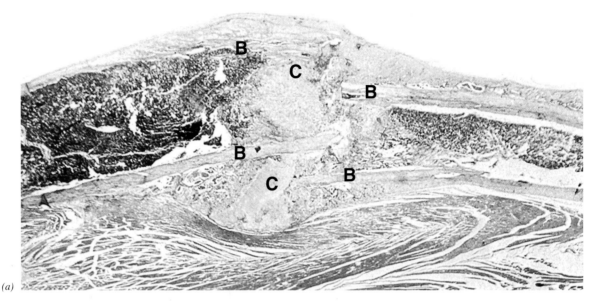

(a)

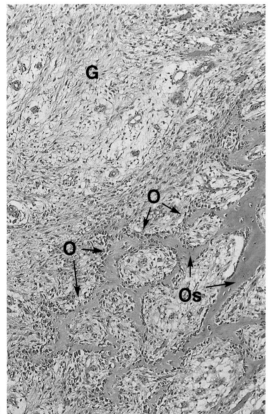

(b)

Fig. 2.12 Specialised repair: healing in bone
(a) LP (b) HP

In most tissues, fibrous scar forms a functionally adequate, albeit unspecialised, replacement for damaged tissues provided sufficient normal tissue remains. In bone, however, the replacement of damaged tissue by fibrous scar is inadequate for restoration of function and so a specialised form of granulation tissue develops where the final product is new bone.

Following fracture, there is usually bleeding in and around the fracture site resulting in a mass of coagulated blood, termed a *haematoma*. An initial acute inflammatory response is rapidly followed by organisation of the haematoma with formation of granulation tissue in much the same way as described in Figure 2.9. In the case of bone fracture, this granulation tissue is termed *provisional callus* **C** and forms around the broken ends of the bone **B** loosely uniting them; this is seen at low magnification in micrograph (a).

In contrast to usual granulation tissue, that of bone contains osteoblasts that produce *osteoid*, the organic matrix of bone. This is seen in micrograph (b) where typical granulation tissue **G** at the top of the field gives way to osteoblasts **O** which surround pink-staining newly formed osteoid **Os**. Osteoid then becomes mineralised to form the *bony callus* between the two fractured ends. This initial bone is haphazardly arranged (known as *woven bone*) and over the next few months undergoes extensive remodelling by osteoclasts and osteoblasts to form lamellar bone with trabecular architecture best suited to resist local stresses. The end result is restitution of normal bony architecture and function.

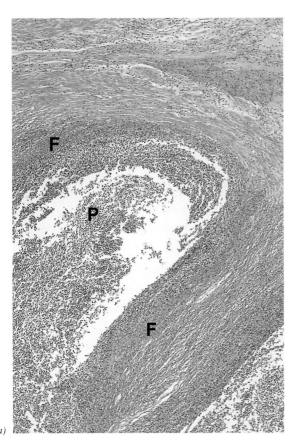

(a)

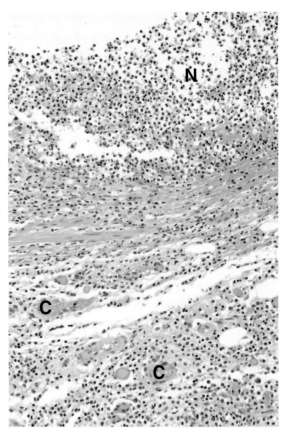

(b)

Fig. 2.13 Abscess formation
(a) LP (b) HP

An abscess is a localised collection of pus, which usually develops following extensive tissue damage by one of the pyogenic bacteria, such as *Staphylococcus aureus*. Such organisms excite an inflammatory exudate in which neutrophils predominate. In these circumstances, large numbers of neutrophils die releasing their lysosomal enzymes and undergoing autolysis; the resulting viscous fluid, *pus*, contains dead and dying neutrophils, necrotic tissue debris and the fluid component of the acute inflammatory exudate with a little fibrin. Pyogenic bacteria often remain viable within the abscess cavity and may cause enlargement of the lesion, which at this stage is described as an *acute abscess*. At an early stage, expansion of the lesion is limited by the processes of organisation and repair at the margins of the abscess. Thus the abscess may become walled off, isolating the bacteria-containing pus and preventing further spread; an

abscess encapsulated by granulation and fibrous tissue is termed a *chronic abscess*. On the other hand, if the bacteria are highly virulent and present in large numbers, such attempts at organisation and repair may be overwhelmed, and expansion of the abscess ensues with destruction of surrounding tissue. The coexistence of active tissue damage and attempts at repair are typical of *chronic inflammation* (see Ch. 3).

Micrograph (a) shows an abscess in the wall of the colon. The centre consists of a collection of pus **P**. At its margin is a pink-staining zone of fibrin **F**. As yet, there is little evidence of organisation at the margins of the abscess; this therefore represents an acute abscess. Micrograph (b) shows the wall and lumen of a chronic abscess at high power, illustrating the neutrophils **N** and tissue debris in the cavity of the abscess, and the capillaries **C** in the inflamed granulation tissue of the wall.

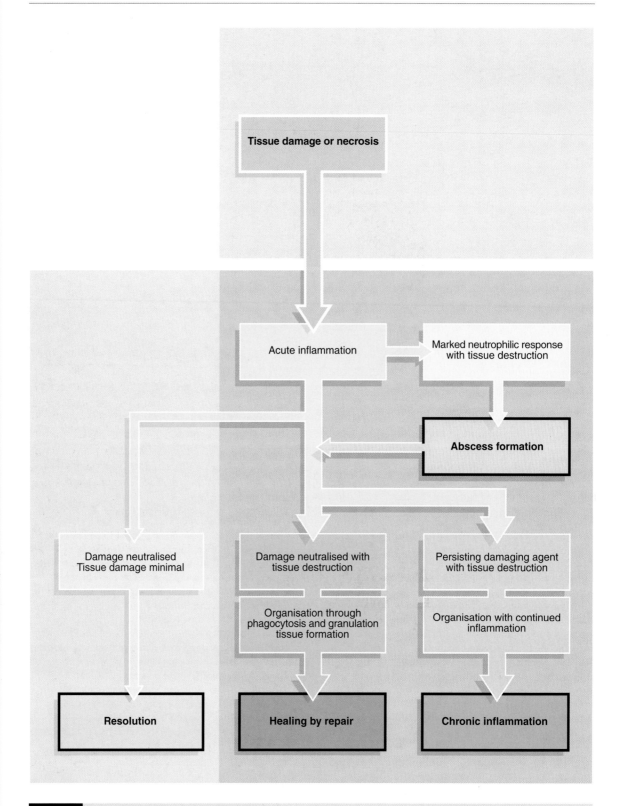

Fig. 2.14 Outcomes of acute inflammation

This flow chart summarises the main outcomes following acute inflammation. Complete resolution is uncommon, the most usual outcomes being either healing by fibrous repair (leaving a collagenous scar) or progression to chronic inflammation.

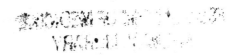

3. Chronic inflammation

Chronic inflammation, by definition, lasts for weeks or months. The term chronic inflammation covers a range of different morphological patterns, which in turn are related to different stimuli and mechanisms. It is important to note, however, that the patterns may be mixed. The hallmark features of chronic inflammation are *ongoing tissue damage* often caused by the inflammatory cells in the infiltrate, a *chronic inflammatory infiltrate* and *fibrosis*. Chronic inflammation may be subdivided as follows:

- *Non-specific chronic inflammation* – arises following non-resolution of acute inflammation
- *Specific (primary) chronic inflammation* – arises *de novo* in response to certain types of injurious agents
- *Granulomatous inflammation* – this is a subset of specific chronic inflammation characterised by the presence of granulomas.

Non-specific chronic inflammation

Chronic inflammation may arise following an episode of acute inflammation (see Ch. 2) where the acute inflammatory response has not been adequate to neutralise or destroy the noxious stimulus. In this situation, tissue damage, acute inflammation, granulation tissue, tissue repair and chronic inflammation coexist. There may be active tissue damage in one area with ongoing acute inflammation, while, in adjacent areas, fibrosis and a chronic inflammatory infiltrate are seen. The chronic inflammatory infiltrate is dominated by tissue macrophages, lymphocytes and plasma cells (see Fig. 3.1) in contrast to the marked preponderance of neutrophils in the acute inflammatory response. This type of chronic inflammation represents a dynamic balance between tissue destruction and repair. The course of the disease might include repeated acute phases when tissue damage is predominant, and intervening chronic phases when chronic inflammation smoulders along with ongoing tissue repair. A good example of this type of chronic inflammation is the chronic peptic ulcer (see Fig. 3.2), which begins as a shallow acute ulcer and may persist over months or even years with alternating periods of acute inflammation with enlargement of the ulcer and chronic inflammation, healing and shrinkage. Another example of this type of chronic inflammation is a chronic abscess.

The outcome of non-specific chronic inflammation depends on whether local and systemic factors favour the injurious agent or the process of healing. Chronic inflammation usually heals by fibrosis.

Factors which impair healing include:
- poor nutrition
- immunosuppression
- persisting tissue damage infection
- retained foreign material
- sequestered dead tissue
- poor blood supply.

Factors which aid the healing of chronic inflammation include:
- administration of appropriate antibiotics
- surgical removal of foreign material
- surgical removal of sequestered dead tissue
- general attempts to improve nutrition, for example by administration of vitamins.

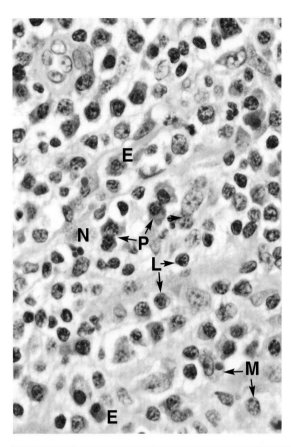

Fig. 3.1 Chronic inflammatory cells (HP)

Chronic inflammatory cells include lymphocytes, plasma cells, eosinophils and macrophages, commonly found infiltrating the tissue as part of the process of chronic inflammation.

This micrograph shows such a chronic inflammatory infiltrate at high magnification. Plasma cells **P** are identified by their amphophilic (purple) cytoplasm and eccentric 'clock face' nuclei. Lymphocytes **L** are seen as dark, rounded nuclei with a thin rim of basophilic cytoplasm. Macrophages **M** are recognised by their oval or kidney-bean-shaped nuclei and pale cytoplasm, which is often foamy as in this case where active phagocytosis of lipid has occurred. Eosinophils **E** have bilobed nuclei and brightly eosinophilic granules in their cytoplasm. Chronic inflammatory cells, often mixed with some neutrophils **N** and many active fibroblasts, are seen in both non-specific and specific chronic inflammation. When the damaging stimulus has been removed and repair is completed, often after weeks or months, these cells will progressively disappear from the tissue.

Fig. 3.2 Chronic peptic ulceration (illustrations opposite)
(a) Entire ulcer (LP) (b) Surface layers of ulcer (MP) (c) Deep layers of ulcer (MP)

A common example which illustrates the principles of non-specific chronic inflammation is the localised chronic ulceration of the stomach or duodenum caused by the damaging effects of acidic gastric secretions, most often in individuals infected by *Helicobacter pylori* (*H. pylori*); such lesions are collectively referred to as ***chronic peptic ulcers***.

Ulceration is caused by an imbalance between damaging factors (gastric acid and peptic enzymes) and protective factors (gastric mucus secretion, local secretion of alkali). *H. pylori* appears to cause direct damage to the epithelial cells as well as secreting enzymes that break down the surface mucus. This allows access of acid to mucosal tissues leading to the formation of an acute ulcer. If the process proceeds unchecked, then the ulcer can erode through the full thickness of the stomach or duodenal wall, leading to perforation and escape of gut contents into the peritoneal cavity (see Fig. 13.8). Most commonly, however, the destructive process is arrested by an acute inflammatory response. Tissue repair then begins with the formation of granulation tissue; repair may be effective if conditions are favourable, leaving a fibrous scar. If tissue destruction continues, the concurrent organisation and repair result in chronic inflammation. A chronic peptic ulcer reflects a dynamic balance between tissue destruction and tissue repair.

A section through a chronic ulcer is shown in micrograph (a). The ulcerated surface is covered in a slough **Sl** composed of a pink-staining layer of necrotic debris (often described as ***necrotic slough***) combined with the fibrin and neutrophils of an acute inflammatory exudate. Beneath the necrotic slough is a zone of vascular granulation tissue **V**; these features are seen at a higher magnification in micrograph (b). Beneath the layer of vascular granulation tissue is a zone of fibrous granulation tissue **F**, seen in detail in micrograph (c). Deeper still in the ulcer base, the fibrous granulation tissue becomes collagenised to form a fibrous scar **Sc**. Also in micrograph (a), note that the muscular wall **M** is completely replaced by the ulcer crater, granulation tissue and scar. A common feature of a chronic peptic ulcer is the presence of one or more large blood vessels (usually arteries) in the ulcer base; erosion of such a vessel leads to bleeding into the stomach lumen, giving rise to the classical symptoms of ***haematemesis*** (vomiting blood) or ***melaena*** (black, tar-like faeces owing to the presence of altered blood).

The outcome of chronic peptic ulceration depends on whether conditions favour the damaging stimulus of the gastric acid or the reparative process of the local tissues. If healing is favoured, then fibrous tissue gradually repairs the ulcer crater and mucosa regenerates from the ulcer margins to cover the epithelial defect and protect the fibrous tissue from further damage. A healed peptic ulcer thus consists of a localised area of fibrous scarring replacing all or part of the thickness of the stomach wall. Internally, the regenerated mucosa is usually puckered because of contraction of the underlying scarred wall.

The most important factors that favour healing of a peptic ulcer are antibiotic treatment to eliminate *H. pylori*, and reduction of gastric acid, for example by H2 receptor antagonist drugs. Factors that favour the destructive process include excessive gastric acid secretion (especially for duodenal ulceration), ongoing infection, and reduced capacity for repair, which may result from corticosteroid therapy and non-steroidal anti-inflammatory drugs.

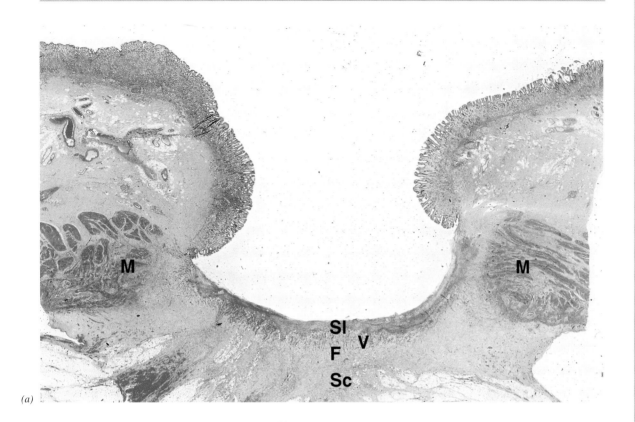

(a)

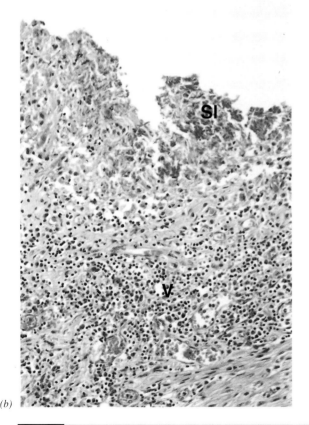

(b)

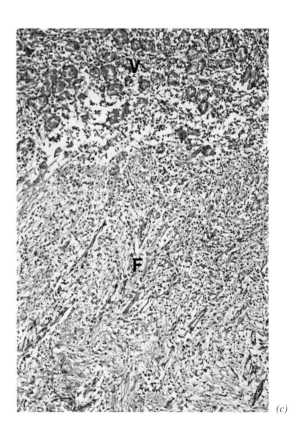

(c)

Fig. 3.2 Chronic peptic ulceration *(caption opposite)*

Fig. 3.3 Bronchiectasis (LP) *(illustration opposite)*

Bronchiectasis is a chronic inflammation of the bronchi associated with destruction of the wall and permanent dilatation.

Damage to the bronchial wall is usually the combined result of repeated episodes of infection coupled with stasis of secretions, leading to progressive destruction of the normal elastic and muscular components of the airway wall. Such damage is particularly likely to occur when airways become partially or completely obstructed. The elastic and muscular components of the bronchial wall are replaced by fibrovascular granulation tissue and later collagenous fibrous tissue. This process weakens the wall, leading to dilatation of the airway, which in turn predisposes to stagnation of secretions and further episodes of bacterial infection.

In this micrograph, two abnormal bronchi are seen, each with the lumen filled with pus **P**. The wall of each affected bronchus is formed of fibrovascular granulation tissue **G,** in which there is a heavy infiltrate of dark-staining cells just visible at this magnification; these cells are a mixture of plasma cells and lymphocytes. Bronchiectasis exemplifies the concept of coexisting tissue damage and attempts at repair which are the hallmark of chronic inflammation.

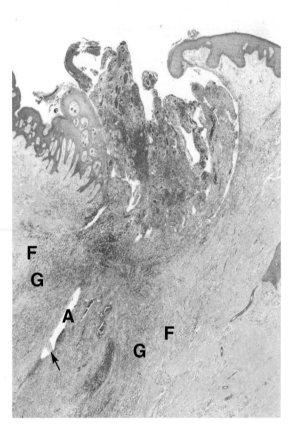

Fig. 3.4 Pilonidal sinus (LP)

A common example of a chronic abscess is the ***pilonidal sinus***. In this condition, a chronic subcutaneous abscess forms, most commonly in the sacrococcygeal area. Hair shafts, derived from locally destroyed follicles and shed body hair, are present in the abscess (arrow) and act as a focus for chronic inflammation. Successful healing and repair are hindered by the persistence of the hairs which are resistant to phagocytosis. Secondary infection may further complicate the process. As part of the attempt at healing, surface epithelium proliferates and comes to line the track leading down into the abscess cavity (not seen in this micrograph); such a track is known as a ***sinus***.

In this micrograph, note the subcutaneous abscess cavity **A**, the wall of which is formed by granulation tissue **G** heavily infiltrated by lymphocytes and plasma cells. There is surrounding fibrosis **F** in the dermis as a result of previous attempts at fibrous repair.

A pilonidal sinus, like any other chronic inflammatory lesion, will only heal if the source of persistent irritation is removed; surgical excision or laying open the complex of sinuses and abscess cavities is usually the only satisfactory method in this situation.

Fig. 3.5 Ulcerative colitis
(a) LP (b) MP (c) HP *(illustrations opposite – below)*

Ulcerative colitis is a relapsing inflammatory disorder of the colon of unknown aetiology. It is characterised by phases of quiescence punctuated by acute exacerbations in which there may be extensive acute inflammation of the mucosa leading to ulceration. Between acute attacks, the mucosa shows infiltration of the lamina propria by chronic inflammatory cells (Fig. 3.1). During an acute attack, confluent areas of mucosal ulceration occur, leaving protruding islands of chronically inflamed mucosa and submucosa that simulate colonic polyps. These so-called ***pseudopolyps*** bear remnants of colonic epithelium.

These three micrographs illustrate longstanding ulcerative colitis. Micrograph (a) shows a pseudopolyp **P** with fragments of surface epithelium **Ep** and surrounded by ulcerated colonic mucosa **U**. In micrograph (b) showing the quiescent phase, the earlier destruction of the colonic crypts can be identified. The crypts are shorter than normal and often crypts are missing. Regeneration is demonstrated by branching of crypts **B**. The chronic inflammatory infiltrate is well demonstrated in micrograph (c), where sheets of plasma cells and lymphocytes infiltrate the lamina propria. In this micrograph, the 'regenerative' appearance of the colonic epithelium is also easily seen. These epithelial cells have larger nuclei than usual, reflecting the less mature state of the actively proliferating cells. This appearance is commonly seen in healing or inflamed epithelia and must be carefully differentiated from ***dysplasia*** (see Chs 6 and 7). Dysplasia of the epithelium may occur in longstanding ulcerative colitis and while not harmful of itself, it may be a precursor of invasive carcinoma, one of the major complications of ulcerative colitis.

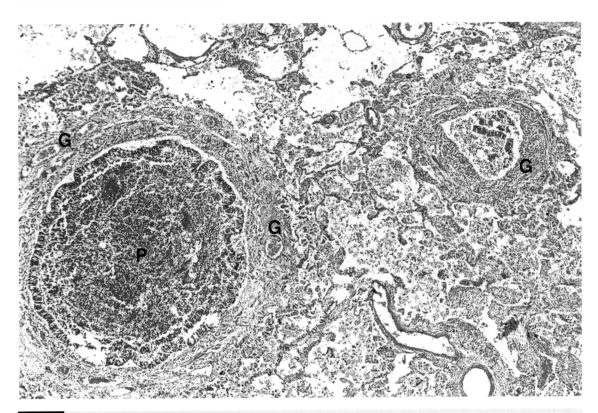

Fig. 3.3 Bronchiectasis (LP) (*caption opposite – top*)

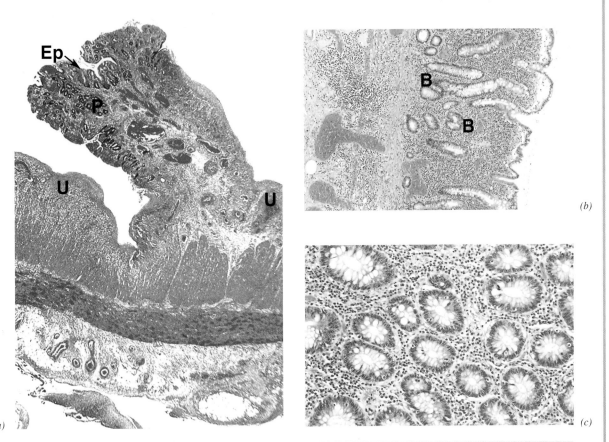

(a)

(b)

(c)

Fig. 3.5 Ulcerative colitis
(a) **LP** (b) **MP** (c) **HP** (*caption opposite – below*)

BASIC PATHOLOGICAL PROCESSES

Specific (primary) chronic inflammation

This type of chronic inflammation arises by different mechanisms from non-specific chronic inflammation. Primary chronic inflammation may be either *granulomatous* or *non-granulomatous*. A key feature in chronic inflammation is the activation of macrophages which orchestrate the chronic inflammatory response. Macrophages may become activated by either immune or non-immune mechanisms. Activated macrophages not only become more efficient at phagocytosis and killing of organisms but secrete a wide range of factors that control the behaviour of other inflammatory cells (e.g. chemotactic factors, lymphokines) and which induce fibrosis (e.g. fibrogenic cytokines, growth factors). The types of agent which can invoke primary chronic inflammation include:

Immunological
- Low toxicity organisms as *Treponema*, the causative organism of *syphilis* and *yaws*
- Infective organisms that grow within cells, e.g. viruses, *Mycobacteria*
- Hypersensitivity reactions such as *extrinsic allergic alveolitis*
- Autoimmune conditions such as *systemic lupus erythematosus*
- Infections by fungi, protozoa and parasites.

Non-immunological
- Foreign body reactions
- Inert noxious materials such as silica, talc, asbestos or beryllium.

Primary chronic inflammation of the immune type may be either granulomatous or non-granulomatous. A good example of the non-granulomatous immune type is *chronic active hepatitis* caused by hepatitis B virus infection (see Fig. 14.5). Virus-infected cells in the liver induce a cell-mediated immune response. The cytotoxic T lymphocytes so activated kill virus-infected hepatocytes. Some individuals mount an effective immune response and clear the infection while in others there is ongoing infiltration of the liver by lymphocytes over months or years. In these people, there is continuing destruction of hepatocytes and fibrosis of the liver tissue, which may lead eventually to cirrhosis. As in many examples of chronic inflammation, the tissue damage is due to the inflammatory cells rather than the virus itself. In non-immune type primary chronic inflammation, the mechanisms are less clear. However, certain materials such as silica can directly activate macrophages to release mediators that induce an inflammatory reaction and fibrosis.

Granulomatous inflammation

The defining feature of granulomatous inflammation is the presence of activated *epithelioid macrophages* and *multinucleate giant cells* derived from macrophages. Epithelioid macrophages are so named because they bear some resemblance histologically to epithelial (squamous) cells. These cells may form well-circumscribed *granulomas* (clusters) which are generally surrounded by lymphocytes, macrophages, fibroblasts and varying degrees of fibrosis. In other conditions, the granulomatous reaction may be rather more diffuse. Granulomatous primary chronic inflammation may arise by either immune or non-immune mechanisms. The immune type, known as the *delayed hypersensitivity response*, is epitomised by tuberculosis (see Ch. 4). T lymphocytes responding to mycobacterial antigens are activated, and divide and mature to produce helper T cells. The helper T cells in turn secrete lymphokines that induce the transformation of macrophages into activated epithelioid macrophages and giant cells.

Non-immune granulomatous inflammation is exemplified by the foreign body reaction, for example in response to suture material after a surgical procedure, or when a rose thorn becomes embedded in the skin. Figure 3.10 is an example of such a reaction and shows plant material (from faeces) embedded in the wall of the bowel. In some granulomatous conditions such as Crohn's disease and sarcoidosis, it is not known whether the mechanism is immune or non-immune. Many researchers have searched in vain for infectious organisms as causes of these conditions, but the question of the causative organism remains unanswered.

The term granuloma needs some clarification. In general, granuloma means a cluster of epithelioid macrophages as opposed to granulation tissue as defined in Chapter 2. However, in the past, 'granuloma' was applied to both a granuloma and granulation tissue and a few examples remain in current terminology where the old usage persists. Examples include an apical granuloma referring to a mass of granulation tissue at the root of a tooth and a pyogenic granuloma (lobular haemangioma), which is a mass of granulation tissue in a healing wound.

Some granulomas develop necrosis in their central area. The classical form is caseating necrosis which is almost always found in tuberculosis (see Ch. 4). Caseous necrosis appears creamy macroscopically (caseous = like cream cheese). By light microscopy caseous necrosis is featureless and eosinophilic, containing few cells. Some other granutomatous conditions such as atypical mycobacterial infection also develop central necrosis but the necrosis is suppurative with plentiful neutrophils. Granulomas which contain this type of necrosis are often called 'suppurating granulomas'. Yet other types of granulomatous inflammation are characterised by their lack of necrosis. Good examples of this type are Crohn's disease and sarcoidosis.

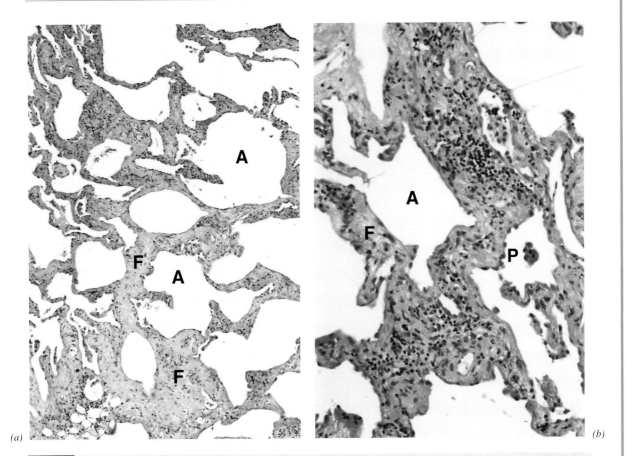

(a) *(b)*

Fig. 3.6 Pulmonary fibrosis (idiopathic)
(a) LP (b) HP

Idiopathic pulmonary fibrosis (or *cryptogenic fibrosing alveolitis*) is a good example of a chronic inflammatory condition which in its earliest phases has a chronic inflammatory infiltrate. At this early stage, it may be called *interstitial pneumonitis* (or *usual interstitial pneumonitis*) where an unknown damaging agent (possibly an aberrant immune response to 'self' antigens, i.e. an autoimmune reaction) triggers the inflammation of the alveolar walls.

The later stages of this process are well illustrated in these micrographs where the alveolar walls are thickened because of the deposition of dense fibrous tissue **F**. The thickened alveolar walls are distorted and less permeable to gases. In the final stages, there may be great distortion of alveoli giving rise to greatly enlarged alveolar spaces **A**, known as *honeycomb lung*. In addition, there is damage to the alveolar lining cells and these are replaced by hyperplastic or regenerating type II pneumocytes. In micrograph (b), the inflammatory infiltrate of lymphocytes and plasma cells is readily seen, as well as type II pneumocyte hyperplasia **P**.

The usual presentation of cryptogenic fibrosing alveolitis is of insidious onset, featuring breathlessness associated with finger clubbing. However, a histologically identical picture may arise as an end stage of *diffuse alveolar damage* owing to oxygen toxicity in premature infants, i.e. *hyaline membrane disease* (Fig. 12.10), and acute viral pneumonitis. The condition may also follow a range of other conditions such as extrinsic allergic alveolitis, drug toxicity, miliary tuberculosis, connective tissue disorders and sarcoidosis. Some of these disorders are associated with granulomatous inflammation in the early stages and this may still be apparent at the end stage.

BASIC PATHOLOGICAL PROCESSES

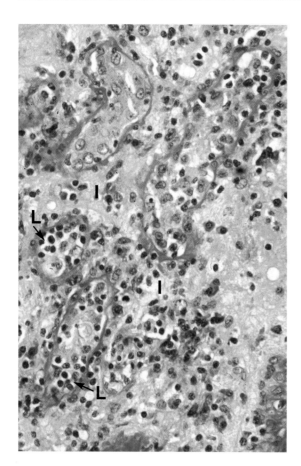

Fig. 3.7 Transplant rejection: kidney (LP)

Organ transplantation introduces non-self antigens into the recipient. Specifically, the **HLA antigens** of the donor are very rarely identical with those of the recipient except in the rare case of transplantation of organs between identical twins. The HLA antigens of the donor excite a **cell-mediated immune response** in the recipient and activated T lymphocytes infiltrate the transplanted organ and attempt to rid the body of the foreign material by killing donor cells. This is, of course, a gross simplification of the many and complex faces of transplant rejection which are dealt with in more detail in Chapter 15. This micrograph illustrates a cell-mediated immune response to a transplanted kidney. There is an infiltrate of lymphocytes, most of which are T cells, in the interstitium **I** of the kidney. The tubules are widely separated (**atrophic**) and there is fibrosis of the interstitium. Lymphocytes **L** can be seen within the tubular basement membrane between the tubular epithelial cells (**tubulitis**). These lymphocytes are attacking the tubular epithelial cells, causing tubular damage and eventual loss of tubules. Loss of any part of the nephron leads to loss of the entire nephron so that the transplanted kidney is unable to function. This process demonstrates that, as in many cases of chronic inflammation, tissue damage is caused primarily by the inflammatory infiltrate. The transplanted kidney makes no attack on the recipient and if left alone by the immnue system does nothing but good. Various combinations of immunosuppressant drugs are used to suppress the cell-mediated immune response to the transplanted kidney to allow it to function in the recipient, thus freeing the recipient from a life of dialysis.

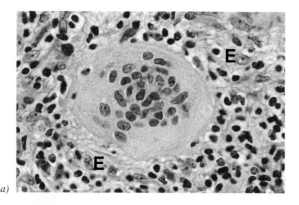

(a)

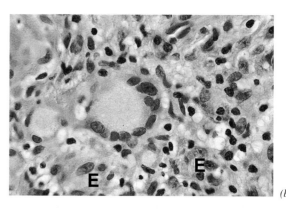

(b)

Fig. 3.8 Giant cells
(a) Foreign body giant cell (HP) (b) Langhans' giant cell (HP)

As described in the introduction, multinucleate giant cells are formed by the fusion of epithelioid macrophages and are a highly characteristic, though not universal, feature of chronic granulomatous inflammation. These micrographs illustrate typical appearances of giant cells. Micrograph (a) is a good example of a **foreign body-type giant cell**, which is characterised by a central group of nuclei similar to those seen in adjacent epithelioid macrophages **E**. These cells may be found in association with implanted foreign material, for example a remnant of a surgical suture or a rose thorn in the skin. These cells are usually found in association with epithelioid macrophages although they may not form the discrete granulomas surrounded by lymphocytes, fibroblasts and fibrosis that may be seen in other types of granulomatous inflammation.

The second important form of giant cell is the **Langhans' giant cell**, said to be characteristic of tuberculosis. As shown in micrograph (b), the multiple nuclei of Langhans' giant cells are arranged in a horseshoe formation around the periphery. Again, epithelioid macrophages **E** are seen in the surrounding tissues.

Both epithelioid macrophages and giant cells are specialised secretory cells, rather than phagocytic cells. The plentiful eosinophilic cytoplasm seen in both cell types is indicative of plentiful rough endoplasmic reticulum as opposed to the pale foamy cytoplasm of phagocytic macrophages. Although Langhans' giant cells and foreign body cells are said to be more or less specific for different types of granulomatous inflammation, in practice this is not so.

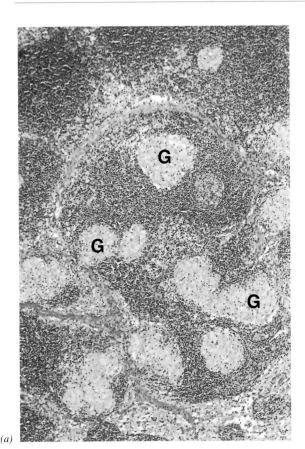

(a)

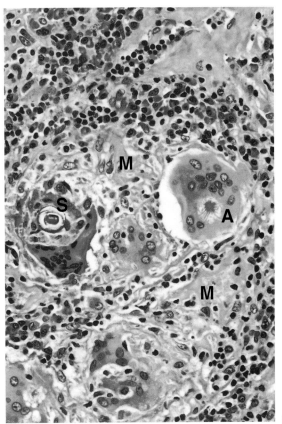

(b)

Fig. 3.9 Sarcoidosis
(a) Sarcoidosis in a lymph node (MP) (b) Sarcoid granulomas (HP)

Sarcoidosis is a chronic granulomatous inflammation of unknown aetiology, characterised by the formation of multiple discrete granulomas in many tissues, similar in many respects to those of tuberculosis (see Ch. 4). In marked distinction to tuberculous granulomas, those of sarcoidosis do not typically undergo central caseous necrosis, although small foci of necrosis may be seen in large granulomas.

Sarcoidosis may occur in any organ or tissue, notably the spleen, liver, skin and lymph nodes, but frequently also involves the lungs which may be peppered with numerous granulomas. In most cases of pulmonary sarcoidosis, the hilar lymph nodes are also grossly enlarged by masses of granulomas; such massive nodes are a useful diagnostic feature when visible on a chest radiograph.

Micrograph (a) illustrates part of a typical lymph node. Note the scattered non-caseating granulomas **G**. Since there is no central mass of caseation, the sarcoid granuloma differs from the tuberculous granuloma by having a much broader zone of epithelioid macrophages. As in tuberculosis, sarcoid granulomas are surrounded by a zone of lymphocytes, although this feature is much less

obvious in sarcoid lesions. In tissues other than lymph nodes, the granulomas are described as being 'naked', i.e. devoid of a rim of lymphocytes and fibroblasts.

Micrograph (b) shows a typical sarcoid granuloma at high magnification. Note the epithelioid macrophages **M**. Multinucleate giant cells are a feature of most of the granulomas. The cytoplasm of sarcoid giant cells may contain inclusion bodies of two types: eosinophilic star-shaped ***asteroid bodies*** **A** or small, laminated calcified concretions called ***Schaumann's bodies*** **S**. In practice, these inclusion bodies are rare. Although characteristic of sarcoid giant cells, such inclusion bodies are not pathognomonic of sarcoidosis (i.e. not exclusive to sarcoidosis) and are occasionally found in other chronic inflammatory granulomas.

Sarcoidosis is most commonly a chronic remitting disease, often exhibiting no symptoms; in persistent cases, the granulomas undergo progressive fibrosis although some giant cells still remain. In the lungs, this may culminate in pulmonary fibrosis and honeycomb lung (see Fig. 3.6) and may lead to chronic respiratory failure.

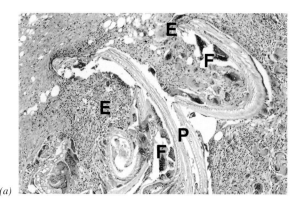

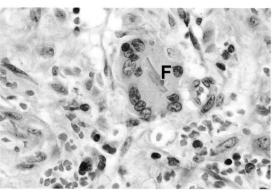

(a)   *(b)*

Fig. 3.10 Foreign body reaction
(a) Foreign body granuloma (LP) (b) Giant cell with inclusion (HP)

The presence of certain non-lysable foreign materials in the tissues may excite a chronic granulomatous inflammatory response similar to that seen in sarcoidosis. Common examples of such *foreign body reactions* are those produced by talc and starch (introduced into the tissues as glove powder during surgical procedures), suture material, wood, metal or glass splinters, and inorganic materials such as silica and beryllium inhaled deep into the lungs during industrial dust exposure. Inhaled materials are of particular clinical importance because of their tendency to produce progressive pulmonary fibrosis similar to that which may occur in cryptogenic fibrosing alveolitis. Many of these foreign

bodies are refractile when viewed with polarised light and can thus be identified within the granulomas or giant cells.

At low magnification, micrograph (a) shows plant material **P** which has become embedded in the wall of the colon in a patient with *diverticulitis*. The pale, incompletely digested plant material is surrounded by aggregates of foreign body giant cells **F** and epithelioid macrophages **E** as well as other inflammatory cells. At high power in micrograph (b), a fragment of foreign material **F** can be easily seen within the cytoplasm of a Langhans' type giant cell.

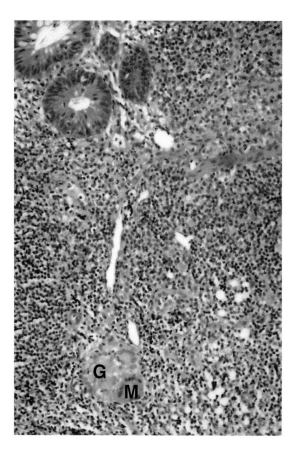

Fig. 3.11 Crohn's disease (HP)

Crohn's disease is another chronic granulomatous disease of unknown aetiology. It typically affects the large and small intestines but may involve any part of the gastrointestinal tract from lips to anus; rarely, it may also involve the skin. The characteristic feature is a chronic inflammatory reaction involving the whole thickness of the wall of the affected bowel segment. The inflammatory infiltrate includes lymphocytes, plasma cells and eosinophils. Granulomas of various sizes are typical but are not always seen.

This high power micrograph shows the mucosa and submucosa of the colon. A few crypts are seen in the mucosa at the top of the micrograph. In the submucosa, there is a well-defined aggregate of epithelioid macrophages forming a small granuloma **G** with multinucleate giant cells **M**. A dense infiltrate of mixed inflammatory cells is seen in the mucosa and submucosa. Granulomas in Crohn's disease are often very scanty but when identified are very helpful in differentiating it from ulcerative colitis. Crohn's disease is described in greater detail in Chapter 13.

4. Infections of histological importance

Introduction

A number of infections may be diagnosed from the characteristic appearances seen in biopsy specimens. In many cases, the diagnosis may be first suspected when a biopsy is examined by light microscopy; in other cases, the clinician suspects an infective agent and seeks confirmation by biopsy as well as by other means. Although histological appearances are often characteristic, it is usually necessary to confirm the presence of the infective agent by other techniques such as microbiological cultures or serology. In addition, the histopathologist may employ a wide variety of techniques such as electron microscopy, immunoperoxidase staining with specific monoclonal antibodies, and a wide range of special stains to confirm the diagnosis. Many infections that are otherwise difficult to diagnose arise in immunosuppressed patients, for example AIDS patients and organ transplant recipients and, as the number of such patients increases, so the role of histopathology in diagnosis of infection expands. Hence, this chapter aims to give an overview of infections which are important in routine histopathological practice, and to illustrate the appearances of these organisms in the tissues and the patterns of tissue damage they cause.

Bacterial infection

Most bacteria cause disease by exciting an acute inflammatory exudative response (pyogenic bacteria), and the inflammatory exudate so formed is responsible for many of the clinical features of the disease (e.g. lobar pneumonia, Fig. 2.4; bronchopneumonia, Fig. 12.5; acute meningitis, Fig. 2.6). The pattern of tissue damage is much the same irrespective of the pyogenic bacteria causing it, and the specific bacterium can only be identified by microbiological methods. Other bacteria cause disease as a direct result of producing toxins which cause necrosis of cells and tissues (e.g. *Clostridium difficile* toxins destroying the surface epithelium of the colon, see Fig. 4.1), and some bacteria initiate a Type IV hypersensitivity reaction (e.g. the *Mycobacteria* group and some Treponemal organisms), producing characteristic histological changes.

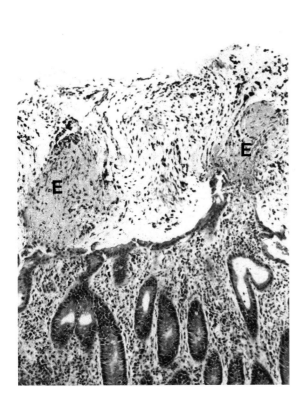

Fig. 4.1 Pseudomembranous colitis

In pseudomembranous colitis, there is focal necrosis of the surface epithelium of the colon, the necrotic epithelium being replaced by an area of 'membrane' composed of a predominantly fibrinous acute inflammatory exudate **E**. It occurs in old people who are taking certain oral antibiotics. The antibiotic destroys the natural bacterial flora, allowing uncontrolled multiplication of *Clostridium difficile*. This bacterium produces a toxin which causes extensive patchy colonic epithelial necrosis, which may be fatal.

The pattern of superficial necrosis of the mucosa is characteristic. There are multiple focal lesions of necrosis with tufts of exudate which have been likened to an erupting volcano. The deep components of the mucosa remain largely intact.

Mycobacterial infections

Infections caused by various Mycobacteria can frequently be diagnosed histologically because of the tissue reaction to their presence. The organisms are difficult and slow to grow in microbiological culture, and biopsy plays an important role in early diagnosis. *Mycobacterium tuberculosis* causes tuberculosis, a disease which is again increasing in incidence because of the emergence of drug-resistant strains, and *Mycobacterium leprae* is the cause of leprosy. There are other pathogenic Mycobacteria (called atypical Mycobacteria) which cause a range of disorders.

Important points to note about the histology of Mycobacterial infections are:

- most show a granulomatous pattern of chronic inflammation
- caseous necrosis (see Fig. 4.2) is particularly associated with *M. tuberculosis* infection
- suppurating granulomas (with neutrophils in the central necrotic area of the granuloma) may occur in infections by atypical Mycobacteria
- the causative organism can sometimes be identified in histological sections by the use of special stains (Ziehl–Neelsen, Wade–Fite).

Fig. 4.2 **Early pulmonary tuberculosis** (*illustrations opposite*)
(a) Early tubercle (MP) (b) Early tubercle (HP) (c) Later tubercle (MP) (d) Later tubercle (HP)

The characteristic histological lesion in tuberculosis is the granuloma which in this case is known as a *tubercle*.

When tubercle bacilli gain access to the lungs by inhalation, they tend to localise in the periphery of the lung where they excite a transient and inconclusive neutrophil response. The organisms survive neutrophil enzyme activity, probably because of their thick and resistant glycolipid cell wall. The tubercle bacilli are then ingested by macrophages where they may initially continue to divide within macrophage cytoplasm. The macrophages present mycobacterial antigen to T lymphocytes which become activated and initiate a cell-mediated (type IV hypersensitivity) response. The sensitised lymphocytes produce various soluble factors (cytokines) which attract and activate the macrophages, enhancing their ability to secrete substances which kill tubercle bacilli. Such activated macrophages become large and develop granular eosinophilic cytoplasm; because of their supposed resemblance to epithelial cells, they are known as epithelioid macrophages (see Ch. 3). These cells form a major component of all granulomas, including tubercles.

Micrograph (a) shows an entire tubercle at an early stage, and (b) illustrates a sector of the same tubercle at higher magnification. At the centre of the tubercle is an area of caseous necrosis **CN** containing tubercle bacilli; these can only be demonstrated by specific staining methods for acid-fast bacilli (Fig. 4.11). The caseous area is surrounded by a zone of epithelioid macrophages **M** with abundant eosinophilic cytoplasm. Some of the macrophages fuse to produce multinucleate giant cells called *Langhans' giant cells* **L**; a typical Langhans' giant cell is shown in more detail in Figure 3.8. Peripheral to the macrophages, there is a rim of lymphocytes.

Progressive central caseous necrosis results in enlargement of the tubercle and the zone of peripheral macrophages and lymphocytes becomes relatively thinner. These changes can be observed by comparing micrograph (a) with micrograph (c) which shows a more advanced tubercle. With further development,

spindle-shaped fibroblasts **F** appear in the peripheral lymphocytic zone of the tubercle where they are stimulated by factors produced by epithelioid macrophages to lay down collagen in the extracellular tissue; this process is evident in micrograph (c) and at higher magnification in (d).

At this stage, further changes in the tubercle can occur in one of two ways. If the tubercle bacilli are virulent and present in large numbers, and particularly if the body's resistance is low (as, for example, in a debilitated or immunosuppressed patient), then the tubercle rapidly enlarges owing to increasing caseous necrosis. The macrophage-lymphocyte-fibroblast defensive reaction is overwhelmed, failing to confine the infection; an example is that of tuberculous bronchopneumonia (Fig. 4.5). On the other hand, if the balance of resistance and attack is reversed, the macrophage-lymphocyte-fibroblast barrier resists enlargement of the tubercle, and proliferation of fibroblasts produces a firm shell confining the infection. Production of collagen by these fibroblasts further strengthens this capsule, imprisoning the necrotic tissue and its contained tubercle bacilli, and isolating the organisms from other susceptible tissue (see Fig. 4.3). Calcium salts may become deposited in the collagenous shell and necrotic centre. In the lung, carbon is also taken up by the macrophages of the granuloma.

In primary tuberculous infection, the initial tubercle in the lung is known as a *Ghon focus* and is usually situated in the subpleural area in the mid-zone of the lung. This lesion rarely attains a large size and undergoes the process of fibrosis described above. Before the lung lesion is walled off, however, tubercle bacilli pass via lymphatics to regional lymph nodes in the lung hilum where tubercles develop in a manner identical to the Ghon focus in the lung. The outcome of the infection depends on what happens to this tuberculous infection of the hilar lymph nodes; possible outcomes are discussed in Figures 4.3 to 4.9.

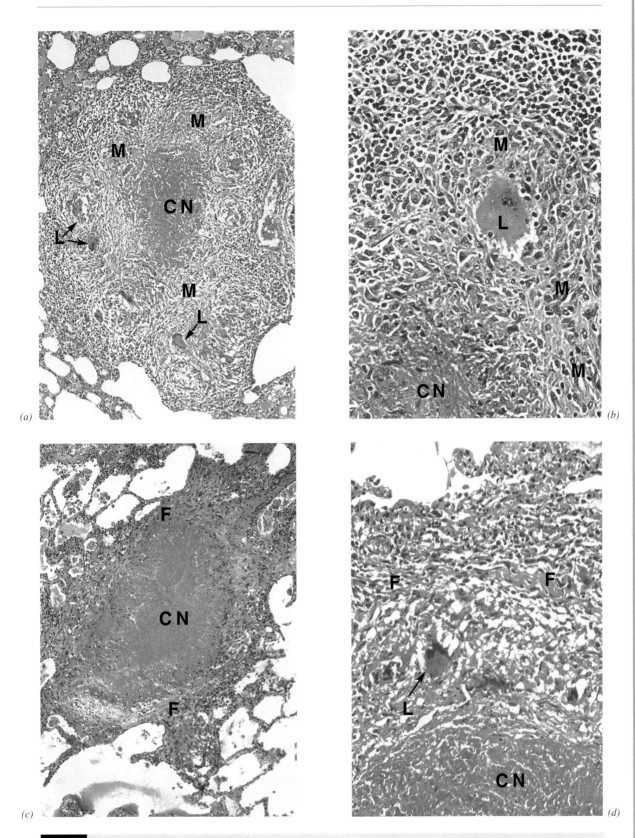

Fig. 4.2 Early pulmonary tuberculosis (*caption opposite*)

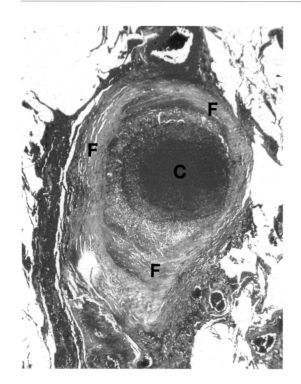

Fig. 4.3 Fibrocaseous tuberculous nodule (LP)

In most individuals with primary tuberculosis, mainly children, the Ghon complex heals by fibrosis leaving a small fibrous nodule which is often calcified. Some individuals, however, are unable to contain the initial infection and develop post-primary tuberculosis. Others contain the initial infection for a time but later, perhaps because of relatively suppressed immunity, get further active infection owing to reactivation of a previously contained infective focus.

In either case, a wide variety of lesions may occur including a localised lesion at the apex of the lung known as an *Assmann focus*. This may progress to further spread of infection or may be contained by chemotherapy giving rise to a fibrocaseous nodule as shown here. A thick fibrous wall **F** completely encircles a mass of caseous necrotic material **C**. In this case, there has been little calcium deposition.

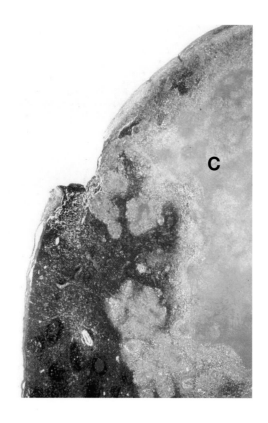

Fig. 4.4 Tuberculous lymph node (LP)

With the formation of a Ghon focus in a child's lung, tubercle bacilli pass via lung lymphatics to regional lymph nodes where they initiate caseous necrosis and tubercle formation similar to that in the lung. The combination of a Ghon focus in the lung and tuberculous regional (peribronchial) lymph nodes is called a *primary complex*, or *Ghon complex*.

The outcome of infection in a child depends on the fate of the lymph node lesion. If the child's defences are strong (as in most cases), healing of all the tubercles occurs by fibrosis as described previously; all that remains is a small fibrocalcific nodule in the lung periphery and similar lesions in the regional lymph nodes. On the other hand, if the patient's defence mechanisms are inadequate, the lymph node tubercle enlarges as a result of extensive caseous necrosis, tending to overwhelm the surrounding macrophage-lymphocyte-fibroblast reaction. The lymph node enlarges until its capsule is breached, then ruptures, discharging caseous material heavily populated by tubercle bacilli, into surrounding tissues. The enlarging node may ulcerate into nearby bronchi causing tuberculous bronchopneumonia (see Fig. 4.5), or into blood vessels (see Fig. 4.6), leading to extensive blood stream spread of the tubercle bacilli. In this micrograph, the tubercle has greatly enlarged so that the lymph node has almost been destroyed by caseous necrosis **C**, and the zone of cellular reaction around it is very thin and insignificant. The necrosis has almost reached the lymph node capsule; rupture is imminent.

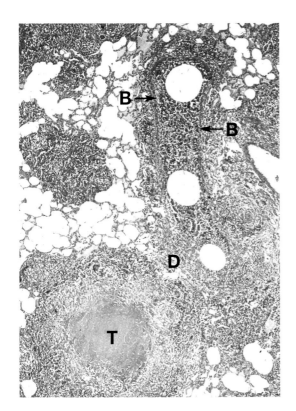

Fig. 4.5 Tuberculous bronchopneumonia (MP)

When the wall of a bronchus is eroded by an enlarging tuberculous node or an apical Assmann focus, tubercle bacilli pass into the bronchial lumen from which they may be spread in various ways. If coughed up in sputum, the infection may be transmitted to other susceptible persons by droplet infection, sometimes infecting the patient's larynx (*tuberculous laryngitis*) on the way. Infected sputum may be swallowed and subsequently produce *tuberculous oesophagitis* or *ileitis*. Infected sputum may also gravitate to lower areas of the same or opposite lung where, by destruction of a bronchiolar wall, the organism may invade peribronchial lung tissue to form further caseating tubercles. This is called *tuberculous bronchopneumonia*.

In this example of an early lesion in tuberculous bronchopneumonia, note a segment of bronchiole containing infected material; the walls of the bronchiole are indicated by the arrows marked **B**. A segment of the bronchiolar wall has been destroyed **D**, permitting access of bacilli which have initiated a caseating tubercle **T** in the nearby lung parenchyma. Large numbers of such lesions may form, merging with one another to produce a wide area of rapidly enlarging caseation, usually in the lower lobes of the lungs. This is the pathogenesis of the once dreaded 'galloping consumption'.

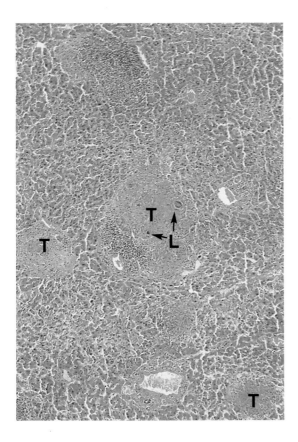

Fig. 4.6 Miliary tuberculosis (MP)

If a ruptured tuberculous lymph node (or a rapidly enlarging focus of post-primary tuberculosis) erodes a blood vessel wall, masses of tubercle bacilli are discharged into the circulation and are carried along in the blood until they lodge in the microcirculation. When the eroded vessel is a branch of the pulmonary artery, the organisms are passed to other areas of the lung; when a pulmonary venous tributary is involved, they are spread in the systemic circulation to many organs, notably the liver, kidney and spleen. In this way, vast numbers of new tubercles may be produced throughout the body. Such multiple lesions rarely attain any great size because this occurrence usually produces rapid clinical deterioration and death; because the gross appearance of individual lesions resembles millet seeds, this condition is known as *miliary tuberculosis*.

This illustration shows several miliary tubercles **T** in the liver, recently formed as a result of blood-borne spread from pulmonary tuberculosis. Two of the tubercles exhibit Langhans' giant cells **L**; the larger tubercles show early central caseous necrosis.

BASIC PATHOLOGICAL PROCESSES

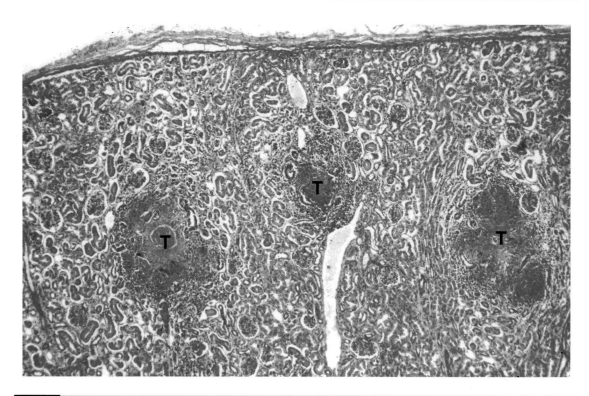

Fig. 4.7 Renal tuberculosis (MP)

Most episodes of pulmonary tuberculous infection are well enough contained by local and systemic defence mechanisms such that gross, blood-borne (miliary) tuberculosis is a relatively uncommon outcome. Nevertheless, it appears that a relatively small number of organisms can be disseminated by the bloodstream to a variety of other organs.

For many reasons, probably including low bacterial virulence and high host resistance, most of these blood-borne bacteria are neutralised without initiating the formation of significant lesions in the organs in which they lodge. It seems that, in certain tissues, some organisms remain viable but quiescent, only to become reactivated at a later date when the host's immune status is temporarily or permanently impaired; this is often long after the initial pulmonary lesion has healed. Active tuberculosis, with the formation of characteristic caseating granulomas, may then reappear in tissues

remote from the original lesion and often many years later. This phenomenon is known as *metastatic* or *isolated organ tuberculosis* and most commonly involves the kidneys, adrenals, meninges, bone, Fallopian tubes, endometrium and epididymis.

This micrograph illustrates renal involvement with the formation of small tubercles **T** in the renal cortex. The granulomas exhibit the classical central caseation of tuberculosis, with larger tubercles tending to become confluent with adjacent lesions. Continuation of this process results in destruction of much of the renal cortex and medulla, with eventual rupture of large confluent tubercles into the pelvicalyceal system which becomes distended with caseous material; this condition is known as *tuberculous pyonephrosis*. In more advanced cases, the infection spreads to involve the ureter and bladder. Renal tuberculosis is frequently bilateral and may result in renal failure.

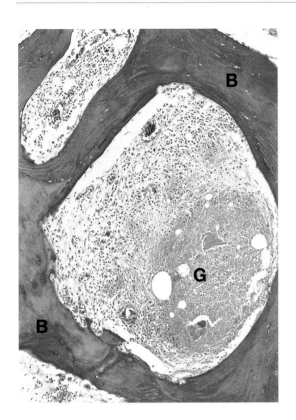

Fig. 4.8 Tuberculosis of bone (MP)

Bone tuberculosis (*tuberculous osteomyelitis*) most frequently affects the long bones and associated joints, and the vertebrae; involvement of vertebrae often leads to spontaneous collapse and is known as *Potts disease*. In long bones, the infection may produce a localised, painful, tumour-like swelling which may drain to the skin to form a chronic sinus. Joint involvement (*tuberculous arthritis*) is most common in children and often affects the hips or joints associated with the vertebrae (*tuberculous spondylitis*) as part of Pott's disease of the spine.

As in other tissues, the characteristic tuberculous lesions are caseating granulomas **G** which cause progressive destruction of the bony trabeculae **B**. The infection tends to spread extensively in the cancellous medullary bone, leading to necrosis of surrounding cortical bone.

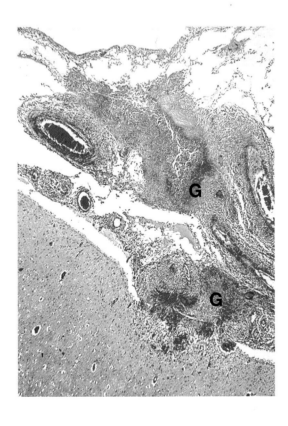

Fig. 4.9 Tuberculous meningitis (MP)

Tuberculous meningitis is a commonly fatal, though uncommon, complication of pulmonary tuberculosis. Most commonly, it affects the meninges around the base of the brain and the spinal cord.

Tuberculous granulomas **G**, with characteristic central areas of caseation, develop in the leptomeninges and adjacent brain tissue where they may damage cranial and spinal nerves.

Langhans' giant cells are relatively sparse in the granulomas, but a heavy infiltrate of lymphocytes is almost always present. The presence of numerous lymphocytes in CSF obtained from lumbar puncture is useful in distinguishing tuberculous meningitis from purulent (bacterial) meningitis; in the latter, neutrophils are predominant (compare with Fig. 2.6a).

BASIC PATHOLOGICAL PROCESSES

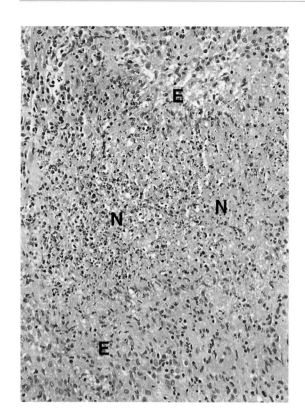

Fig. 4.10 Atypical mycobacterial infection involving lymph node (MP)

Infection with organisms of the ***Mycobacterium avium-intracellulare-scrofulaceum*** (**MAIS**) group is not uncommon in the cervical lymph nodes of young children. Another group at risk from these organisms are AIDS patients who, because of their severe immunosuppression, commonly develop widespread infections, especially involving the liver, lymph nodes and spleen. In these patients, there is usually a deficient immune response and the histological appearance may simply be of aggregates of epithelioid cells or even foamy macrophages in the tissue with no lymphocytic component.

This micrograph shows a lymph node from an otherwise healthy child with *Mycobacterium avium-intracellulare-scrofulaceum* infection. The lymphoid tissue is replaced with a granulomatous inflammatory response consisting of confluent sheets of epithelioid macrophages **E**. In contrast to *M. tuberculosis*, the granulomas in MAIS infection show suppurative necrosis with aggregates of neutrophils **N**, rather than caseous necrosis. Giant cells, as in this example, may be sparse.

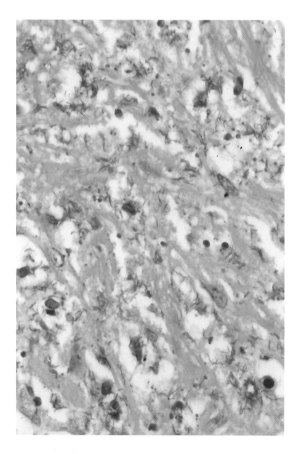

Fig. 4.11 Mycobacteria on Ziehl–Neelsen stain (HP)

Mycobacterium tuberculosis and the atypical mycobacteria are not visible on the routine H&E stains. To demonstrate the presence of mycobacteria in tissue, the Ziehl–Neelsen (ZN) staining method is employed. The stain is taken up by the cell walls of the mycobacteria and remains despite treatment with acid; this is the origin of the other term, ***acid-fast bacilli***, used in describing mycobacteria. In this very high power micrograph, groups of magenta-coloured bent rods can be seen in a background of epithelioid cells. In an immunocompetent individual, these organisms may be very sparse and difficult to find, but even a single organism in the appropriate background of a caseating granuloma is diagnostic. In immunosuppressed individuals and also in MAIS infection (as shown here), the organisms are often much more numerous.

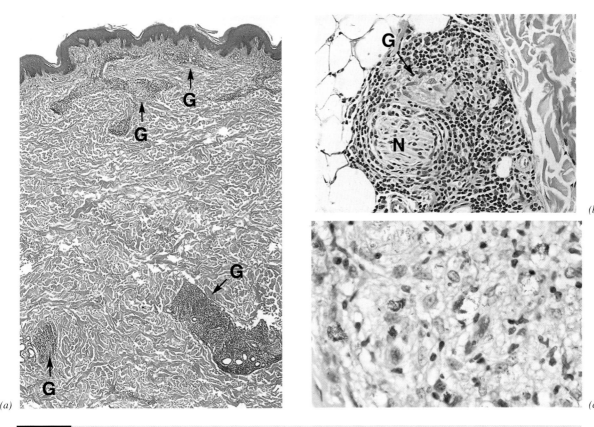

(a)   *(b)*   *(c)*

Fig. 4.12 Leprosy

(a) Dermal infiltration (LP) (b) Nerve involvement (HP) (c) Wade–Fite stain in lepromatous leprosy (HP)

Leprosy is a disease caused by infection with *Mycobacterium leprae*. The tissue reaction to the bacillus depends on the immune response of the infected person. In the ***tuberculoid form*** of the disease, there is an active cell-mediated immune response and granulomas are formed similar to those seen in tuberculosis but without evidence of caseation. In the ***lepromatous form***, there is no effective cell-mediated immune response and tissues are infiltrated with macrophages colonised by large numbers of bacteria. Intermediate forms of leprosy exist with both tuberculoid and lepromatous features.

Clinically, people with the lepromatous form of the disease have nodular dermal and subcutaneous deposits of macrophages filled with bacteria and lipid. The disease affects the face, ears, arms, knees and buttocks, as the leprosy bacilli require cooler areas of the body for proliferation. In contrast, the tuberculoid form of the

disease gives rise to macular or plaque-like skin lesions and in addition causes extensive inflammatory destruction of peripheral nerves, giving rise to anaesthesia in limbs which become prone to damage through repeated non-perceived injury.

Micrograph (a) is from the skin of a person with tuberculoid leprosy. Histiocytic granulomas with a heavy surrounding lymphocytic infiltrate **G** are present at all layers throughout the dermis but particularly in relation to small nerves; this is seen in the higher magnification micrograph (b) where a small nerve **N** is seen surrounded by lymphocytes with an associated granuloma **G**. Micrograph (c) of lepromatous leprosy shows the Wade–Fite stain, which is similar to the ZN stain for tuberculosis, in that it stains the organisms red. The similarity in appearance between *M. tuberculosis* and *M. leprae* can be readily appreciated.

BASIC PATHOLOGICAL PROCESSES

Treponemal infections

The major Treponemal infection worldwide is syphilis, due to *Treponema pallidum*; yaws and pinta are Treponemal infections which are rare other than in specific tropical regions.

Fig. 4.13 Syphilis
(a) **Syphilitic gumma of the liver (LP)**
(b) **Syphilitic aortitis (MP –** *illustration opposite***)**

Although now relatively uncommon, late stage syphilis is still regarded as one of the classic examples of specific chronic inflammation. The infecting organism, the spiral-shaped *Treponema pallidum*, resists usual tissue defences and excites a progression of fascinating pathological and clinical phenomena which represent typical chronic inflammatory responses with superimposed hypersensitivity reactions mounted by the immune system. Classically, the condition proceeds through three stages extending over a long period.

In brief, the organism usually gains access to the body by penetrating the genital mucosa where it produces a single, small *primary lesion* known as a *chancre*. The chancre is a raised, reddened nodule caused by an intense local accumulation of plasma cells and lymphocytes in the sub-epithelial connective tissue. The chancre may ulcerate at this stage, but it is often painless and may easily pass unnoticed. By the time the chancre has developed, the organism has multiplied extensively and has been disseminated via local lymphatics to regional lymph nodes and thence into the bloodstream causing a generalised bacteraemia. The chancre and concomitant bacteraemia (*primary syphilis*) are followed some weeks or months later by a transient *secondary stage* characterised by a widespread variable skin rash, often with moist warty genital lesions and ulceration of the oral mucosa. These various mucosal lesions are histologically similar to the primary chancre and are full of Treponemal organisms. The disease is now at its most contagious, yet the patient usually feels well and the only other evidence of a generalised infection is a widespread lymphadenopathy and positive serological findings.

In most untreated cases, the infection is effectively resolved by body defences, and in many of these even serological evidence of previous infection disappears. Unfortunately, a proportion of untreated cases proceed from the secondary stage to develop *tertiary syphilis* after a variable interval of from one to many years. The lesions of tertiary syphilis may be either focal or diffuse, and it is the focal lesion of tertiary syphilis, known as the *gumma*, which exhibits many of the features of a granulomatous inflammation. Tertiary lesions may occur in almost any organ or tissue, and the clinical consequences vary enormously. The diffuse form of tertiary syphilis most notably involves the cardiovascular system, particularly the ascending aorta, and less commonly the central nervous system; the well known *tabes dorsalis* and *general paralysis of the insane* (GPI) are two of the manifestations of neurosyphilis. In the

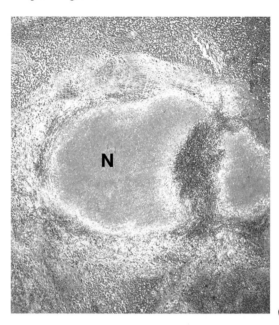

(a)

focal form of tertiary syphilis, gummas may develop in the liver, bone, testes and other sites, the clinical outcome depending on the nature and extent of local tissue destruction.

Micrograph (a) illustrates the classical appearance of a gumma. The active gumma has a central area of homogeneous coagulative necrosis **N** surrounded by a zone of epithelioid macrophages, lymphocytes, plasma cells and plump fibroblasts. Fibrous healing of liver gummas may produce a pattern of coarse deep scars dividing the liver surface into numerous irregular lobules; this condition is known as *hepar lobatum*.

Micrograph (b) illustrates syphilitic aortitis, the most common form of diffuse tertiary syphilitic lesion. The characteristic feature of diffuse tertiary syphilis, and also of primary and secondary syphilitic lesions, is a low grade chronic vasculitis of small vessels which exhibit thickening of the wall, particularly the endothelium, and a perivascular cuff of lymphocytes and plasma cells, known as *endarteritis obliterans*. In the aorta, the vasculitis affects the vasa vasorum of the tunica adventitia and their smaller branches which extend into the tunica media; the blue-stained areas in the tunica media represent lymphocytic cuffing around numerous small vessels. The smooth muscle and elastic fibres of the media degenerate, probably because of ischaemia, and the aortic wall is replaced by collagen. Residual elastin **E** is stained deep pink. The loss of elasticity and contractility in the aortic wall allows progressive stretching with the formation of an *aortic aneurysm*, usually in the ascending aorta or aortic arch.

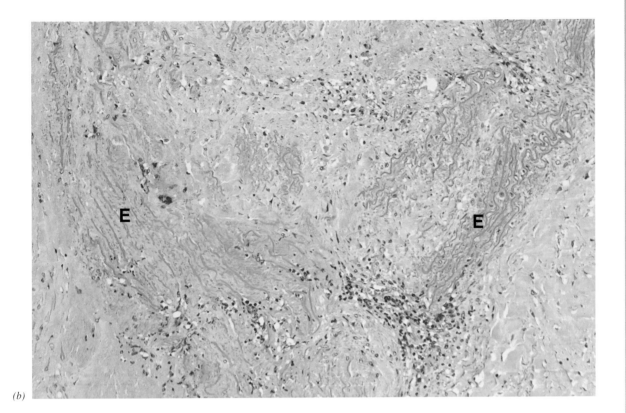

(b)

Viral infections

Viruses cause disease in three main ways:

- By causing death of the cell they infect, either by a direct effect or by modifying the genome such that the host cell is recognised as foreign and is destroyed by the host's own immune system.
- By causing excessive proliferation of the infected cell line. This may be an important factor in the eventual development of malignant tumours in the affected cell line. Human papilloma virus (HPV) is important in this respect.
- By integrating themselves in the cell nucleus where they produce latent infection.

Although viral culture and the demonstration of rising titres of antibodies against the virus remain the mainstay of diagnosis, some viral infections can be diagnosed by characteristic histological appearances. Individual viruses are too small to be seen by light microscopy, but when congregating together in enormous numbers within the host cell, they are visible as viral inclusion bodies and may be either intranuclear, intracytoplasmic, or both. Inclusion bodies provide a histological clue to the causative virus, and this can be confirmed by electron microscopy and immunohistology.

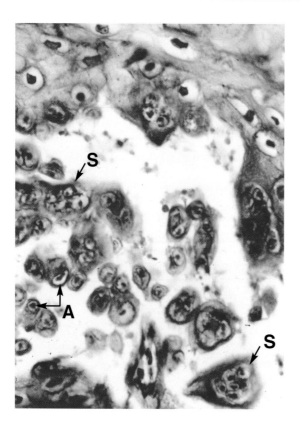

Fig. 4.14 Herpes virus infection of skin (HP)

Herpes simplex virus types 1 and 2 (HSV-1 and HSV-2) cause the common skin eruptions known as 'cold sores' and genital Herpes, whilst the chicken pox virus (*Herpes zoster*) is responsible for 'shingles'. In immunocompetent individuals, the Herpes viruses are able to remain latent in nerve cells with intermittent episodes of reactivation when the virus replicates within and destroys epidermal cells or the epithelial cells of mucous membranes. Clinically, this gives rise to the typical appearance of groups of vesicles on an erythematous background. The vesicles are caused by hydropic degeneration and necrosis of epithelial cells.

This micrograph shows a biopsy specimen from a patient with *Herpes zoster* infection. Intranuclear inclusion bodies **A** which are large and pink-purple in colour can be seen within the nuclei, pushing the hyperchromatic host chromatin to one side. They consist of masses of intact and disrupted virus particles. Another characteristic feature is the fusion of epithelial cells to form multinucleate syncytia **S** which are well demonstrated in this micrograph. Infected cells are often much increased in size with proportionately enlarged nuclei.

Most lesions heal spontaneously although the latent viral DNA remains in the nerve cells from where it will emerge in subsequent clinical episodes.

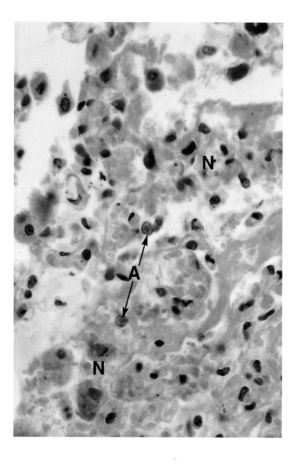

Fig. 4.15 Herpes pneumonitis (HP)

In immunosuppressed patients such as those with AIDS or those on immunosuppressive treatment, Herpes viruses may result in widespread skin or visceral infections rather than a localised, self-limiting rash as in the immunocompetent. Similar histological features are seen.

This micrograph shows a section of lung from an AIDS patient with *Herpes simplex* pneumonitis. Occasional cells with intranuclear inclusion bodies **A** are seen; these may be sparse and difficult to find. In addition, there is necrosis **N** of lung tissue and a mild infiltrate of lymphocytes into the tissue.

The brain, oesophagus and liver are other common sites of infection in immunosuppressed patients. Another group at risk of disseminated infection are neonates who can become infected during passage through the birth canal in which there is active infection. Neonates are relatively immunologically incompetent and may succumb to a generalised infection of the lymph nodes, spleen, lungs, liver, adrenals and central nervous system.

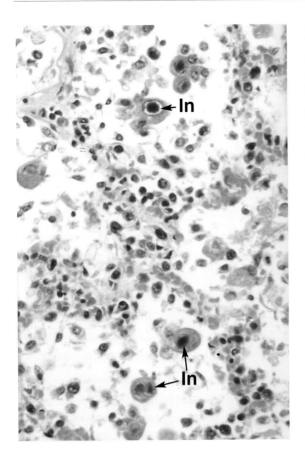

Fig. 4.16 Cytomegalovirus infection (HP)

Cytomegalovirus (CMV), another of the Herpes virus group, causes a mild, non-specific infection in immunocompetent individuals. Most adults will have been exposed to this virus by late middle age and will have specific serum antibodies. CMV infects white blood cells and may remain latent in leucocytes for many years. If the individual then becomes immunosuppressed for any reason, widespread systemic infection may result. Common sites of infection include the lungs, brain, retina, gastrointestinal tract and kidney.

CMV pneumonitis is shown in this micrograph. The characteristic feature is markedly enlarged cells with large dark-staining intranuclear inclusion bodies **In**. These are surrounded by a clear halo. Cytoplasmic inclusions are also sometimes seen but are not illustrated in this micrograph. Focal necrosis is also sometimes present but there is usually minimal, if any, inflammation. Cytomegalic inclusions are usually seen in epithelial cells, endothelial cells and in macrophages, and as is the case in other Herpes virus infections, they may be sparse.

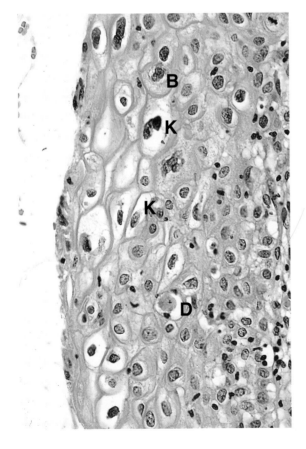

Fig. 4.17 Human papilloma virus (HP)

Human papilloma virus (HPV) is the causative agent of the common viral warts on the skin and genital warts. It has also been shown to be very closely associated with *cervical intraepithelial neoplasia* (**CIN**) and with invasive squamous cell carcinoma of the cervix, vagina, vulva and other sites.

HPV infects squamous epithelial cells and causes characteristic changes in the epithelial morphology. The epithelium is usually thickened (acanthotic) or may have the papillary appearance of an exophytic wart (*condyloma acuminatum*). Infection of cells in the upper layers of the epithelium produces enlargement of the nuclei which are hyperchromatic and have a folded appearance. A prominent cytoplasmic halo is also seen. These cells are called *koilocytes* **K**. In addition, the epithelium contains binucleate cells **B** and dyskeratotic cells **D** (i.e. individual cell keratinisation).

Such changes as those above are usually seen in association with low grade CIN, as in this specimen from a woman with CIN I. In high-grade CIN, these changes are not usually apparent, being overshadowed by more advanced dysplastic changes; HPV infection can, however, be demonstrated by molecular techniques in almost all high grade CIN lesions (see also Fig. 17.4).

BASIC PATHOLOGICAL PROCESSES

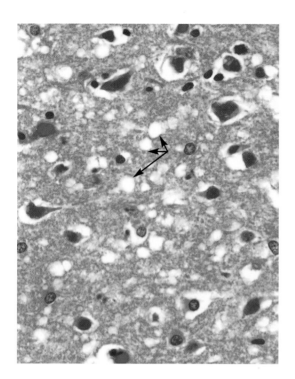

Fig. 4.18 Spongiform encephalopathy caused by prion disease (HP)

The spongiform encephalopathies are caused by an unconventional protein-only agent (containing no nucleic acid) called a ***prion***, which can be transmissible. In these diseases there is an excessive accumulation of a modified normal cell membrane protein called ***prion protein* (*PrP*)** in the brain. It is believed that disease develops when normal prion protein is progressively converted into an abnormal conformation by contact with the abnormal form.

The commonest disease is ***Creutzfeldt Jakob disease* (*CJD*)** in which there is rapidly progressive dementia, causing death within two years. ***Variant CJD*** is currently believed to be caused by transmission of abnormal prions through the ingestion of beef products from cattle with ***bovine spongiform encephalopathy***.

The dominant histological feature is vacuolation in the cerebral cortex, termed spongiform change (arrows). There is also neuronal degeneration and loss, and astrocytic gliosis. Immunohistochemical methods show accumulation of abnormal prion protein in the brain, sometimes in the form of amyloid plaques (see Fig. 23.8).

Fungal infections

Fungal infections range from minor localised skin infections to major systemic life-threatening diseases in immunosuppressed patients. The inflammatory reaction in fungal infections may have one of three patterns. The classic appearance is of a granulomatous inflammation which may in some sites exhibit central suppurative necrosis. A second pattern is of an acute inflammatory response with a tissue infiltrate consisting primarily of neutrophils; this pattern is seen in *Candida* infection of the oesophagus. The third is a very minimal inflammatory response, as in superficial infections in the skin by dermatophytic fungi.

Fungi are not usually obvious on routine H&E staining but the thick cell walls are highlighted by special stains such as PAS with diastase stain or silver stains. Some fungi are easily recognised histologically because of the characteristic shape and structure of the hyphae, and the pattern of budding of the yeast cells. However, culture techniques are preferable for definitive identification of fungal species. Figures 4.19 to 4.23 illustrate a few fungi which are commonly encountered in routine histopathology practice. An important diagnostic point is that the presence of fungal yeast forms such as *Candida* at a mucosal surface or on the skin does not necessarily indicate active infection, as these agents are common commensals. Evidence of active invasion must be demonstrated such as the presence of hyphae and, in most cases, an appropriate inflammatory response.

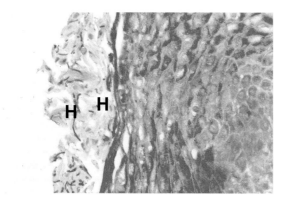

(a)

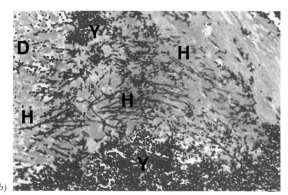

(b)

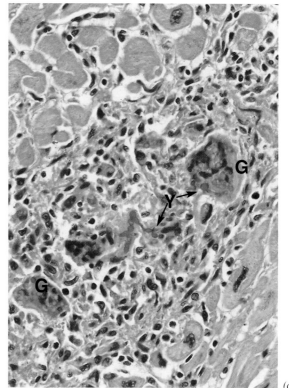

(c)

Fig. 4.19 Candidiasis

(a) Oral candidiasis (PAS – MP) (b) Oesophageal candidiasis (PAS – HP) (c) Myocardial candidiasis (PAS – HP)

Candida albicans is a ubiquitous commensal fungus on the epithelial surfaces of the skin, mouth and genital tract, and exists in both a hyphal/mycelial form, and also as rounded yeasts. Although usually commensal, it can become pathogenic, usually producing reddening and soreness of the affected epithelium, often with a whitish surface membrane comprising excess keratin production and fungal hyphae. The common sites for this are the mouth (oral Candidiasis or thrush) and the vulvo-vaginal region (Candidal vulvo-vaginitis). Both may be precipitated by debilitation or as a complication of systemic antibiotic therapy destroying the normal bacterial flora and allowing overgrowth of the fungus.

More severe infections can occur in patients who are immunosuppressed: surface epithelial infections are more extensive and symptomatic, with large numbers of organisms in both hyphal and yeast forms (see micrograph b). Organisms may also gain access to the bloodstream and in immunosuppressed patients may produce disseminated Candidiasis with organisms in many organs (see micrograph c).

Micrograph (a) shows Candidal infection, mainly in hyphal forms **H,** on the surface of the buccal epithelium from a case of oral thrush in a patient taking antibiotics.

Micrograph (b) shows abundant Candidal infection, both in hyphal **H** and yeast **Y** forms in the oesophagus of an elderly man debilitated by terminal cancer. There is also abundant necrotic debris **D** forming a thick surface membrane. The infection had started as severe oropharyngeal thrush, but had spread down his oesophagus.

Micrograph (c) shows *Candida* yeast forms **Y** in giant cells **G** in the myocardium, forming a small granuloma. Often, bloodstream spread of *Candida* produces small abscesses filled with neutrophils (pus), but this patient was severely immunosuppressed and was unable to mount an acute inflammatory reaction.

BASIC PATHOLOGICAL PROCESSES

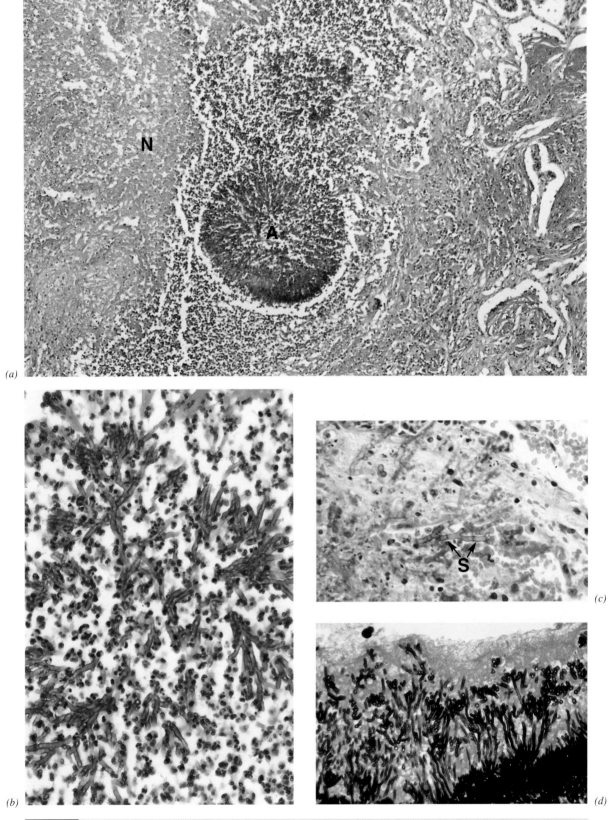

(a)

(b)

(c)

(d)

Fig. 4.20 Pulmonary aspergillosis *(caption opposite – above)*

Fig. 4.20 Pulmonary aspergillosis
(a) MP (b) HP (c) HP (d) Silver stain (HP) *(illustrations opposite)*

Aspergillus is a ubiquitous fungus which may cause an allergic pulmonary response in otherwise healthy individuals. This is known colloquially as brewer's lung and belongs to the group of diseases known by the term ***extrinsic allergic alveolitis***. In this case, the *Aspergillus* does not colonise or invade the lung. Asthmatic individuals may have their bronchial tree colonised by *Aspergillus* without invasion. They are then likely to suffer from an exacerbation of their asthma as a result of ***allergic bronchopulmonary aspergillosis***. That is to say they develop a hypersensitivity response to *Aspergillus* antigens to which they are constantly exposed. *Aspergillus* may also colonise pre-existing abscess cavities, classically old tuberculous cavities, where it may form a ***fungus ball (Aspergilloma)***. Invasive

Aspergillus infections occur in individuals who are immunosuppressed.

Micrograph (a) shows a medium-power view of invasive *Aspergillus* infection in the lung. A mass of *Aspergillus* hyphae **A** is surrounded by an inflammatory infiltrate consisting mainly of neutrophils. Adjacent to this is a zone of necrotic lung tissue **N**.

At high power, micrograph (b) shows the mass of *Aspergillus* hyphae. These characteristically branch at an acute angle as is shown in micrograph (c). The hyphae are also ***septate***, i.e. the hyphae have divisions or septae **S** which divide them into segments. The typical appearance of *Aspergillus* on a silver stain is shown in micrograph (d) which shows the fungal hyphae clearly.

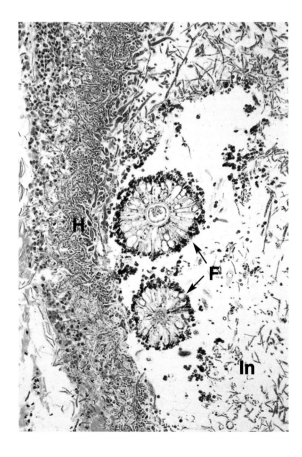

Fig. 4.21 Aspergillus niger (MP)

This micrograph shows a mass of hyphae of ***Aspergillus niger*** **H** and inflammatory cells **In** from the external ear canal of a patient with chronic otitis externa. In the centre of the field are two characteristic ***fruiting bodies*** **F** or ***conidia***. These are similar to the fruiting bodies of other *Aspergillus* species except that they are pigmented. The brownish-black pigment is visible around the periphery of the fruiting body and gives rise to the name *Aspergillus niger*. This is a common cause of chronic otitis externa, an infection of the outer ear, mainly the auditory canal.

BASIC PATHOLOGICAL PROCESSES

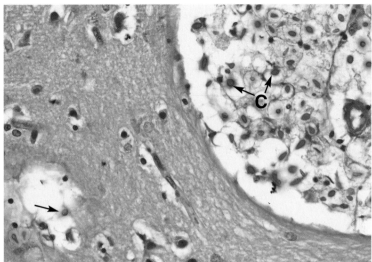

(a)

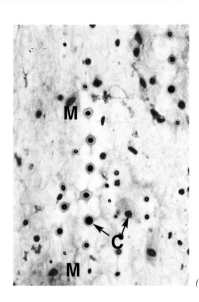

(b)

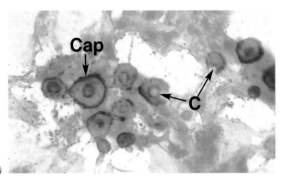

(c)

Fig.4.22 Cryptococcus

(a) Brain (MP) (b) Fine needle aspirate (Giemsa – HP) (c) Needle biopsy (mucicarmine – HP)

Cryptococcus neoformans is another yeast which causes serious infections in many tissues, mainly in immunosuppressed individuals such as patients with AIDS, haematological malignancy, and transplant recipients. Occasionally, however, it may cause meningitis, meningoencephalitis or lung infection in an otherwise well individual.

Micrograph (a) shows the typical appearance of *Cryptococcus* in the brain. The organisms are seen forming a cyst in a Virchow–Robin perivascular space. These lesions are known as 'soap bubble' lesions. The *Cryptococci* **C** stain magenta with the PAS stain and the thick surrounding capsule of the organism appears as a clear space. A few organisms (arrowed) can be seen invading the adjacent brain tissue which is oedematous. Typical of this organism, there is a minimal inflammatory response which may be due to the immunosuppressed state of the patient. However, in chronic infections in non-immunosuppressed individuals, the organisms may incite a granulomatous response.

In the lung, *Cryptococcus* may cause a diffuse infection; however, it may also form a solitary mass lesion in previously healthy individuals. In this case, the lesion is in fact a large granuloma with a jelly-like centre formed by a mass of organisms surrounded by a thick layer of macrophages, lymphocytes and giant cells.

Micrographs (b) and (c) are from such a lesion which presented as a solitary mass on chest X-ray in a previously well smoker. Bronchogenic carcinoma was suspected and fine needle aspiration biopsy (FNAB) performed; rather than the expected clusters of malignant cells, the smear, shown in micrograph (b), contained large numbers of *Cryptococcus* organisms **C** which appear as purple-stained cells in this Giemsa preparation, each surrounded by a clear capsule. A few macrophages **M** with foamy cytoplasm are seen in the background. A needle biopsy taken at the same time is shown in micrograph (c). Stained with mucicarmine, it demonstrates the *Cryptococci* **C**, each comprising a bright carmine-stained cell with a less intensely stained outer capsule **Cap**.

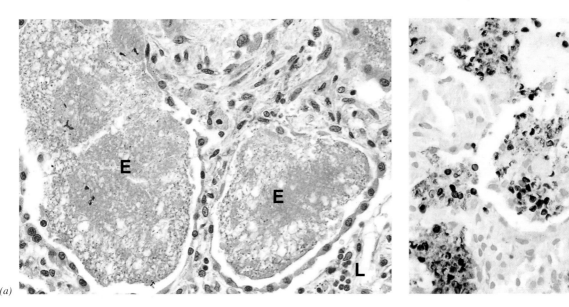

(a)   *(b)*

Fig. 4.23 Pneumocystis in lung
(a) H&E (MP) (b) Silver stain (MP)

The organism ***Pneumocystis carinii*** was previously classified as a protozoan, but more recently it has become clear that it is more likely to be a member of the fungal family. It is a ubiquitous organism and can be demonstrated in the lungs of most normal individuals where it causes no disease. *Pneumocystis* has, however, been brought into the spotlight by the AIDS epidemic, although it may infect patients with immunosuppression from other causes.

In AIDS patients, *Pneumocystis* causes a diffuse patchy pneumonia which may be the presenting feature of full-blown AIDS and is often fatal. Diagnosis may be difficult and transbronchial lung biopsy is often required. With routine H&E staining, as in micrograph (a), the organisms may not be apparent. The alveoli are often filled by a foamy, acellular exudate **E** with an interstitial infiltrate of lymphocytes **L** in the alveolar wall. The inflammatory infiltrate may be minimal or more severe, showing features of diffuse alveolar damage (see Fig. 12.10) with hyaline membranes, capillary dilatation and exudation of red cells. Demonstration of the organisms requires a silver stain as shown in micrograph (b). The organisms are cup-shaped and measure 4–6 μm. Giemsa and toluidine blue stains may also be employed. The above stains may also be carried out on sputum samples and bronchial washings. AIDS patients frequently have concurrent infections with other organisms such as *Cytomegalovirus* (see Fig. 4.16).

Protozoa and helminths

Of the wide range of protozoa which are of pathological importance, only a few are usually diagnosed histologically. Many of these organisms are major causes of morbidity and mortality in particular geographic regions in the Third World but with the advent of widespread travel and migration they are increasingly being seen elsewhere.

Protozoa are unicellular organisms which may reproduce asexually or sexually. Many have a complex life cycle involving one or more animal hosts. ***Giardia lamblia*** is a common protozoan infecting the small intestine in communities worldwide and is discussed in Chapter 13. Malaria and amoebiasis are described in this chapter.

A wide variety of helminths infect humans, many primarily infecting the gut although they may pass through other anatomic sites en route. Some helminths such as the nematodes ***Enterobius vermicularis*** and ***Toxocara canis*** are found worldwide, while others such as ***Wucheria bancrofti*** and ***Loa loa*** have a more limited tropical distribution. ***Schistosomiasis*** is of particular histological importance and is thus illustrated in this chapter.

BASIC PATHOLOGICAL PROCESSES

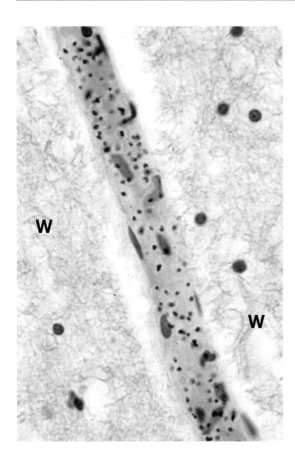

Fig. 4.24 Cerebral malaria (HP)

Malaria, which is caused by four species of the protozoan *Plasmodium*, is common in the tropics and subtropics and is a major cause of mortality. After entering the blood via the proboscis of a mosquito, the merozoites enter erythrocytes. Further cycles of division occur within the erythrocytes which rupture, allowing further cycles of infection. The sexual phase of the life cycle occurs within the mosquito. *Falciparum malaria* is the most virulent species of malaria with cerebral involvement being a major cause of death. The cerebral tissue is characteristically congested, as shown in this micrograph, where a dilated small blood vessel is packed with erythrocytes within which the malarial parasites can be seen as dark brown dots. Falciparum malaria has the property of causing erythrocytes to adhere to endothelium, thus obstructing blood flow. The surrounding white matter **W** is oedematous and the congested vessels often rupture to cause 'ring haemorrhages' (not shown here).

Without specific treatment, cerebral malaria is almost always fatal and the increasing incidence of drug resistance makes it difficult to treat. Malarial parasites can be seen within erythrocytes in any other tissues and the diagnosis is usually made by examination of a blood smear. The different species can be identified by their characteristic appearance. The other species which cause malaria, namely *P. vivax, P. ovale* and *P. malariae*, cause a much milder illness which may be recurrent. *P. falciparum* may cause severe anaemia, pulmonary oedema, renal failure, shock and hypoglycaemia in addition to cerebral disease.

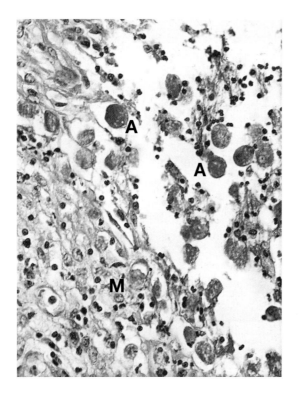

Fig. 4.25 Amoebiasis (PAS – HP)

Infections with *Entamoeba histolytica* occur worldwide. The organism is restricted to man and it has been estimated that about 10% of the world's population (i.e. 550 million people!) carry the organism in the colon. However, less than 20% of those colonised develop clinical infection. The most common form of infection is *amoebic dysentery* where the *Entamoeba* invades the mucosa of the colon and rectum, causing painful bloody diarrhoea. Pathologically, the mucosa is breached and extensively undermined producing typical flask-shaped ulcers; occasionally, this leads to perforation.

This micrograph shows organisms **A** adherent to an area of ulcerated colonic mucosa **M**. The *Entamoebae* are slightly larger than a macrophage. They characteristically phagocytose erythrocytes which may be identifiable histologically (not in this micrograph). There is a mixed inflammatory response with plentiful neutrophils and plasma cells but no granuloma formation. The organisms may invade and obstruct colonic arteries causing superimposed ischaemic necrosis.

The organism may spread to the liver causing an **amoebic abscess** and thence to the lung or pleural, peritoneal or pericardial cavities. Venereal infections of the cervix and penis also occasionally occur.

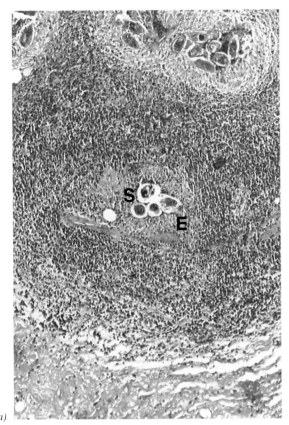

(a)

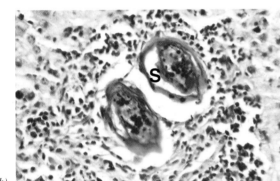

(b)

Fig. 4.26 Schistosomiasis
(a) MP (b) HP

Schistosomiasis is a systemic parasitic infection caused by the organism *Schistosoma*, a genus of trematode worm (flukes). Three species are of pathological importance. Their life cycle includes water snails (the intermediate host), with man (the definitive host) becoming infected by bathing or working in water containing the larvae or ***cercaria*** released from snails. The cercaria penetrate the skin, in the process converting to ***schistosomules***, and then migrate via the venous system to the pulmonary vessels where they mature for 4 weeks before entering the systemic circulation. From here they migrate to the hepatic branches of the portal vein (*S. mansoni* and *S. japonicum*) or the pelvic veins (*S. haematobium*) where they mature and may persist for several years or even more. In their chosen location, the adult worms mate with the females producing up to 3000 eggs per day. Some eggs leave the body in urine or faeces and, on reaching still or gently flowing fresh water, hatch into a ciliated form called ***miracidia*** and thus reach their intermediate snail hosts. Other eggs lodge in the tissues (*S. mansoni* and *S. japonicum* in the small and large intestine and thence to the liver; *S. haematobium* in the bladder and rectum) exciting a florid granulomatous reaction progressing to extensive fibrosis. In the liver, there is severe fibrosis of the portal tracts where the eggs lodge; schistosomiasis is the major cause of portal hypertension worldwide. *S. haematobium* causes a similar reaction in the bladder with a number of manifestations including papillomas, ulcers and bladder contractures. Chronic inflammation predisposes to dysplasia and malignancy. Eggs may also be found at many other sites such as the lungs and CNS.

Micrograph (a) shows a low-power view of schistosome eggs **S** in the colon. The groups of eggs are surrounded by epithelioid cells **E**, giant cells and eosinophils.

Micrograph (b) shows two schistosome eggs **S** at high power. The eggs of each species can be identified by their size and the position of the spine, which in this case is terminally located and therefore likely to come from *S. haematobium*.

BASIC PATHOLOGICAL PROCESSES

5. Amyloidosis

Introduction

Amyloidosis is a condition characterised by the extracellular deposition of abnormal fibrillar proteins, termed *amyloid*. These may be deposited in many tissues and organs, termed *systemic amyloid*, or in a single organ, *localised amyloid*. Amyloid is defined by its staining characteristics with certain stains such as Congo red and its ultrastructural appearance where it is seen to form rigid fibrils, 10–15 nm in diameter. These are made up of different peptides, as outlined in Figure 5.2, and comprise about 90–95% of the deposited material in amyloid. The important characteristic of these peptides is that they form a *β-pleated sheet* protein structure. This is similar to the structure of silk and makes the peptides very resistant to proteolysis. These peptides then assemble into the fibrillar structure seen ultrastructurally (Fig. 5.1). In addition, all types of amyloid contain a small amount of *amyloid protein P*, a glycoprotein which makes up about 5–10% of the total material.

The peptides which form amyloid are derived from normal body proteins. By way of example, *AL amyloid protein* consists of the variable segment of immunoglobulin light chains produced in abnormal quantities by a clone of malignant plasma cells in multiple myeloma. *AA amyloid protein* is derived from a normal serum protein, an acute phase protein, which is produced in excess in certain chronic inflammatory conditions. There are also a number of heredo-familial amyloidoses caused by polymorphisms in genes coding for a variety of proteins.

Amyloidosis has traditionally been classified as *primary* or *secondary* according to whether there was a pre-existing disease which was known to be associated with amyloid or not. This classification has been superseded since the peptide structure of amyloid has now been elucidated and classification according to peptide structure is more clinically useful.

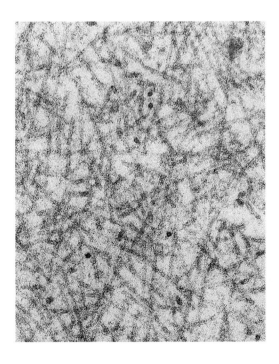

Fig. 5.1 Amyloid ultrastructure (EM)

Electron microscopy is a useful method for the detection of amyloid in tissues, particularly when it is present in small quantities and hence does not show up with special stains. This electron micrograph shows amyloid deposited in renal glomeruli and resulting in proteinuria (excess protein leaking into the urine). A renal biopsy was performed and at light microscopy revealed thickening of the basement membrane of the glomeruli. Ultrastructural examination of a portion of the thickened basement membrane revealed the deposition of amyloid.

The amyloid is seen to have a fibrillar ultrastructure, each fibril being composed of the precursor peptide arranged as finer filaments of a β-pleated sheet.

In this instance, the amyloid was deposited as a result of long-standing rheumatoid disease and was presumably of the serum amyloid A protein type (see Fig. 5.2).

Distribution and classification of amyloid

Amyloid is deposited in the extracellular compartment of tissues, and in H&E preparations is seen as uniformly eosinophilic (pink-staining) material. It can be highlighted in histological sections by use of special stains such as Congo red and Sirius red. Congo red staining is commonly used for diagnostic purposes, amyloid staining orange-red in colour and exhibiting a characteristic green coloration when viewed with polarised light.

Amyloidosis may involve many tissues in the body but most commonly affects kidneys, spleen, liver, adrenals and heart (Figs 5.3 to 5.6). It has a particular predilection for deposition in blood vessel walls (Fig. 5.8) and basement membranes. The progressive accumulation of amyloid leads to cellular dysfunction, either by preventing normal diffusion through extracellular tissues or by physical compression of functioning parenchymal cells.

Fig. 5.2 Classification of amyloid

Localisation	Clinical association	Fibril protein
Systemic amyloid	Multiple myeloma, B-cell lymphoma	Immunoblobulin light chain variable region (AL)
	Chronic inflammation	Serum amyloid A protein (AA)
	Familial Mediterranean fever	Serum amyloid A protein (AA)
	Familial neuropathy	Transthyretin (pre-albumin)
	Dialysis associated	β-2-microglobulin
Localised amyloid	Senile cardiac amyloid	Transthyretin (pre-albumin)
	Medullary carcinoma of thyroid, insulinoma	Calcitonin gene-related peptide (CGRP)
	Type II diabetes	Amylin
	Alzheimer's disease, Down's syndrome	β APP
	Cerebal angiopathy	β APP

Amino acid sequencing of amyloid proteins in different disease states has enabled a classification of amyloid to be made on biochemical grounds as shown in Figure 5.2.

Amyloid associated with monoclonal proliferation of plasma cells or B-lymphocytes is made up of the variable segment of immunoglobulin light chains (*AL protein*); examples of such disease include multiple myeloma, plasmacytoma and non-Hodgkin's B-cell lymphoma.

AA type amyloid occurs in a minority of cases of chronic inflammatory disease. The end result is deposition of amyloid derived from serum amyloid A protein (AA), an acute phase protein which is produced by the liver in response to inflammation and circulates in the serum. Examples of diseases leading to this type of amyloid include tuberculosis, rheumatoid arthritis, bronchiectasis and chronic osteomyelitis. Why some individuals have deposition of amyloid and others do not is unknown.

Certain familial types of amyloid involve the deposition of transthyretin-derived amyloid (transthyretin is so named as it transports thyroxine and retinol in plasma; this was formerly termed pre-albumin). *Transthyretin amyloid* in the familial types is associated with amino acid substitutions in the protein which predispose to the formation of the β-pleated sheet amyloid structure.

Tumours of peptide-secreting endocrine cells may form amyloid from an abnormal form of the hormone peptide. A well-known example is the localised deposition of **calcitonin-derived amyloid** in medullary carcinoma of the thyroid (Fig. 5.7).

The central nervous system provides perhaps the most common example of localised amyloid deposition in Alzheimer's disease (Fig. 23.3) derived from a peptide termed *βAPP* (amyloid precursor peptide) which is derived from a normal neuronal protein termed APP, the gene for which is found on chromosome 21. This may relate to deposition of the same protein in Down's syndrome (trisomy 21).

BASIC PATHOLOGICAL PROCESSES

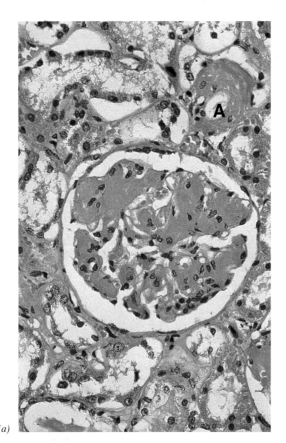

(a)

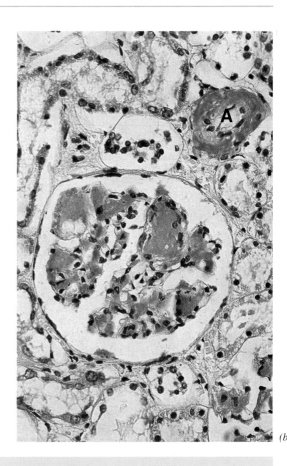

(b)

Fig. 5.3 Renal amyloidosis
(a) H&E (HP) (b) Sirius red (HP)

The kidneys are the organs most commonly involved by systemic amyloidosis, and renal failure is one of the most serious clinical complications, accounting for the majority of deaths from the disease. These sections from the same glomerulus are from an autopsy specimen taken from a 58-year-old woman with a 20-year history of rheumatoid arthritis; the sections have been stained with contrasting histological methods to illustrate the principal features.

Amyloid deposition usually begins in the glomerular mesangium and around capillary basement membranes, leading to progressive obliteration of capillary lumina, destruction of glomerular endothelial, mesangial and podocyte cells, and eventually complete replacement of the glomerulus by a confluent mass of amyloid. Concurrently, the walls of renal arterioles and arteries **A**

may become infiltrated by amyloid, causing impairment of the blood supply to the glomeruli. Interstitial spaces between renal tubules may also become infiltrated, further compromising tubular function. With H&E staining, amyloid appears as a homogeneous eosinophilic (pink) material, difficult to distinguish from collagen or hyaline deposition. Staining methods such as Congo red or Sirius red, as in micrograph (b), readily distinguish amyloid which stands out as red-stained material, in this case in the glomerulus and an affected afferent arteriole.

Amyloid of the kidney usually presents with proteinuria, often severe enough to produce the nephrotic syndrome. As increasing amyloid deposition leads to glomerular ischaemia and tubular atrophy, chronic renal failure supervenes.

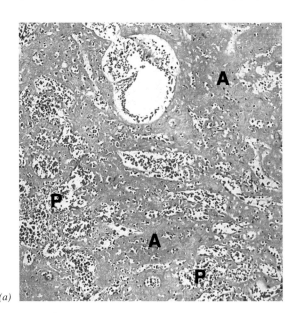

(a)

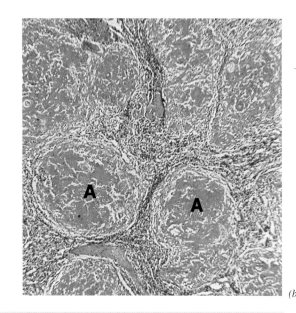

(b)

Fig. 5.4 Splenic amyloidosis
a) Diffuse type (MP) (b) Nodular type (MP)

There are two patterns of amyloid deposition seen in the spleen, described as either *diffuse* or *nodular*.

Micrograph (a) shows the more common diffuse pattern. Splenic amyloidosis most commonly begins with deposition in the walls of splenic sinuses progressing until the deposits coalesce to form large diffuse masses **A**; little red pulp **P** and lymphoid tissue (white pulp, not seen in this specimen) remains. This form is sometimes termed 'lardaceous' because of the waxy firmness of the spleen when the specimen is cut.

Less commonly, amyloid deposition results in the formation of the so-called 'sago' spleen as illustrated in micrograph (b). In this pattern, the amyloid **A** becomes deposited in the periarteriolar lymphoid sheaths (white pulp), giving the appearance of discrete deposits on the cut surface of the gross specimen. Note the small vessels in the centre of the pink-staining nodular amyloid deposits.

Amyloid deposition in the spleen can give rise to clinically palpable splenic enlargement.

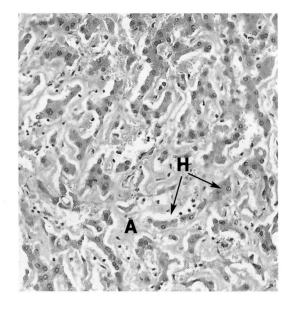

Fig. 5.5 Hepatic amyloidosis (HP)

In the liver, amyloid is deposited in the space between sinusoidal lining cells and hepatocytes. With progressive deposition, hepatocytes become compressed by sheets of amyloid and undergo atrophy.

Amyloid is visible as ribbon-like, pink-staining deposits **A** within hepatic sinusoids. Hepatocytes **H** have become compressed and are atrophic.

Clinically, hepatic amyloidosis may be a cause of hepatomegaly (enlargement of the liver). However, even when liver involvement is severe, there is rarely significant clinical evidence of impaired liver function.

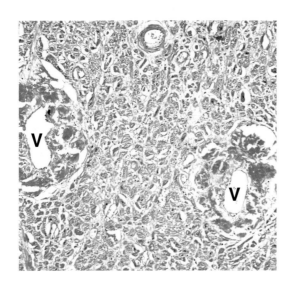

Fig. 5.6 Cardiac amyloid (MP)

Amyloid involvement of the heart may be an incidental finding at autopsy in the elderly, and in such cases is usually a manifestation of senile cardiac amyloid derived from transthyretin (pre-albumin).

The most severe form of cardiac amyloid is seen in systemic heredo-familial amyloidosis derived from serum amyloid A protein, as in familial Mediterranean fever. Cardiac involvement may also occur in cases of systemic AA amyloidosis.

Myocardial amyloidosis leads to intractable cardiac failure with enlargement of the heart; subendocardial deposition of amyloid may interfere with the conducting system resulting in cardiac arrhythmias.

In the case illustrated here, amyloid has accumulated in the walls of myocardial vessels **V** and is extending to form masses within the myocardium.

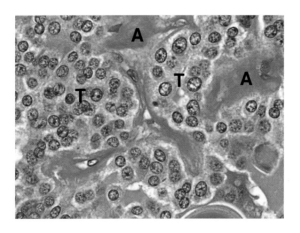

Fig. 5.7 Amyloid in medullary carcinoma of the thyroid (MP)

An example of localised amyloid is seen in tumours derived from the calcitonin-secreting cells of the thyroid, namely medullary carcinomas. Large islands of pink-stained amyloid **A** are present in between zones of tumour cells **T**. The amyloid is derived from pro-calcitonin secreted by the tumour. Amyloid is present only within the tumour and is not deposited in other tissues. Another example of localised amyloid is seen in insulinomas, which are tumours arising from the islets of Langerhans in the pancreas. In this case, it appears that the amyloid is also formed from a peptide similar to calcitonin.

In contrast, systemic amyloidosis may occur in association with certain tumours such as renal adenocarcinomas (derived from serum amyloid A protein), and multiple myeloma and certain B-cell lymphomas (derived from immunoglobulin light chain).

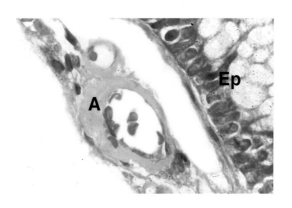

Fig. 5.8 Vessel amyloid in rectal biopsy (HP)

The diagnosis of systemic amyloidosis can be confirmed by tissue biopsy, and the rectum is the commonest biopsied site.

In rectal biopsies, amyloid can be detected in the submucosal vessels in 60–70% of cases of generalised amyloidosis. This photomicrograph, taken at very high magnification, shows rectal glandular epithelium **Ep** with a small blood vessel in the adjacent lamina propria. The vessel wall is thickened by homogeneous pink-staining amyloid **A**. Amyloid in small vessels such as this may be subtle, and it is usual to confirm the diagnosis by a special stain such as Congo red.

6. Disorders of growth

Introduction

Cells respond to environmental changes in several fundamentally different ways depending on the nature of the stimulus. As briefly discussed in Chapter 1, if the stimulus is overwhelming then the cells undergo degeneration or cell death. However, many less noxious stimuli cause cells to adapt by altering their pattern of growth. This may occur in three main ways:

- change in the size of cells
- change in the differentiation of cells
- change in the rate of cell division.

In an organ composed of different types of cell, only one of the cell types may be affected leading to a marked change in tissue appearance and function.

In all tissues there is a population of undifferentiated cells (*stem cells*) which retain the capacity to divide and differentiate into specialised cell types. Normal tissues may be divided into three types by the way in which their stem cells maintain the differentiated cell population:

- stem cells divide continuously to maintain a constantly replenished population of differentiated cells, e.g. intestinal epithelium
- stem cells do not normally divide and differentiate, but are capable of doing so in response to certain demands, e.g. after partial hepatectomy (*facultative dividers*)
- stem cells which have only been shown to divide in experimental situations; for example, the myocardium and brain have no capacity for functional regeneration (*non-dividers*).

Extrinsic to the cell, factors such as blood supply, innervation, hormonal stimulation, physical stress or biochemical alterations will determine the normal pattern of cell growth in an organ or tissue. Depending on the intrinsic characteristics of a particular cell type, a change in environment may result in a change in the growth pattern. Such responses are now recognised as being under the control of various growth factors which act upon specific cell surface receptors. Alterations in the concentrations of growth factors or the expression of growth factor receptors will result in altered cell growth.

Increased cell mass

Certain organs may respond to environmental stimulation by an increase in functional cell mass. There are two mechanisms by which this occurs:

- increase in cell number as a consequence of cell division; this is termed *hyperplasia*
- increase in the size of existing cells; this is termed *hypertrophy*.

An important feature of these forms of increased cell mass is that, following removal of the environmental stimulus, the altered pattern of growth ceases and often the tissue reverts to its former state. Hypertrophy and hyperplasia can, in many circumstances, be regarded as normal physiological adaptations, as exemplified by exercise-induced skeletal muscle hypertrophy, and hyperplasia and hypertrophy of the myometrium during pregnancy. Many pathological stimuli invoke the responses of hypertrophy and hyperplasia, and it appears that these responses occur in many cases by the same mechanism which induces the normal physiological response. Thus, in the first part of the menstrual cycle, the endometrium proliferates with elongation of glands and increased numbers of epithelial cells. When an excessive concentration of oestrogen acts in the endometrium, such as at the menopause or owing to injudicious hormone replacement therapy, similar but more pronounced changes occur leading to crowding of endometrial glands. Hyperplastic tissue is not of itself neoplastic but it does carry with it an increased risk of neoplastic change. Thus endometrial hyperplasia is more likely than normal endometrium to progress to cancer and this risk is increased further when the hyperplasia is combined with dysplasia (termed *atypical hyperplasia*).

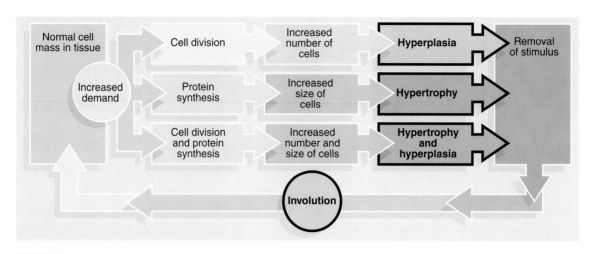

Fig. 6.1 Increased functional mass

For poorly understood reasons, the process of hyperplasia may not be uniform throughout an organ or tissue, and in these instances, nodules of excessive cell growth arise in between areas of unaltered cell growth. This phenomenon, known as ***nodular hyperplasia***, is seen in the thyroid gland (Fig. 20.5), the adrenal gland (Fig. 20.8) and the prostate gland (Fig. 19.9).

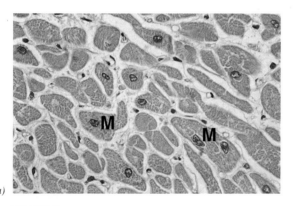

(a)

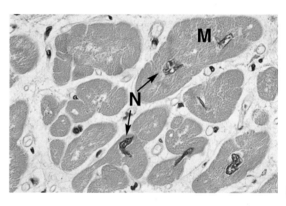

(b)

Fig. 6.2 Hypertrophy
(a) Normal myocardium (MP) (b) Hypertrophic myocardium (MP)

Pure hypertrophy without coexisting hyperplasia is virtually only seen in muscle where the stimulus is an increased demand for work. A good example is the adult myocardium. Myocardial cells are incapable of division and are therefore unable to undergo hyperplasia. The myocardium becomes hypertrophic when it is subjected to an increased haemodynamic load over a period of time, such as when there is systemic hypertension or valvular stenosis or incompetence. Micrograph (a) shows normal myocardium **M** while micrograph (b), which is at the same magnification, shows enlargement of myocardial cells **M** and of their nuclei **N**. This

enlargement is due to increased synthesis of proteins and filaments, permitting an increased workload; thus the size and weight of the heart are increased.

Other examples of muscular hypertrophy include that of bowel wall smooth muscle in chronic obstruction of the bowel by a tumour, that of the bladder detrusor muscle by chronic prostatic obstruction and that in regularly exercised skeletal muscles. It is interesting to note that athletes desirous of achieving increased muscle bulk supplement the effects of increasing muscle load by taking androgenic hormones.

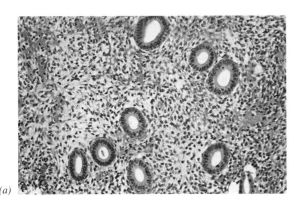 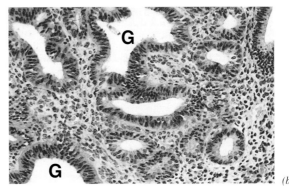

(a) *(b)*

Fig. 6.3 Hyperplasia
(a) Normal proliferative-phase endometrium (HP) (b) Hyperplasia of endometrium (HP)

Endometrial hyperplasia occurs when there is abnormal oestrogenic stimulation. Micrograph (a) shows normal proliferative-phase endometrium responding to normal ovarian oestrogenic stimulation. In contrast, in micrograph (b), the endometrial glands are markedly hyperplastic and continued increase in the number of cells in each gland has resulted in some glands **G** showing cystic dilatation. In addition there is irregularity and crowding of the glands and crowding of the epithelial cells lining the glands. This example is from a woman

on hormone replacement therapy where the effects of oestrogen were not counterbalanced by progestogens, resulting in persisting growth of the endometrium. Similar changes may also be seen in the endometrium of women with oestrogen-secreting ovarian tumours. Thus hyperplasia results from exaggeration of a normal physiologic mechanism.

In such examples, removal of the abnormal oestrogenic stimulation restores the normal pattern of endometrial growth.

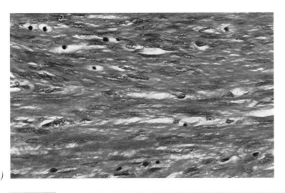 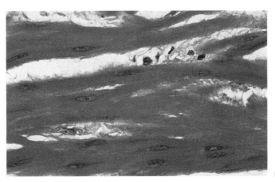

(a) *(b)*

Fig. 6.4 Hyperplasia with hypertrophy
(a) Normal myometrium (HP) (b) Myometrium during pregnancy (HP)

Hypertrophy and hyperplasia commonly occur together in response to increased functional requirements. When compared to the normal myometrial fibres seen in micrograph (a), the fibres of the pregnant uterus (b), at the same magnification, are greatly enlarged; their larger nuclei reflect increased protein synthesis.

Within the uterus as a whole, the number of smooth muscle cells is increased by hyperplasia. Occasionally in the uterus a mitotic figure may be seen where a myometrial cell is in the process of cell division.

Following pregnancy, the uterus returns to normal size by physiological atrophy, which by convention is termed *involution*.

Reduction in functional cell mass

When the functional cell mass in a tissue is reduced, the tissue is then said to have undergone *atrophy*. The mechanisms of atrophy may involve reduction in cell volume or in cell number, both leading to a reduction in functional capacity. Grossly, the appearance of the tissue depends on whether the functional cells lost are replaced by other tissue. Commonly, when atrophy occurs, the lost cells are replaced by either adipose or fibrous tissue, often maintaining the overall size of the organ; when adipose or fibrous replacement does not occur, then the overall size of the organ is reduced. Examples are the testis in the elderly (Fig. 6.5) and the adrenal gland when suppressed by exogenous steroid administration (Fig. 20.8). Atrophy may occur as a physiological event, when it is usually termed *involution*. An example is the normal involution of the thymus gland during adolescence.

Atrophy must be distinguished from *hypoplasia*, a condition where there is incomplete growth of an organ, and *agenesis*, where there is complete failure of growth of an organ during embryological development. In general, conditions opposite to those causing hypertrophy or hyperplasia result in atrophy. Thus disuse of skeletal muscle will result in a loss of cell mass. Removal of endocrine stimulation causes atrophy in target organs. Reduction in blood supply to a tissue may result in loss of functional cells; this is termed *ischaemic atrophy* and is seen commonly in the kidney.

In many atrophic tissues, a brown pigment called *lipofuscin* accumulates within the shrunken cells. This is thought to represent degenerate lipid material in secondary lysosomes produced by breakdown of the cell membranes and organelles. Lipofuscin accumulates particularly in the atrophic myocardial fibres of the hearts of elderly people and gives rise to the term *brown atrophy*.

Hyaline is a term used to describe replacement of tissue by an amorphous pink-staining material similar to basement membrane matrix; it is a common end result of atrophy or cell damage, being frequently accompanied by fibrosis. It is a feature of end-stage kidney (Fig. 15.1).

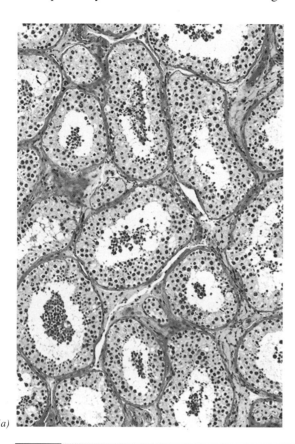

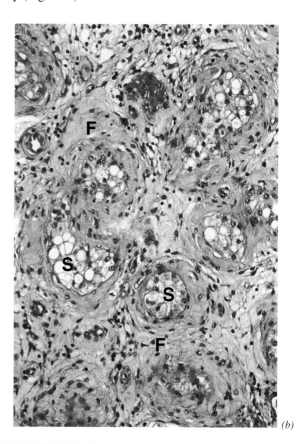

(a)   *(b)*

Fig. 6.5 Atrophy
(a) Normal testis (HP) (b) Atrophic testis (HP)

Micrograph (b) illustrates atrophy of the testis in a man aged 94. When compared with the normal testis in micrograph (a), the seminiferous tubules of the atrophic testis show almost no spermatogenic activity; however the Sertoli cells **S** are still easily identified. The basement membranes of the tubules are thickened and pink-stained, a process known as *hyalinisation*. The interstitial tissue shows an increased deposition of fibrous tissue **F**. Atrophy of a tissue occurs by shrinkage of cells, with reduction of cytoplasmic components such as organelles and enzyme proteins, and also by loss of cells by apoptosis.

Change in cell differentiation

When cells adapt to a change in environment by altering their differentiated appearance, this is termed *metaplasia*. The characteristic feature is that fully differentiated cells of one type replace the type usually found in that tissue. Metaplasia is thought to be an adaptive response which produces cells better equipped to withstand a (usually pathological) environmental change. For example, in the bronchi, the respiratory epithelium may be replaced by squamous epithelium under the influence of chronic irritation by cigarette smoke (*squamous metaplasia*). Similarly, in response to environmental changes during the reproductive cycle, the normal columnar endocervical epithelium is replaced by a stratified squamous epithelium (Fig. 6.6a). Also, in response to acid reflux into the lower oesophagus, the normal stratified squamous epithelium may be replaced by gastric or small intestinal mucosa (Fig. 6.6b).

The basic alteration appears to occur in the stem cells of the tissue in question, so that rather than differentiating into a squamous cell, for instance, they mature instead into a mucus-producing columnar cell which is better able to protect itself from an acid environment. When the stimulus is removed, the stem cells may revert to producing differentiated cells of the original type.

Metaplasia most commonly occurs in epithelial tissues but may also be seen in mesodermal tissues; for example, areas of fibrous tissue exposed to chronic trauma may form bone (*osseous metaplasia*). Metaplasia may coexist with hyperplasia and, more importantly, dysplasia.

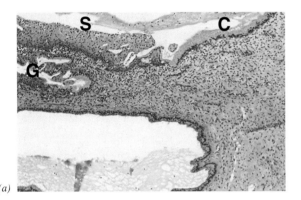

(a)

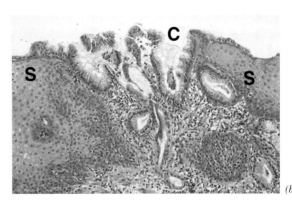

(b)

Fig. 6.6 Metaplasia
(a) Squamous metaplasia of cervix (MP) (b) Gastric metaplasia of lower oesophagus (MP)

Squamous metaplasia of the cervix is so common that it may almost be regarded as physiologically normal. During a woman's reproductive life, the shape of the cervix changes cyclically, exposing the endocervical columnar epithelium to the environment of the vagina. This *ectropion*, often incorrectly referred to as an 'erosion', is apparent macroscopically as an area of velvety pink epithelium at the external os. In consequence, the endocervical epithelium is replaced by stratified squamous epithelium as shown in micrograph (a). On the left, the surface is covered by mature stratified squamous epithelium **S** which overlies endocervical glands lined by the normal mucus-secreting columnar epithelium **C** which is also present at the surface on the right. In time, the metaplastic squamous epithelium may extend into the glands. Inflammation of the cervix accelerates this process. In micrograph (b), the reverse change is occurring in the lower oesophagus where normal native squamous epithelium **S** at the right and left is being replaced by gastric-type columnar epithelium **C** which is able to produce mucous to protect the epithelium from acid reflux. This is known as *Barrett's oesophagus*.

Cellular atypia and dysplasia

Sometimes cells have an increased rate of cell division, and this means that the cells do not have time to reach complete maturation (with full development of cytoplasmic specialisation) before another cycle of cell division supervenes. This leads to a population of cells which are structurally abnormal. They have a high nuclear to cytoplasmic ratio, with large nuclei containing abundant dark-staining chromatin and prominent nucleoli which are sometimes multiple. The nuclear changes are associated with evidence of incomplete maturation of the cytoplasm, which is relatively scanty and lacking in the specialised structures normally seen in that cell type, such as mucin vacuoles or surface cilia. This is called *failure of differentiation*, and the cells are said to show *atypia*.

Cellular atypia may be a consequence of rapid multiplication of cells as a response to cell destruction due to a persistent damaging stimulus. In this case, the atypia is a result of high turnover of the cells attempting to regenerate damaged epithelium. When the damaging stimulus is removed, these cell abnormalities should revert to normal and full differentiation of the cells occur. However, sometimes the cellular atypia is persistent and not simply the result of regeneration; in these cases experience shows that the population of atypical cells may eventually be the focus from which invasive cancer develops. This type of persistent cellular atypia is called *dysplasia* and is regarded as a precursor of invasive cancer. Cytological examination of cells scraped from the surface of the uterine cervix may reveal dysplastic epithelial cells, the earliest indication of the possibility of a developing cancer (Fig. 17.4).

The problem for the pathologist is in distinguishing between the cellular atypia which is merely a reactive regenerative response to tissue damage from that which is indicative of early pre-cancer, i.e. dysplasia. There is no simple answer. Dysplasia often arises in metaplastic tissues and it is likely that the stimuli which cause dysplasia are also responsible for metaplastic change. Thus metaplastic epithelium in the cervix and Barrett's oesophagus are at risk of dysplasia and subsequent neoplasia. In dysplastic cells, molecular biological techniques have demonstrated some of the genetic abnormalities of cellular oncogenes and tumour suppressor genes found in invasive neoplasms. Because of the sinister association of dysplasia with the subsequent development of neoplasia, treatment of dysplastic conditions is undertaken to minimise the risk of subsequent development of a malignancy. Recognition of dysplastic changes by cytological examination of cervical smears forms the basis of screening for cancer of the cervix (Fig. 17.4).

Fig. 6.7 **Dysplasia** (*illustrations opposite*)
(a) Normal cervix (HP) (b) Dysplasia in the cervix (HP) (c) Normal skin (HP) (d) Dysplastic skin (HP)

Dysplasia is a morphological feature characterised by increased cellular proliferation with incomplete maturation of cells. It occurs commonly at the uterine cervix and in the skin, and in both cases is thought to predispose to neoplastic change. Micrograph (a) illustrates normal stratified squamous epithelium from the cervix. Cellular proliferation is confined to the basal layer **B** where the stem cells are small, uniform and darkly stained. As the cells mature towards the surface, their cytoplasm expands and becomes more eosinophilic (pink-stained). Near the surface, the cells become progressively flattened; the ratio of nucleus to cytoplasm diminishes as the cells pass from the basal to the surface layers. In contrast, micrograph (b) shows dysplastic cervical epithelium where there is disruption of the normal orderly maturation sequence. Cells in all strata now exhibit larger than normal nuclei, some with prominent nucleoli; mitotic figures **M** may be seen well above the basal layer. The nuclei of the cells are more variable in shape and size than is normal (*pleomorphism*)

and the nuclear to cytoplasmic ratio is greater than normal. It is the presence of such surface cells with large nuclei which alerts the cytologist to underlying dysplasia when they are scraped off in a cervical smear.

Micrographs (c) and (d) demonstrate similar differences between normal and dysplastic skin respectively. Note how the normal cellular stratification is disrupted in the dysplastic specimen by cells with large, darkly staining nuclei and multinucleate cells **N** extending far up into the middle strata. In addition, a disturbed pattern of maturation is reflected in the development of a thick layer of keratin which contains purple-stained nuclear remnants (*parakeratosis*). It is this keratin layer which becomes clinically evident as thickening and scaling of the skin over such areas of dysplasia. Mitotic figures **M** are also apparent above the basal layers. Both of these conditions have a greatly increased tendency to develop into invasive carcinoma and when severe are referred to as *carcinoma in situ*.

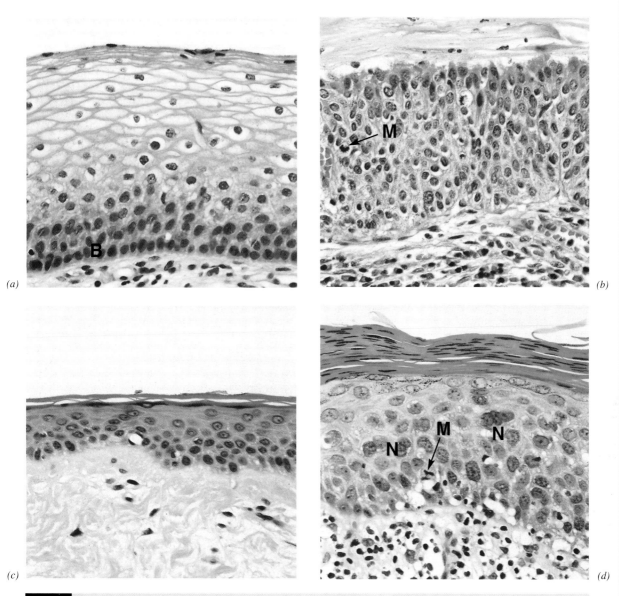

(a)   *(b)*

(c)   *(d)*

Fig. 6.7 **Dysplasia** *(caption opposite)*

7. Neoplasia

Introduction

In a neoplasm, cellular proliferation and growth occur in the absence of any continuing external stimulus. The term **neoplasia** therefore describes a state of autonomous cell division, and the abnormal mass of cells that results is termed a **neoplasm**. The state of neoplastic growth contrasts with **hyperplasia**, discussed in the preceding chapter, where although there is abnormal proliferation of cells, this ceases with removal of the causative stimulus.

By convention, a neoplastic mass of cells is termed a **tumour**; the Latin derivation used to refer to any tissue swelling, although this literal use has largely gone out of fashion.

As well as abnormal cell proliferation, neoplasia is characterised by abnormal maturation of cells. A feature of normal tissue growth is the maturation of constituent cells into a form adapted to a specific function; this adaptation may involve the acquisition of specialised structures such as mucin vacuoles, neurosecretory granules, microvilli or cilia. This process of structural and functional maturation is termed **differentiation**. A fully mature cell of any particular cell line is said to be **highly differentiated**, whereas its primitive precursor or **stem cells** are described as being **undifferentiated**. In any given tissue, the normal cells have a characteristic state of differentiation. In contrast, neoplastic cells exhibit variable states of differentiation and commonly fail to achieve a highly differentiated state. Neoplasms are divided clinically into two main groups:

- **benign neoplasms** grow slowly and remain localised to the site of origin
- **malignant neoplasms** grow rapidly and may spread widely.

There is a broad correlation between histological appearances and biological behaviour, allowing prediction of the likely prognosis. In general, the cells of benign neoplasms are well differentiated. In the case of malignant neoplasms, there is a variable degree of differentiation. At one end of the spectrum, the constituent cells may closely resemble the tissue of origin, in which case the tumour is described as being a **well-differentiated malignant neoplasm**; alternatively, the constituent cells may bear little resemblance to the tissue of origin, in which case the neoplasm is described as being **poorly differentiated**. At the extreme end of the spectrum, neoplasms which exhibit no evidence of differentiation are termed **anaplastic neoplasms** and in many cases it may not be possible to identify the cell of origin on morphological grounds alone. Generally, the degree of differentiation of a neoplasm is related to its behaviour. A poorly differentiated neoplasm tends to be more invasive and more aggressive than a well-differentiated neoplasm.

Fig. 7.1 **Degrees of tumour differentiation: colon** (*illustrations opposite – above*)
(a) Normal mucosa (HP) (b) Benign neoplasm (HP)
(c) Well-differentiated malignant neoplasm (HP) (d) Poorly differentiated neoplasm (HP)

This series of micrographs demonstrates the variable degree of differentiation that may be seen in tumours arising from the same cell of origin, in this case the mucus-secreting columnar epithelium of the colon. There is a spectrum of change from normal through benign to poorly differentiated malignant neoplasms.

Note the similarity between normal colonic mucosa in micrograph (a) and a benign neoplasm (tubular adenoma) in micrograph (b); in both cases, the epithelial cells **E** are tall, columnar and regular in form. The main points of difference are that the cells of the benign neoplasm contain less mucin **Mu** and their nuclei are larger and more crowded.

The cells of the well-differentiated malignant neoplasm shown in micrograph (c) are also tall and columnar, but the nuclei are more irregular in shape and arrangement; there is no mucin secretion, most of each cell being occupied by the nucleus. The nuclei are crowded and exhibit **stratification**, i.e. they are no longer arranged along the basal parts of the cells. The nucleoli are also large and irregular in size and shape. In contrast, in the poorly differentiated colonic neoplasm shown in micrograph (d), the cells bear little resemblance to the tissue of origin and are arranged haphazardly instead of in even rows lining glandular spaces. The cells show a great variability in size and nuclear shape; mitoses **M** are seen, and there is little evidence of mucin secretion.

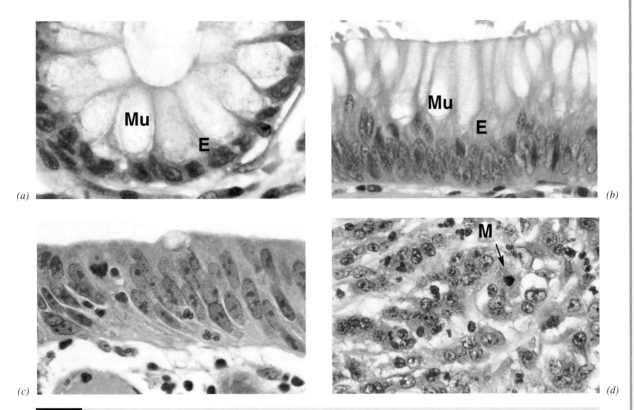

(a)   *(b)*

(c)   *(d)*

Fig. 7.1 **Degrees of tumour differentiation: colon** *(caption opposite)*

Fig. 7.2 **Cytological features of malignancy**

Pleomorphism, nuclear hyperchromicity and abnormal mitotic activity are features of malignant neoplasms and are not usually seen in benign neoplasms. The malignant tumour illustrated shows considerable variation in cell size and shape (*cellular pleomorphism*) and nuclear size and shape (*nuclear pleomorphism*); in addition, many nuclei are very darkly stained (*nuclear hyperchromatism*). The chromatin pattern in nuclei is typically coarsely clumped. Nucleoli are also prominent and some cells may have multiple nucleoli. Large numbers of cells in mitosis are seen in many conditions in which there is excess cellular proliferation (e.g. hyperplasia), but in malignant lesions many of the mitotic figures are abnormal; note two ring mitotic figures **M**. Multiple mitoses may also be seen in malignant tumours.

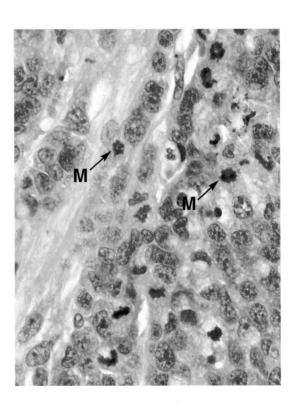

BASIC PATHOLOGICAL PROCESSES

General characteristics of neoplasms

As mentioned before, neoplasms may be divided into two broad groups according to their behaviour:

- If the margins of the tumour are well defined and cell growth is entirely local, then the neoplasm is termed **benign**.
- If the margins of the neoplasm are poorly defined and the neoplastic cells extend into and destroy surrounding tissues or spread to a distant location (metastasis), then the neoplasm is termed **malignant**.

The property whereby a malignant tumour can grow into and at the expense of surrounding tissue is termed **invasion**. A further property of malignant neoplasms is distant spread of neoplastic cells away from the main neoplasm (termed the **primary tumour**) to form subpopulations of neoplastic cells which are not in continuity with the primary tumour. The property of distant spread of tumour is termed **metastasis**; the **secondary tumours** which result are often termed **metastases**.

In general terms, a benign tumour will behave in a relatively innocuous manner, and a malignant tumour will have deleterious effects often leading to death. There are, however, exceptions to these generalisations, and factors other than the biological growth pattern of a tumour may be important in influencing the outcome. Of these, the most notable is the location of the tumour; for example, a benign tumour of the brain stem may lead to rapid death, whereas a malignant tumour of the skin may progress slowly over many years.

Systemic symptoms such as weight loss, loss of appetite, fever and general malaise frequently accompany malignant tumours; in most cases, the pathophysiology is poorly understood but includes effects of secreted cytokines such as **tumour necrosis factor**. Some tumours, benign and malignant, retain the function of their organ of origin; if this happens to be an endocrine function, then the tumour may exert harmful effects by secretion of excess hormone. Other tumours secrete hormones not usually secreted by that tissue, for example the secretion of parathormone by lung carcinomas; this is known as **ectopic hormone secretion** and the clinical manifestations are described as **paraneoplastic phenomena**.

Modes of spread of malignant neoplasms

There are four main modes of tumour spread:

- **Local invasion**. Invasive tumours tend to spread into surrounding tissues by the most direct route. Examples include carcinoma of the breast invading into overlying skin or deeply into underlying muscle, and carcinoma of the cervix invading into rectum or bladder.
- **Lymphatic spread**. Tumours may spread via lymphatic vessels draining the site of the primary tumour; neoplastic cells are conducted to local lymph nodes where they become trapped and set up secondary tumours, e.g. breast cancer spreading to lymph nodes in the axilla, or carcinoma of the tongue spreading to lymph nodes in the neck.
- **Vascular spread**. Tumours can spread via the venules and veins draining the primary site; gut tumours tend to spread via the portal vein to the liver where secondary tumours are very common. In the systemic circulation, neoplastic cells may be trapped in the capillaries of the lung to form pulmonary metastases.
- **Trans-coelomic spread**. Certain tumours can spread directly across coelomic spaces, for example across the peritoneal or pleural cavities. Carcinoma of the ovary may spread transcoelomically to produce large numbers of metastatic deposits on the peritoneal surfaces.

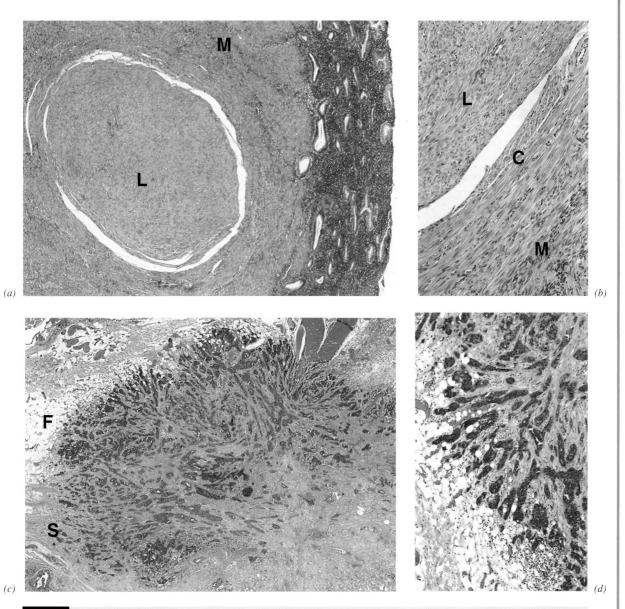

Fig. 7.3 Local invasiveness
(a) Benign neoplasm of myometrium (LP)   (b) Margin of lesion in (a) (MP)
(c) Malignant neoplasm of breast (LP)   (d) Margin of lesion in (c) (MP)

These micrographs compare the local invasive behaviour of benign and malignant neoplasms within solid organs. Micrograph (a) shows a benign neoplasm of the uterine smooth muscle, a leiomyoma **L**, surrounded by normal myometrium **M**. The tumour margin is shown at higher magnification in micrograph (b). Note that the neoplasm is well circumscribed and shows no evidence of local invasion. This neoplasm has expanded symmetrically and compressed the supporting stroma of the myometrium to form a *pseudocapsule* **C**.

Micrograph (c) illustrates a malignant neoplasm of female breast epithelium; note that the neoplasm has an irregular outline with tongues of neoplastic cells invading the fatty tissue **F** and collagenous stroma **S** of the breast. There is no tendency to form a capsule. The ill-defined tumour margin is illustrated in micrograph (d) in which hyperchromatic malignant cells can be seen infiltrating the surrounding adipose tissue.

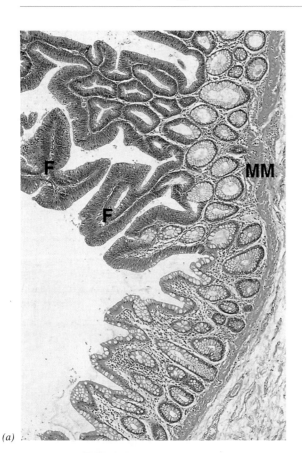

(a)

Fig. 7.4 Invasive characteristics of surface neoplasms: colon
(a) Benign neoplasm: villous adenoma (MP)
(b) Malignant neoplasm: adenocarcinoma (LP)

Benign neoplasms of surface epithelia usually grow in the form of warty, papillary or nodular outgrowths and show no tendency to infiltrate downward into the submucosa. Micrograph (a) shows one form of benign colonic neoplasm; this *villous adenoma* has grown into the lumen in the form of papillary fronds **F** with a stromal core covered by moderately dysplastic epithelial cells. The underlying muscularis mucosae **MM** is intact and there is no downward tumour spread.

Malignant neoplasms not only form a mass in the lumen, but also spread across the epithelial basement membrane into subepithelial tissues. In micrograph (b) of a colonic *adenocarcinoma*, the tumour cells **T** have grown in complex, abnormal gland formations **G** within the mucosa; malignant glands are also seen invading into the submucosa **SM**, having breached the muscularis mucosae **MM**, and have spread beneath the adjacent normal mucosa **Muc**. Even at low power, it is obvious that the malignant cells are disorganised, crowded together and are less differentiated than are the cells of the benign adenoma. Note the nuclear hyperchromatism of both benign and malignant lesions in comparison to the normal. Higher power micrographs of similar neoplasms are shown in Figure 7.1.

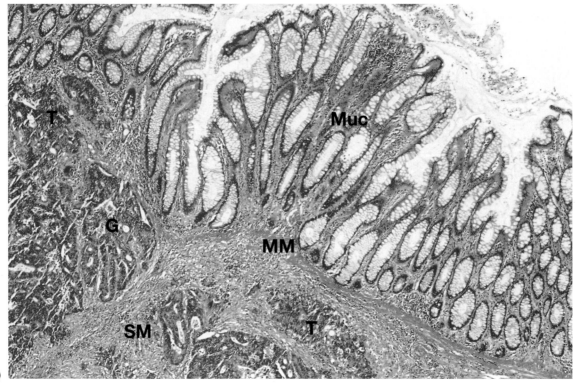

(b)

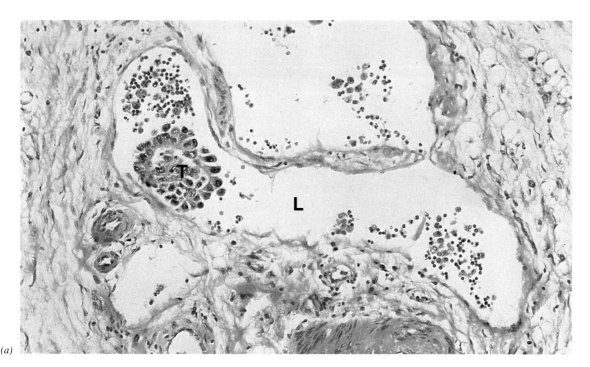

(a)

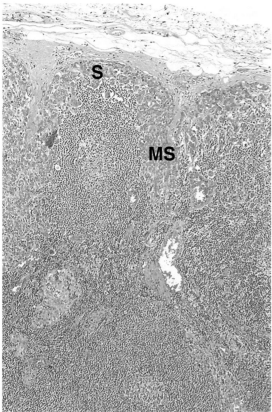

(b)

Fig. 7.5 Lymphatic spread of malignant neoplasm
(a) **Tumour in lymphatic vessel (HP)**
(b) **Metastasis in a lymph node (MP)**

Malignant tumours may invade through the walls of lymphatics, and tumour may then spread along lymphatic channels either by growth of solid cores along the lymphatic lumina, or by fragments breaking off the intralymphatic tumour mass to form emboli which pass in the lymph drainage to regional lymph nodes. Micrograph (a) illustrates a large, valved lymphatic **L** containing an embolic clump of malignant tumour cells **T** *en route* to a lymph node. Tumour spread via lymphatics to regional lymph nodes is a very common mode of spread in malignant tumours of epithelial origin.

Micrograph (b) shows a lymph node draining a primary malignant tumour of the breast. Tumour cells, which arrive via afferent lymphatics, lodge and proliferate in the subcapsular sinus **S**. From here, the malignant cells infiltrate down the medullary sinuses **MS** and go on to form solid masses in the parenchyma of the node (not illustrated here).

BASIC PATHOLOGICAL PROCESSES

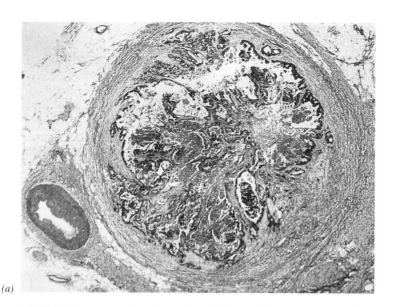

(a)

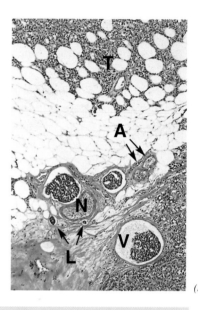

(b)

Fig. 7.6 Haematogenous spread of malignant neoplasms
(a) Malignant colonic neoplasm (MP)   (b) Malignant breast neoplasm (MP)

The thin-walled vessels of the venous system provide a ready means of spread for many types of malignant tumour; invasion of arterial vessels is rare and tends to result in haemorrhage or infarction rather than tumour spread. Malignant cells may grow along veins in solid cores from which fragments may break off to form tumour emboli which tend to lodge in the first capillary beds encountered. The lungs and liver are frequent sites of metastatic deposition. From here, tumour cells may pass through the heart and into the arterial system and spread throughout the body. Brain and bone marrow thus become other common sites for metastatic deposits.

Micrograph (a) shows a large serosal vein from a colon in which there was an extensive malignant

neoplasm; a solid mass of blue-staining tumour is growing along the vessel lumen. The site of invasion of the vessel wall was proximal to this section and therefore cannot be seen.

Venous invasion by carcinoma of the breast is seen in micrograph (b). Solid masses of tumour cells **T** infiltrate the fatty tissue of the breast. Tumour emboli are seen within three small venules **V** and also two small lymphatics **L**, adjacent to a nerve **N**. The arterioles **A** close by are not affected. Vascular and lymphatic invasion by tumour is an important factor in the prognosis of many types of tumour.

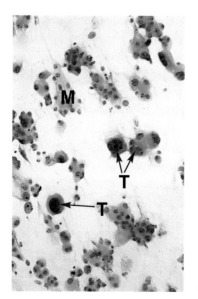

Fig. 7.7 Trans-coelomic spread of malignant neoplasms (HP)

Malignant tumours may spread into coelomic spaces by direct extension from adjacent organs. Tumour emboli may then break free from the tumour to float in the small amount of fluid normally present in these spaces and thus spread to other areas of the mesothelial surface. Thus breast and lung tumours commonly involve the pleural space; ovarian and gastric tumours are usually responsible for peritoneal involvement. In response to tumour growth in these serous spaces, there is commonly an inflammatory response in the lining with accumulation of protein-rich fluid and inflammatory cells, proliferation of mesothelial cells and often haemorrhage to form a ***malignant pleural effusion*** or ***malignant ascites***.

This example is a smear of ascitic fluid from a patient with metastatic breast carcinoma. The tumour had spread through the pleural space and reached the peritoneum probably via the diaphragm. Aspiration of the fluid serves to relieve symptoms and to confirm the diagnosis cytologically (***diagnostic paracentesis***). Tumour cells **T** are present as single cells and small aggregates. They are pleomorphic with large hyperchromatic nuclei and prominent nucleoli. Reactive mesothelial cells **M** are also present, and in contrast to the tumour cells are smaller with bland nuclear features. In this example, inflammatory cells are sparse.

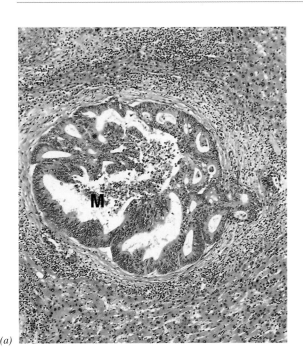

(a)

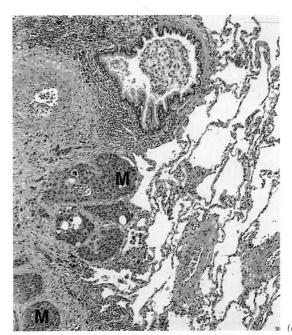

(b)

Fig. 7.8 Metastatic tumour deposits in solid organs
(a) Liver (LP) (b) Lung (LP)

Metastatic deposits of tumour are frequently encountered in liver, lung, bone marrow and brain as a result of haematogenous spread. Other tissues are less common sites for deposition of metastatic tumour (e.g. heart and skeletal muscle); however, metastases can occur in any tissue or organ. Certain types of tumour have characteristic patterns of spread; for example malignant tumours of the prostate gland have a propensity to spread to bone. It is thought that the malignant cells and the target organ must express mutually compatible receptors and cell-surface adhesion molecules which facilitate cellular anchorage and subsequent growth promotion.

Micrographs (a) and (b) show examples of hepatic and pulmonary blood-borne metastases **M**, respectively. Hepatic metastases often arise from organs drained by

the portal system; the lesion in micrograph (a) is from a moderately differentiated adenocarcinoma of the colon. Lung metastases on the other hand arise from tumour emboli from the systemic venous circulation, and micrograph (b) is an example of secondary spread from a primary breast carcinoma. Note that both tumours have induced a stromal reaction in the host organ in the form of fibrous connective tissue containing blood vessels and inflammatory cells. Without this ability to induce the formation of a vascular supply (*angiogenesis*), the growth of metastases would not be possible. The inflammatory cells are thought to represent an immunological response to the abnormal tumour cells and may in rare cases cause total regression of a malignant tumour; this is the rationale behind various types of tumour immunotherapy.

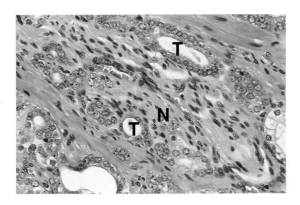

Fig. 7.9 Perineural spread (HP)

Spread along the course of nerve bundles is a common feature of some tumours such as adenocarcinoma of the prostate but which may be seen occasionally in other tumour types. This micrograph shows perineural invasion by a well-differentiated prostatic adenocarcinoma. Tumour cells **T** in a glandular conformation are seen infiltrating around and between bundles of nerve fibres **N**.

Staging of malignant tumours

The extent of local, regional and distant tumour spread is an important determinant of tumour management and prognosis. Several systems have been devised for defining these characteristics in a standardised fashion; this is known as *staging* of a tumour. The *TNM system* is the most widely used method and involves scoring the extent of local **T**umour spread, regional lymph **N**ode involvement and the presence of distant **M**etastases. Despite advances in diagnostic techniques, the stage of a tumour is generally a very good indicator of likely prognosis. Tumour stage assessment is also important in planning therapy; tumours at an advanced stage (extensive spread) may require aggressive treatment, while early stage tumours (localised) can be treatable by more conservative measures such as surgical excision alone. Staging is usually performed by a combination of histopathology, radiology and clinical assessments.

By way of example, the TNM method of breast cancer staging is as follows:

T0 = breast free of tumour   N0 = no axillary nodes involved   M0 = no metastases
T1 = local lesion < 2 cm in size   N1 = mobile nodes involved   M1 = demonstrable metastases
T2 = lesion 2–5 cm in diameter   N2 = fixed nodes involved   MX = suspected metastases
T3 = lesion >5 cm in diameter   N3 = ipsilateral internal mammary
T4 = skin and/or chest wall involved   node involved

Histological assessment of neoplasms

Histological assessment of a tumour provides a useful guide to tumour behaviour, i.e. whether the tumour is benign or malignant, and provides a rational basis for treatment. Histological assessment should establish the following features:

- The type of tumour. This is based on the presumed tissue of origin and/or differentiation of the tumour.
- The degree of differentiation. This is known as *grading* and takes into account some or all of the following features:
  — the similarity of the tumour to the supposed tissue of origin both architecturally and cytologically (*differentiation*)
  — the degree of variability of cellular shape and size (*pleomorphism*)
  — the proportion of mitotic figures (dividing cells).
- The extent of spread of tumour (*staging*) is partly assessed histologically, particularly:
  — size of the primary tumour
  — histological assessment of local invasion, and vascular, lymphatic and perineural invasion
  — the presence of metastatic tumour deposits, for example in lymph nodes and bones.
- The presence or absence of other prognostic factors; for instance, the presence of oestrogen receptors in breast carcinoma cells confers an improved prognosis. The expression of certain oncogenes is increasingly being related to prognosis in some tumours.

The histological features which distinguish benign and malignant tumours are summarised in Figure 7.10.

Fig. 7.10 Summary of histological features of neoplasms

	Benign	Malignant
Behaviour	Expansile growth only; grows locally Often encapsulated	Expansile and invasive growth; may mestastasise Not encapsulated
Histology	Resembles cell of origin (well differentiated) Few mitoses Normal or slight increase in ratio of nucleus to cytoplasm Cells are uniform through the tumour	May show failure of cellular differentiation Many mitoses, some of which are abnormal forms High nuclear to cytoplasmic ratio Cells vary in shape and size (cellular pleomorphism) and/or nuclei vary in shape and size (nuclear pleomorphism)

In situ neoplasia (carcinoma in situ)

These terms are used when an epithelial tissue shows the cytological and histological features of a carcinoma (architectural and cytological abnormalities, such as cell crowding, pleomorphism, increased and abnormal mitotic activity, i.e. severe dysplasia, see Ch. 6), but there is no evidence of any invasion. The basement membrane bounding the abnormal epithelial tissue is intact, and there is no encroachment of the atypical cells into underlying stroma. Thus, the epithelial cells show the cytological, but not the behavioural, characteristics of malignancy. However, many forms of *in situ carcinoma* will become invasive if left untreated.

Certain benign epithelial tumours may progress to form an invasive malignant tumour by development and selective persistence of mutations in key oncogenes. A sequence from benign neoplasm through increasing dysplasia to in situ carcinoma, and on to invasive carcinoma is well recognised in certain sites (e.g. the colon).

In situ neoplasia occurs particularly in skin (intra-epidermal carcinoma, see Fig. 2.15), uterine ectocervix (cervical intra-epithelial neoplasia, CIN III, see Fig. 17.6), vulval skin and mucosa (VIN), and other sites. In situ neoplasia also occurs in solid glandular organs, most notably the breast (see Fig. 18.9).

Two other terms are used in this context: some ovarian carcinomas, which show the cytological features of malignancy but no histological evidence of invasion, are said to be '*of borderline malignancy*', and some soft tissue tumours, which show limited cellular and nuclear pleomorphism with increased mitotic activity, yet are bounded with a discrete capsule, are said to be '*of low malignant potential*'.

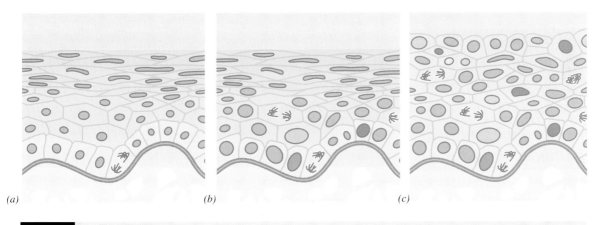

(a)   *(b)*   *(c)*

Fig. 7.11 In situ neoplasia

Diagram (a) shows the regular architecture of a normal stratified squamous epithelium. The layered epithelium is formed by mitotic replication of the basal layer, producing layers of regular cells which differentiate and flatten as they get near the surface (stratification). The cells are regular in shape and size, as are the nuclei, and mitotic activity is confined to the basal layer.

Diagram (b) shows an epithelium in which there is dysplasia in the lower layers. The cells and their nuclei are irregular in shape and size, and the nuclei occupy more of the cell. Mitoses are present in layers other than the basal layer. The cells still differentiate and mature, eventually, near the surface.

Diagram (c) shows fully developed in situ neoplasia. The dysplastic epithelial cells now occupy the full thickness of the epithelium, and stratification and differentiation are largely lost; mitoses can be present in

any of the layers, even in surface cells. Although all the cells in this epithelium show cytological characteristics of malignancy (cellular and nuclear pleomorphism, high nucleus/cytoplasm ratio, nuclear hyperchronicity and increased abnormal mitotic activity), the epithelial cells as yet show no tendency to invade across the basement membrane into the stroma.

The changes shown in (b) are regarded as an early stage in the development of in situ neoplasia. In certain locations, this is acknowledged by applying a numerical value. Hence, in the squamous epithelium of the uterine cervix, the changes in (c) would be called CIN III (cervical intra-epithelial neoplasia III), whereas those in (b) would be called CIN II. A similar scheme exists in the nomenclature of dysplastic/in situ neoplastic changes in the vulva (VIN), anus (AIN) and vagina (VAIN), with gradings of I, II and III.

Tumour nomenclature and classification

The classification and nomenclature of neoplasms have developed from gross morphological, histological and behavioural observation. Ideally, the name given to a tumour should convey information about the cell of origin and the likely behaviour (either benign or malignant). While this is so for the majority of tumours of epithelial and connective tissues, there are many tumours which are given eponymous or semidescriptive names out of either poor understanding of pathogenesis or long-established tradition. Some tumours have several different names which are synonymous but derive from different classifications.

Tumours of epithelial origin

- Benign neoplasms of surface epithelia, for example skin, are termed ***papillomata*** (singular ***papilloma***). This term is preceded by the cell of origin, for example squamous papilloma of skin, squamous papilloma of larynx.
- Benign neoplasms of both solid and surface glandular epithelia are termed ***adenomata*** (singular ***adenoma***). This is prefixed by the tissue of origin, for example thyroid adenoma, salivary gland adenoma. Frequently, a benign tumour of surface glandular epithelium (almost always in the large bowel) assumes a papillary growth pattern when it is termed a ***villous adenoma***.
- A malignant tumour of any epithelial origin is termed a ***carcinoma***. Tumours of glandular epithelium (including that lining the gut) are termed ***adenocarcinomas***. Tumours of other epithelia are preceded by the cell type of origin, for example squamous cell carcinoma, transitional cell carcinoma. To classify a carcinoma further, the tissue of origin is added, for example adenocarcinoma of prostate, adenocarcinoma of breast, squamous cell carcinoma of larynx.

The nomenclature of epithelial tumours is summarised in Figure 7.12.

Fig. 7.12 Nomenclature of epithelial tumours

Tissue of origin	Benign	Malignant
Surface epithelium	Papilloma/adenoma	Carcinoma
Examples		
Squamous	Squamous cell papilloma	Squamous cell carcinoma
Glandular (columnar)	Adenoma (villous or tubular)	Adenocarcinoma
Transitional	Transitional cell papilloma	Transitional cell carcinoma
Solid glandular epithelium	Adenoma	Adenocarcinoma
Examples		
Thyroid	Thyroid adenoma	Thyroid adenocarcinoma
Kidney	Renal adenoma	Renal adenocarcinoma
Liver	Hepatic adenoma	Hepatic adenocarcinoma

Tumours of connective tissue origin

In connective tissues, there is a simpler and more descriptive classification of neoplasms. First, the tissue of origin is designated, with the addition of the suffix ***-oma*** for a benign tumour, or ***-sarcoma*** for a malignant tumour. As an example, a benign tumour of adipose tissue is termed a lipoma, whilst a malignant tumour of the same origin is termed a liposarcoma. A summary of other connective tissue tumours is shown in Figure 7.13.

Fig. 7.13 Nomenclature of connective tissue tumours

Tissue of origin	Benign	Malignant
Fibrous	Fibroma	Fibrosarcoma
Bone	Osteoma	Osteosarcoma
Cartilage	Chondroma	Chondrosarcoma
Adipose	Lipoma	Liposarcoma
Smooth muscle	Leiomyoma	Leiomyosarcoma
Skeletal muscle	Rhabdomyoma	Rhabdomyosarcoma
Blood vessel	Haemangioma	Haemangiosarcoma

Nomenclature of other tumours

There are other neoplasms which do not fit into either the epithelial or the connective tissue category described above and these are grouped according to their tissue of origin. The main categories are as follows:

- **Lymphomas**: tumours of solid lymphoid tissue (Ch. 16).
- **Leukaemias**: tumours derived from haemopoietic elements which circulate in the blood and only rarely form tumour masses (Ch. 16).
- **Tumours of childhood**: these are believed to derive from primitive embryonal 'blastic' tissue (also called *small round cell tumours of childhood*); the most common are nephroblastoma of the kidney (Fig. 15.14) and neuroblastoma of the adrenal medulla (Fig. 20.11).
- **Gliomas**: tumours derived from the non-neural support tissues of the brain (Ch. 23).
- **Germ cell tumours**: tumours derived from germ cells in the gonads (Chs 17 and 19). This category includes *teratomas* which contain elements of all three embryological germ cell layers, i.e. ectoderm, endoderm and mesoderm; these are most commonly found in the testis and ovary. They vary in malignancy from benign to extremely malignant and are commonest in young people. Teratomas represent complex forms of germ cell tumours.
- **Neuroendocrine tumours**: tumours derived from cells of the neuroendocrine system and which secrete polypeptide hormones or physiologically active amines. Examples include phaeochromocytoma of the adrenal medulla (Fig. 20.10), carcinoid tumour of the small intestine (Fig. 13.17) and medullary carcinoma of the thyroid Fig. 5.7). Certain of these tumours used to be grouped under the term APUD tumours in recognition of functional amine precursor uptake and decarboxylation, but they are now more often named according to the hormones they produce, for example, insulinoma, glucagonoma.

In addition to the system described above, individual tumours may also be known by other names according to histological appearance (e.g. oat cell carcinoma), or by an eponym (e.g. Hodgkin's disease).

Finally, there is a group of tumour-like lesions known as *hamartomas* which represent non-neoplastic overgrowths of tissues indigenous to the site of their occurrence. These are thought to be developmental abnormalities. A common example is the 'port-wine stain' of the skin composed of blood vessels and known as a haemangioma; note that the suffix '-oma' erroneously implies that this is a benign neoplasm. An example of a haemangioma in the liver is shown in Figure 11.14.

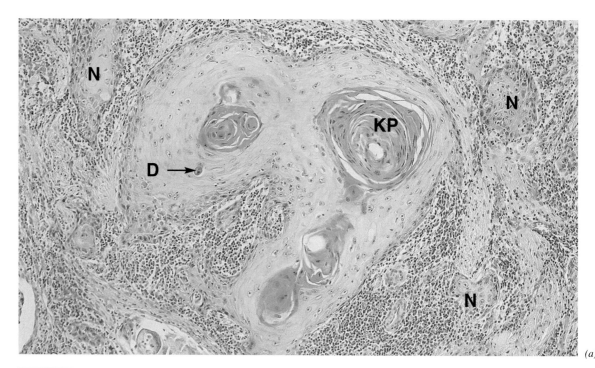

(a)

Fig. 7.14 Squamous cell carcinoma
(a) Well differentiated (HP)
(b) Poorly differentiated (HP)

Squamous cell carcinomas may arise in any site of native stratified squamous epithelium, for example skin, oesophagus, tongue. They may also arise in stratified squamous epithelium which has formed by the process of metaplasia, for example bronchus, urinary bladder.

The degree of differentiation varies widely. Well-differentiated tumours as seen in micrograph (a) have cytological features similar to the prickle cell layer of normal stratified squamous epithelium; the cells are large and slightly fusiform in shape. The nuclei exhibit a moderate degree of pleomorphism, and mitotic figures are not very abundant. The cells are commonly arranged in broad sheets and large nests **N**; at very high magnification, intercellular bridges (typical of normal prickle cells) may be visible. The most characteristic feature of well-differentiated squamous carcinomas is the formation of keratin which may be seen within individual cells, known as dyskeratosis **D**, but which more often forms lamellated pink-stained masses known as keratin pearls **KP**.

In contrast, poorly differentiated squamous carcinomas as in micrograph (b) lose most of their resemblance to normal prickle cells and have a high nuclear to cytoplasmic ratio. Keratin pearl formation is not seen, although individual *dyskeratotic cells* **D** may be present. In the most anaplastic squamous carcinomas, the only evidence of cell of origin may be intercellular bridges which are only visible at high magnification after careful search, or the detection of certain types of cytokeratin by monoclonal antibodies.

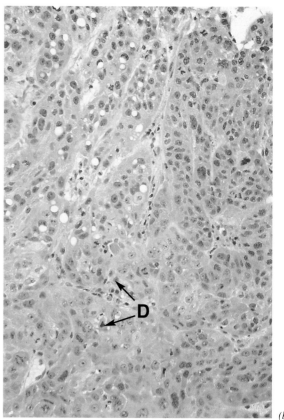

(b)

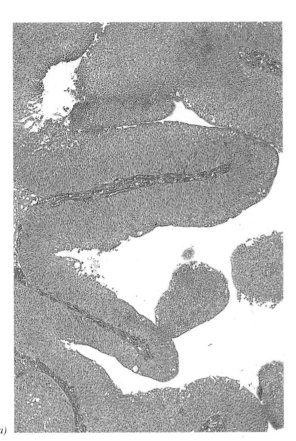

(a)

These tumours arise almost exclusively from native transitional epithelium in the urinary tract.

Well-differentiated lesions usually adopt a papillary growth pattern (see Fig. 15.19) and the cytological features may be almost indistinguishable from those of normal transitional epithelium. Micrograph (a) shows a typical papillary tumour resembling normal urothelium but with slight nuclear pleomorphism and minimal evidence of mitotic activity.

As transitional cell carcinomas become less differentiated, the growth pattern becomes more solid, and nuclear pleomorphism becomes more marked. In anaplastic tumours, it may not be possible to determine the tissue of origin except by knowing that the tumour has arisen in the urinary tract. Micrograph (b) shows a poorly differentiated solid tumour from the bladder wall; note the nests of highly pleomorphic tumour cells **T** invading between bundles of smooth muscle **M**.

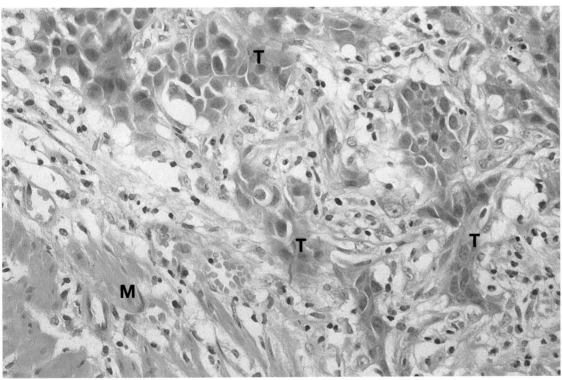

(b)

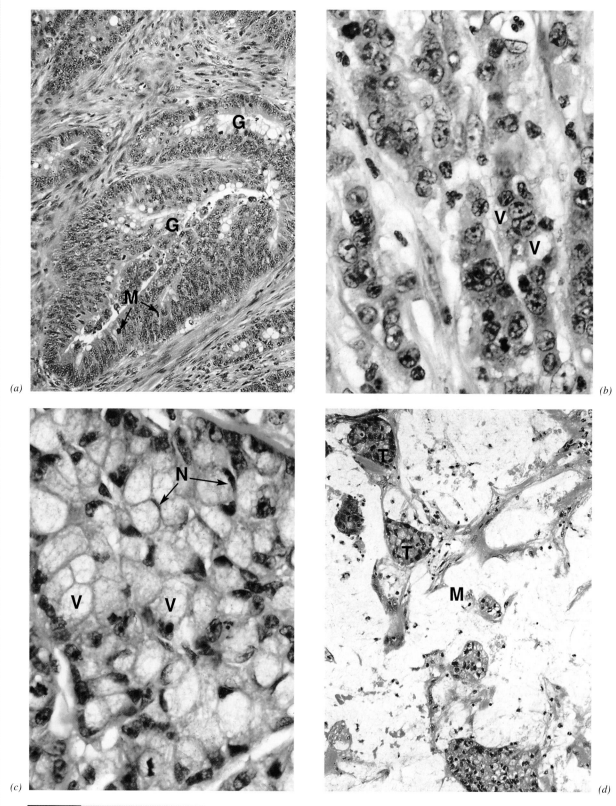

Fig. 7.16 **Adenocarcinomas: colon** (*caption opposite*)

Fig. 7.16 Adenocarcinomas: colon *(illustrations opposite)*
(a) Well differentiated (MP)   (b) Poorly differentiated (HP)   (c) Signet ring (HP)   (d) Mucinous (MP)

Carcinomas which derive from surface glandular epithelium such as large bowel and stomach tend to exhibit a glandular pattern of growth and are known as *adenocarcinomas*. The same is true of carcinomas arising in solid glandular tissues such as kidney, breast and prostate, and of tumours of the liver (which in embryological terms develops as an outgrowth of primitive gut epithelium).

Micrograph (a) illustrates a typical well-differentiated adenocarcinoma from the colon. Although it is a carcinoma, it still exhibits a glandular pattern **G** reminiscent of normal colon; the cell nuclei are, however, hyperchromatic, with a high nuclear to cytoplasmic ratio, and numerous mitoses **M** are seen. Unlike the normal colon, the glandular pattern is irregular and there is little evidence of mucin secretion.

Poorly differentiated adenocarcinomas, as shown in micrograph (b), display minimal tendency to form a glandular pattern and the cells are extremely pleomorphic. The only evidence of glandular origin is the presence of occasional cells with a secretory vacuole **V** containing mucin.

Two other patterns of adenocarcinoma, seen much more commonly in other tissues than in colon, are signet ring cell and mucinous forms. In *signet ring cell carcinoma* as shown in micrograph (c), the tendency to produce mucin-filled cytoplasmic vacuoles is greatly exaggerated such that the majority of cells have their nuclei **N** pushed to one side by a mucin-filled vacuole **V**. This pattern is much more common in the stomach (see Fig. 13.11) than in the colon although focal areas of this pattern may be seen in adenocarcinomas from a wide variety of tissues. In contrast, in a *mucinous carcinoma* as shown in micrograph (d), excessive secretion of mucin **M** results in so-called 'lakes' of mucin in which small nests of tumour cells **T** are found. This pattern of adenocarcinoma is not uncommon in the colon and is also well recognised in the breast where it is also known as *colloid carcinoma* (Fig. 18.10).

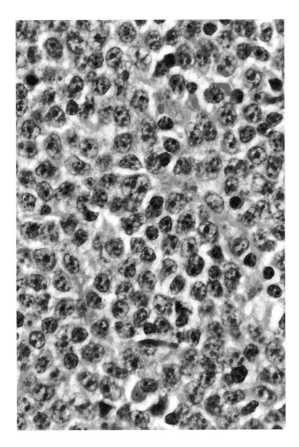

Fig. 7.17 Lymphoma (HP)

Lymphomas are solid tumours derived from cells of the lymphoreticular system. The majority arise in lymphoid organs such as lymph nodes, spleen and bone marrow, but may spread to other tissues, particularly the skin, liver and CNS. Primary lymphomas may also arise at extranodal sites, often in tissues where a long-standing chronic inflammatory or autoimmune response is present, for example the small intestine in coeliac disease, the thyroid in Hashimoto's thyroiditis.

Histologically, lymphomas consist of sheets of lymphoid cells arranged either diffusely or in a follicular pattern. These neoplasms can be divided into good prognosis and poor prognosis types on the basis of cytological features and differentiation. Lymphomas are discussed in detail in Chapter 16.

This micrograph illustrates a poor-prognosis malignant lymphoma composed of diffuse sheets of large lymphoid cells with no evidence of follicle formation. Such tumours may have a rapidly progressive clinical course.

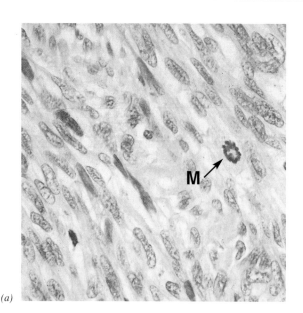

(a)

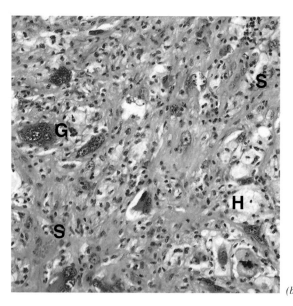

(b)

Fig. 7.18 Sarcomas

(a) Leiomyosarcoma (HP)   (b) Malignant fibrous histiocytoma (HP)

Sarcomas are malignant tumours derived from connective tissues including adipose tissue, bone, cartilage and smooth muscle. Many sarcomas resemble the tissue of origin either cytologically, structurally or by producing characteristic extracellular materials such as collagen and ground substance. For example, fibrosarcomas produce collagen, liposarcomas have intracellular lipid vacuoles and chondrosarcomas produce cartilaginous ground substance.

Micrograph (a) shows a sarcoma derived from uterine smooth muscle. The tumour cells are spindle-shaped and resemble normal smooth muscle cells. However, they have large pleomorphic nuclei with evident mitoses

including an abnormal ring-form mitotic figure **M**; this is therefore a leiomyosarcoma.

Micrograph (b) shows a common sarcoma of soft tissue known as a ***malignant fibrous histiocytoma***; this is probably not derived from histiocytes but more likely represents an extremely poorly differentiated sarcoma. This category of sarcoma was previously called spindle cell sarcoma or undifferentiated sarcoma. These tumours are characteristically large and aggressive and consist of various combinations of spindle cells **S**, cells resembling histiocytes **H** with pale foamy cytoplasm and malignant giant cells **G**. Mitotic figures are usually plentiful.

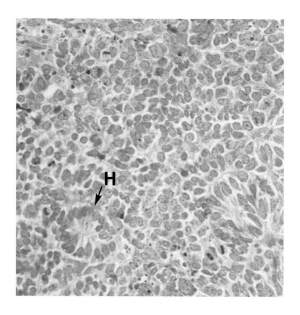

Fig. 7.19 Neuroblastoma (MP)

This is one of a group of tumours known as ***small round cell tumours of childhood*** which also includes retinoblastoma, nephroblastoma (Wilms' tumour), medulloblastoma and hepatoblastoma. These tumours are derived from cells similar to various embryonal tissues. They usually present in childhood and may be rapidly growing and highly malignant.

This micrograph shows a neuroblastoma arising in an adrenal gland. The tumour is composed of sheets of small cells with dark-staining nuclei and little cytoplasm resembling primitive neuroblasts. Foci of differentiation are present in the form of ***Homer–Wright rosettes*** **H** where tumour cells are arranged in a circular formation with fibrillary cytoplasmic extensions filling the central area. These formations may be absent, making the tumour difficult to differentiate from other small round cell tumours.

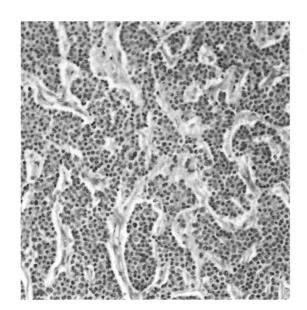

Fig. 7.20 Neuroendocrine tumour (HP)

The neuroendocrine cell system is composed of a diverse group of cells which synthesise and secrete peptide and amine hormones. *Neuroendocrine tumours* may be benign or malignant and mainly arise in the gastrointestinal tract, pancreas, adrenal and thyroid glands. A functional classification is applied where the secretory product can be identified, for example insulinoma, gastrinoma and glucagonoma; however, many neuroendocrine tumours have no identifiable secretory product. By long usage, the neuroendocrine cell tumours which secrete 5-hydroxytryptamine are termed *carcinoid tumours* and may give rise to the *carcinoid syndrome*.

Neuroendocrine tumours have certain common histological features. As shown in this micrograph of a typical carcinoid tumour, the cells are relatively small and uniform with prominent, round nuclei and characteristic granular cytoplasm owing to the presence of secretory granules; these may be demonstrated using special stains or immunohistochemistry (Fig. 13.17). Electron microscopy may also be used to identify cells according to the ultrastructural features of the secretory granules.

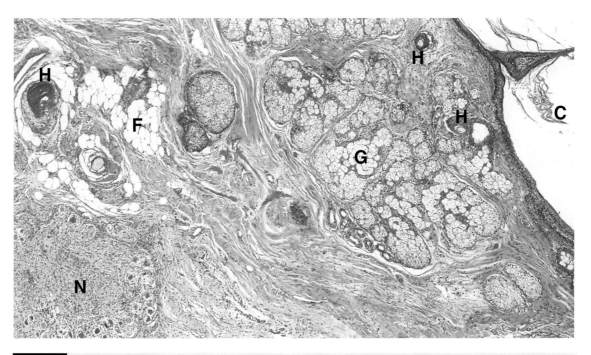

Fig. 7.21 Teratoma (MP)

Teratomas are tumours derived from germ cells and most commonly arise in the testis or ovary. The tumours contain neoplastic tissues derived from all of the three germ cell layers, i.e. endoderm, mesoderm and ectoderm (including neuroectoderm), and thus can contain tissues as diverse as skin, teeth, thyroid, brain and muscle. The tumours range from benign to highly malignant.

A benign teratoma of the ovary is shown in this micrograph. Epidermis-type epithelium, including hair follicles **H** and sebaceous glands **G**, has formed a cystic space **C**. Connective tissue elements including fat **F** are also seen. Neural tissue **N** is present in the form of well-differentiated clusters of ganglion cells. Teratomas arising in the ovary are usually benign while those in the testis are usually malignant and contain more primitive, immature tissue such as primitive mesenchyme.

8. Atherosclerosis

Introduction

The walls of arterial vessels are composed of smooth muscle, elastin and collagen which together make up a resilient system for maintaining vascular tone. Alterations in the relative amounts of these specialised elements lead to hardening, thickening and loss of elasticity of vessel walls and are a major cause of illness and death, particularly in affluent societies. The term **arteriosclerosis** is often used as a general descriptive term for such diseases.

The commonest type of arteriosclerosis is that affecting large and medium-sized arteries in which the underlying histopathological lesion is **atheroma**; this form of arteriosclerosis is thus known as **atherosclerosis**. Other forms of arteriosclerosis occur, such as thickening of the walls of arterioles in association with hypertension (Figs 11.9 and 11.10); from a histopathological and clinical point of view, however, atherosclerosis is the condition of overwhelming importance.

To some extent, atherosclerotic changes can be demonstrated in large and medium-sized arteries in almost all adults; however, clinical consequences mainly occur in association with severe atherosclerosis. The factors predisposing to severe lesions with a high incidence of complications are now well recognised and can be divided into **constitutional factors**, those which have a major effect on atheroma formation (**major risk factors**), and those with a weaker association with the development of atheroma (**minor risk factors**); these are summarised in Figure 8.1. In addition to epidemiological risk factors, many of the cellular pathogenic mechanisms giving rise to arterial wall disease have now been determined.

Fig. 8.1 Risk factors in atherosclerosis	
Constitutional risk factors	
Age	Incidence of severe disease rises with each decade up to 85 years
Sex	Higher risk in males up to the age of 75
Genetic	Some families have increased risk independent of other risk factors
Major risk factors	(Large contribution to incidence; potentially avoidable or treatable)
Hyperlipidaemias	Particularly hypercholesterolaemia
Hypertension	Especially after the age of 45
Smoking	Predominant atherogenic effects in the aorta and coronary vessels
Diabetes	Particularly in coronary, cerebral and peripheral arteries
Minor risk factors	(Small contribution to incidence in statistical studies)
Lack of regular exercise	
Obesity	
Stressful lifestyle	

Fig. 8.2 Stages in atheroma formation

Diagram (a) shows a normal artery, in this case an elastic artery with a distinct internal elastic lamina. The artery is lined internally by a smooth flat cellular endothelium which lies on a thin tunica intima, a delicate fibroelastic loose connective tissue containing occasional multifunctional myointimal cells. Beneath the intima is a strong internal elastic lamina, beneath which is the tunica media, a layer of smooth muscle containing some elastic fibres. On the outer surface is the loose tunica adventitia (not shown in these diagrams).

Diagram (b) shows the early *fatty streak stage*. Lipid (mainly cholesterol, cholesterol esters and triglycerides) enters the intima, probably from the blood across a damaged endothelium. Much of the lipid is phagocytosed by foam cells (probably blood-derived macrophages and myointimal cells) but some eventually becomes free, and more free lipid accumulates when bloated foam cells undergo cell death.

Diagram (c) shows the *fibro-lipid plaque stage*. The presence of the lipid in the intima initiates the formation of fibrocollagenous tissue. Cytokines secreted by macrophages stimulate the proliferation of myointimal cells and switch the function of some of them toward active collagen synthesis, to form a thick collagenous cap. As the intimal deposit of atheroma enlarges, the underlying muscular media begins to atrophy and thin as smooth muscle cells are lost.

Diagram (d) shows *complicated atheroma*. By now, the atheromatous intimal plaque is extensive, and there is marked atrophy of the associated tunica media, with contractible muscle being replaced by collagen. The lipid deposits in the intima frequently acquire deposits of calcium salts, and the fibro-lipid plaque becomes progressively calcified. Ulceration of the overlying endothelium predisposes to the deposition of thrombus on the exposed atheromatous plaque (see Ch. 9).

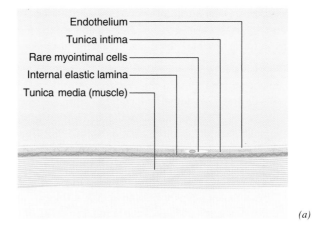

(a)

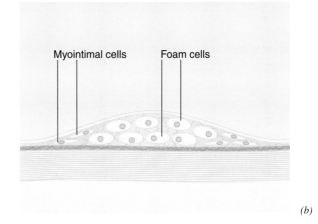

(b)

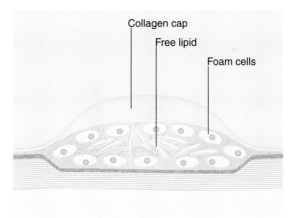

(c)

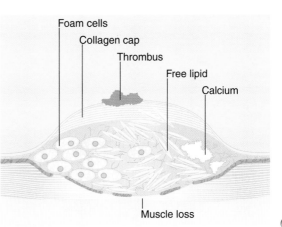

(d)

Consequences of atheroma

Atherosclerosis may affect all arterial vessels, but the aorta, coronary, cerebral, carotid, renal and ilio-femoral arteries tend to be most severely affected and are the most common sites of significant clinical disease.

The most important pathological and clinical sequelae of atherosclerosis are as follows:

- **Occlusion:** narrowing of the arterial lumen produces partial or complete obstruction to blood flow; this may result in ischaemia and *infarction* of the tissue supplied by the atheromatous vessel (Ch. 10).
- **Thrombosis:** endothelial ulceration stimulates formation of an overlying thrombus. This may occlude the vessel at the site of *thrombosis*, or fragments of thrombus may become detached to form *emboli* which block one or more smaller vessels distally (Ch. 9).
- **Aneurysm:** loss of muscle and elastin from the media causes weakening of the vessel wall, predisposing to a localised area of dilatation; such a dilatation is known as an *aneurysm*. Rupture of the weakened and dilated artery wall, leading to a fatal haemorrhage, is a further serious complication and is seen most commonly in the abdominal aorta. Aneurysms may also lead to thrombus formation (see Ch. 9) because of areas of stasis in some areas of the aneurysm cavity.

The main histopathological complications are shown in Figures 8.5 to 8.8.

Fig. 8.3 **Arteriosclerosis and early atheromatous lesions** (*illustrations b and c opposite*)

(a) **Arteriosclerosis (LP)**
(b) **Early atheromatous plaque (LP)**
(c) **Foam cells and lipid (HP)**

Intimal thickening of arteries and arterioles is extremely common with increasing age. This may form part of the spectrum of atherosclerotic disease or may simply represent a physiological adaptation which occurs with increasing age. Micrograph (a) shows a small artery exhibiting eccentric intimal proliferation **P**. The thickened intima, clearly defined by the internal elastic lamina **IEL**, can be seen to consist of multiple cell layers and involves approximately half the circumference of the vessel. In contrast to the early atheromatous lesion shown in micrograph (b), there is no evidence of lipid deposition in this case.

Micrographs (b) and (c) opposite show the early changes of atheroma in the aorta. Micrograph (b) shows a pale-staining area of thickening in the intima **In** representing an early atheromatous lesion. It consists of aggregated myointimal cells containing lipid, and some intimal fibrous tissue. Because such lesions appear macroscopically as slightly raised flat areas, they are termed *atheromatous plaques*. Note that the medial layer of the vessel **M** is uniform and appears normal at this stage; early atheroma is a disease confined to the intima.

At higher power in micrograph (c), a detail of the intimal thickening is shown. Foam cells **F** filled with lipid appear as large, pale-staining cells with very vacuolated cytoplasm. These cells may be derived from either myointimal cells or macrophages. As the lesion progresses, some of the foam cells break down and liberate free lipid into the intima where it is represented by non-staining angular clefts **C**. The presence of free lipid appears to induce a fibrous reaction in the surrounding tissues which appear eosinophilic (pink-staining) because of the presence of increased amounts of collagen.

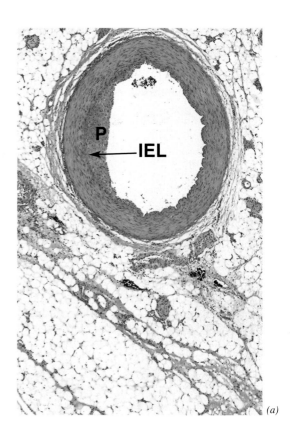

(a)

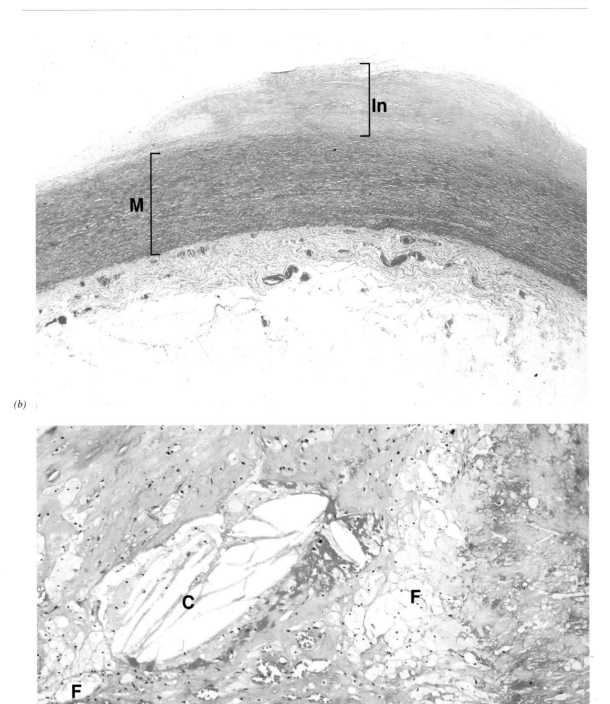

(b)

(c)

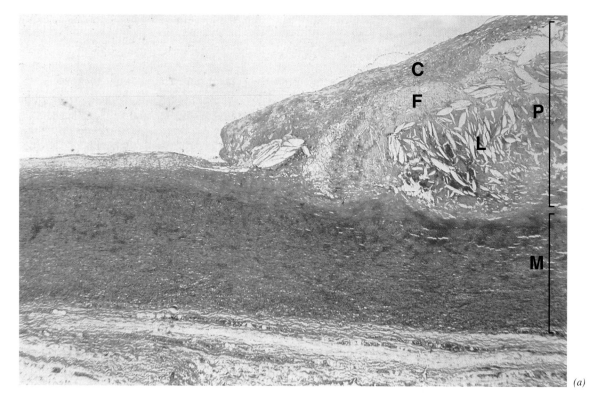

(a)

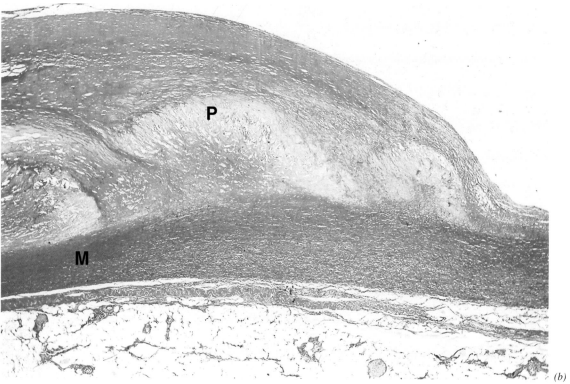

(b)

Fig. 8.4 **Fibrous atheromatous plaques** *(caption opposite)*

Fig. 8.4 **Fibrous atheromatous plaques** (*illustrations opposite*)
(a) **Fibrolipid plaque (LP)** (b) **Fibrous plaque (LP)**

Early intimal atheromatous lesions enlarge by further accumulation of lipid in foam cells and also free within the extracellular intimal tissue. This is associated with a more marked fibrotic response in the intima leading to increased thickening of the plaque. Once a more significant degree of fibrous tissue develops in an atheromatous lesion, it is termed a *fibrolipid plaque*.

Micrograph (a) shows a section of aorta with part of a fibrolipid plaque **P**. Note the areas of non-staining lipid **L** surrounded by pink-staining fibrous tissue **F**, making up the thickened intima. A zone of denser, more intensely stained fibrous tissue, sometimes termed a *fibrous cap* **C**, runs between the endothelial surface and the underlying

fibrolipid aggregate. With progression of the lesion, the fibrous cap thickens and the intimal lesion becomes larger and more raised. Micrograph (b) shows such a plaque **P**, which is composed mostly of fibrous tissue. Note that in both micrographs there is early thinning of the tunica media **M** beneath the plaque compared to the adjacent normal vessel wall. This is the result of loss of supporting elastic tissue, atrophy of smooth muscle cells and progressive medial fibrosis. With time, the medial fibrous tissue stretches owing to loss of elastic recoil in the vessel wall, and the vessel dilates. This dilatation is the basis of the formation of an atheromatous aneurysm.

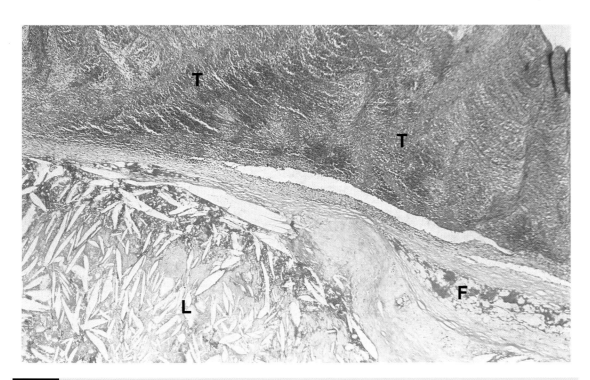

Fig. 8.5 **Complicated atheroma (MP)**

As an atheromatous plaque enlarges, it may become very thick relative to the normal thickness of the vessel wall, and in addition to lipid, foam cells and fibrous tissue, calcium may be deposited in the lesion. With thickening and fibrosis, the blood supply to the abnormal intima may become insufficient and the lesion may undergo necrosis and surface ulceration; this is then described as a *complicated atheromatous lesion*. The normal smooth endothelial lining having gone, the collagen and lipid of the atheromatous lesion are exposed directly to the blood

flow. The coagulation sequence is thus activated and thrombus is formed on the vessel wall at the site of ulcerated atheroma (see Ch. 9).

This micrograph shows the top of an atheromatous plaque with foam cells **F** and free lipid **L**. The surface has ulcerated and is encrusted with thrombus **T** composed of fibrin, platelets and entrapped blood cells. In a small vessel, for example a coronary artery, such a thrombus can occlude the lumen.

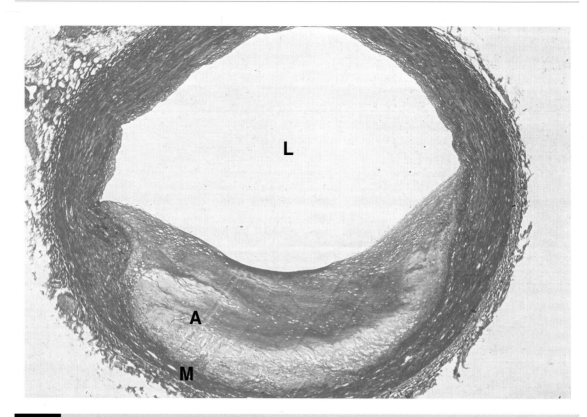

Fig. 8.6 Arterial narrowing by atheroma (LP)

The formation of a large plaque of atheroma **A** in the intima of a small or medium-sized artery, such as the coronary artery branch shown here, can greatly reduce the size of the lumen **L**. The consequent reduction in blood flow leads to ischaemia of the tissues supplied, in this case the myocardium. Note that the media **M** underlying the thickest mass of atheroma is markedly thinned. Such partly occlusive atheroma is very frequent in the coronary arteries of cigarette-smoking males, particularly in the region of the bifurcation of the left coronary artery. A frequent symptom of this arterial narrowing is the condition known as ***angina pectoris***, a gripping pain in the chest particularly experienced on exertion, and settling with rest. This pain is a manifestation of ischaemia of the myocardium, and patients with longstanding angina often show replacement of small areas of myocardial muscle by fibrous scar tissue, the end result of anoxic necrosis of muscle fibres.

Luminal narrowing by atheroma occurs similarly in many other arteries. In the leg arteries, such changes can produce severe calf pain on walking (***intermittent claudication***) and may eventually lead to the development of gangrene of the lower leg. In the vertebrobasilar arterial system which supplies the cerebellum and brain stem, severe atheroma can produce transient ischaemia manifest clinically as dizziness, loss of balance and occasional unconsciousness (***vertebro-basilar syndrome***).

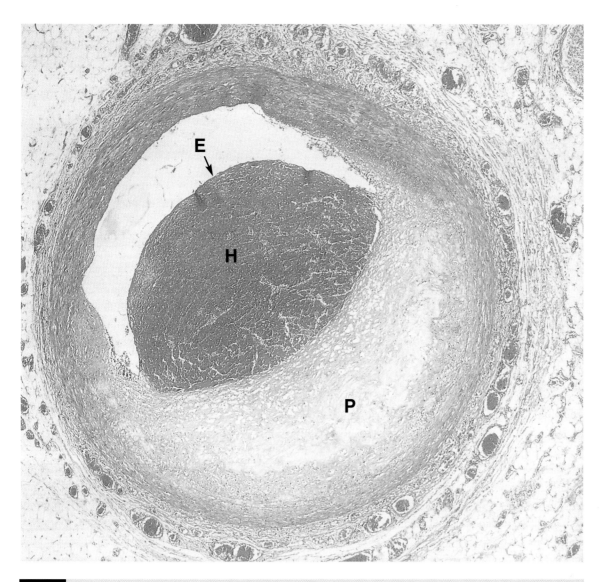

Fig. 8.7 Haemorrhage into atheromatous plaque (LP)

There are two possible mechanisms for the development of haemorrhage in an atheromatous plaque. First, the rigid fibrotic plaque may split under the constant trauma of pulsatile movements and allow blood from the vessel lumen to greatly expand the plaque lesion; such a process is termed *plaque fissuring*. Alternatively, small capillary vessels which develop in established plaques may rupture and lead to haemorrhage. Whatever the mechanism, because of the confined space in which such apparently trivial haemorrhage occurs, the consequences can be disproportionately devastating. In this micrograph, a small haemorrhage **H** has occurred in the superficial area of fibrolipid atheromatous plaque **P**; the accumulated

blood has tracked beneath the non-ulcerated endothelium **E**, causing it to bulge markedly into the artery. This has led to even greater narrowing of a lumen already reduced to about half its normal size by the pre-existing atheromatous plaque. Such an abrupt reduction in arterial flow leads to acute ischaemia in the supplied tissues.

In this patient, the lesion was situated in the anterior descending branch of the left coronary artery and resulted in acute ischaemia of a substantial area of the anterior wall of the left ventricle and the anterior half of the interventricular septum. Necrosis of heart muscle ensued, a process known as *myocardial infarction*, resulting in this patient's death (Fig. 10.2).

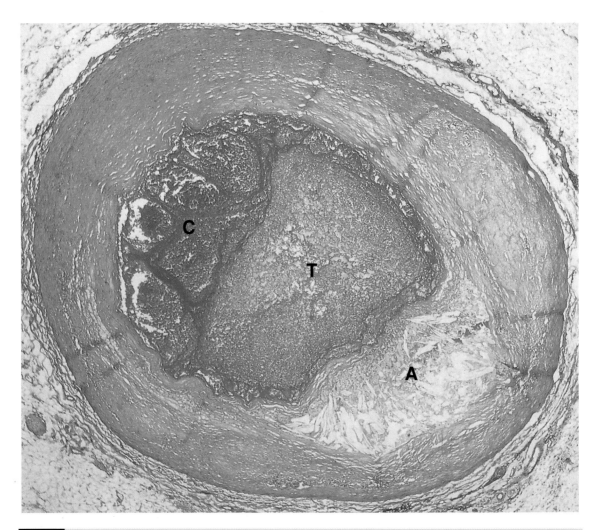

Fig. 8.8 Thrombus formation on atheroma (LP)

The most important complication of atheroma in small and medium-sized arteries is the development of a *thrombus* on the surface of an atheromatous plaque; the process of thrombus formation is discussed in detail in Chapter 9. Thrombus, which consists of a mass of platelets and insoluble fibrin, tends, in the arterial system, to form on any intimal surface which is denuded to expose the underlying tissues. Endothelial ulceration over an atheromatous plaque is the commonest cause of thrombosis in the arterial system, although plaque fissuring as discussed in Figure 8.7 can also initiate thrombosis.

This micrograph of a coronary artery shows an ulcerated atheromatous plaque **A** which has already significantly constricted the arterial lumen. A thrombus **T** has then developed on the ulcerated surface largely obliterating the remaining lumen. The thrombus is deep pink in colour, and is composed of fibrin and platelets

with entrapped red blood cells. The residual lumen is occupied by bright red postmortem blood clot **C** composed entirely of tightly packed red blood cells. The naked eye distinction between genuine antemortem thrombus and postmortem clot is important; thrombus is pinkish red, granular and firm, whereas clot is predominantly dark red, shiny and jelly-like.

When thrombus formation occurs on an atheromatous lesion in a large diameter artery, such as the aorta or carotid arteries, the thrombus may be small and cause little significant obstruction to blood flow at the site. Fragments of thrombus may, however, become detached and pass into the peripheral circulation to block a smaller vessel and cause ischaemia or infarction in its area of distribution. This phenomenon is known as *thromboembolism* and is described more fully in Chapter 9.

9. Thrombosis and embolism

Thrombosis

The vascular system normally contains fluid blood: however, it is often necessary for blood to coagulate to prevent bleeding following injury to vessel walls. To control haemostasis, there are interacting systems which either promote or inhibit the process of blood coagulation. Under certain pathological circumstances, these dynamics may be disrupted leading to the formation of a solid mass of blood products in a vessel lumen; this process is known as *thrombosis*, and the mass of blood products is referred to as a *thrombus*. It is important to distinguish thrombosis, a dynamic process occurring in flowing blood, from coagulation which is a process that takes place in static blood to form a blood *clot* and involves coagulation factors only.

Thrombus consists of aggregates of platelets bound together by fibrin strands with variable numbers of erythrocytes and leucocytes trapped in the tangled mass and contributing to the bulk of the thrombus. Thrombosis may occur in any part of the circulation but most particularly in large veins, large arteries, in the heart chambers and on heart valves. Three major factors, alone or in combination, predispose to thrombosis. These are often referred to as *Virchow's triad*:

- *Damage to the vessel wall*, particularly the endothelium, is the main cause of arterial and intracardiac thrombosis; in arteries it is due to atheroma, in the heart to endocardial damage (Fig. 9.3).
- *Disordered blood flow*. Relative stasis is important in initiating thrombus in slow-flowing blood such as in veins. Turbulent blood flow predisposes to thrombus formation in arterial vessels and the heart.
- *Abnormally enhanced haemostatic properties of the blood*. Increased platelet concentration or stickiness, or factors promoting blood clotting or diminished fibrinolysis contribute to both arterial and venous thrombosis. Changes in blood viscosity such as occur in dehydration, major illness, disseminated carcinoma and the postoperative state are included in this category.

A thrombus has a defined architecture and consistency which reflects the manner and stages of its formation and the nature of blood flow in the vicinity. For example, thrombus formed in an artery is usually dense and composed mainly of aggregated platelets and fibrin, whereas thrombus formed in slowed or static blood more closely resembles clotted blood in that it contains masses of erythrocytes and leucocytes.

BASIC PATHOLOGICAL PROCESSES

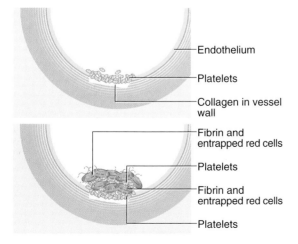

Endothelium — Platelets — Collagen in vessel wall — Fibrin and entrapped red cells — Platelets — Fibrin and entrapped red cells — Platelets

Fig. 9.1 Early thrombogenesis

(1) Following endothelial injury, platelets adhere to exposed subendothelial collagen (mediated by von Willebrand factor) and become activated, liberating ADP and thromboxane A2 which mediate further platelet aggregation.
(2) Platelets undergo degranulation and their products, together with released tissue factors, activate the coagulation cascade. This results in generation of thrombin which converts soluble fibrinogen to insoluble fibrin. Red cells become passively entrapped in the resultant fibrin–platelet mesh, the number depending on the circumstances of thrombus formation. In arteries, there are few red cells and more platelets and fibrin; in veins, where blood flow is slower, there are generally many more red cells.

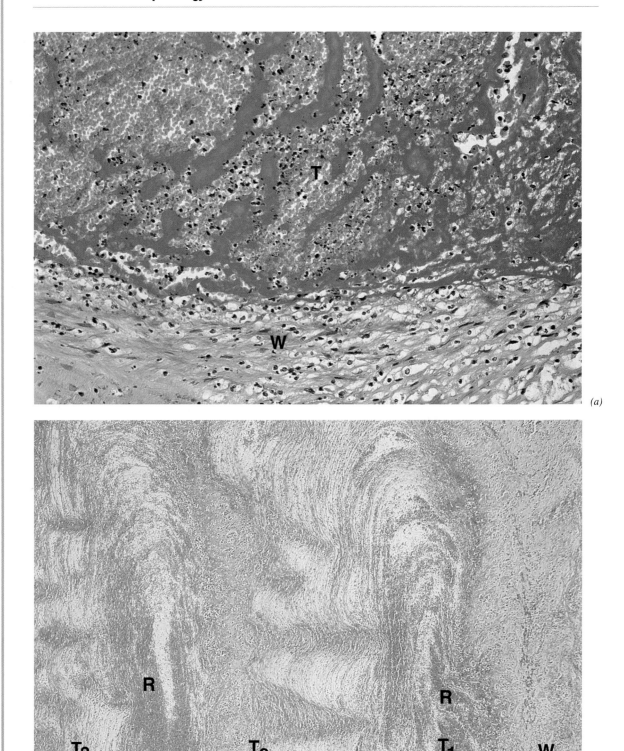

(a)

(b)

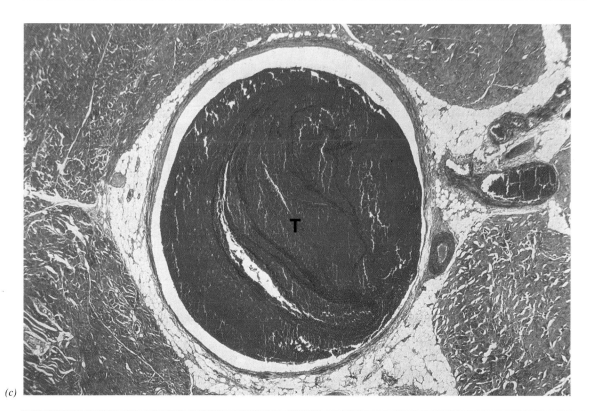

(c)

Fig. 9.2 **Thrombus formation** *(illustrations a and b opposite)*
(a) Early thrombus (HP) **(b) Enlargement of thrombus (MP)** **(c) Thrombosis in a vein (LP)**

Damage to a vessel wall usually involves damage to the endothelial lining and exposure of intimal collagen resulting in first adherence, and then aggregation, of platelets at the site of damage. Tissue damage and collagen exposure also activate the extrinsic and intrinsic blood clotting systems respectively, the latter system also depending on release of platelet factor 3 from aggregated platelets. The result is activation of prothrombin to thrombin, which in turn catalyses the conversion of soluble plasma fibrinogen into insoluble fibrin. Thus the flimsy platelet aggregates become bound together into a solid resilient mass, the thrombus.

Micrograph (a) illustrates an arterial wall **W** damaged by atheroma. The endothelium has become ulcerated with the formation of thrombus **T** at the site of injury. This thrombus consists of platelet aggregates within a meshwork of eosinophilic fibrin; entrapped erythrocytes and leucocytes are present, but are not themselves involved in the specific haemostatic processes.

Small areas of thrombus formed on vessel walls may be dissolved completely by fibrinolytic mechanisms; however, under appropriate conditions, the thrombus continues to enlarge. Micrograph (b) illustrates this

process. The abnormal vessel wall **W** has become coated by a thin layer of fibrin and platelet thrombus **T₁**, with entrapped red cells **R**. This has formed the basis for the deposition of another layer of fibrin–platelet thrombus **T₂**, again with entrapped red cells. A third layer **T₃** can be seen forming at the left of the picture. Thus thrombi enlarge by the successive deposition of a number of layers, a feature which is apparent to the naked eye in the laminated cut surface seen in an established thrombus (*lines of Zahn*).

In the arterial system, damage to the intimal layer is the most common predisposing factor in thrombus formation, but in the venous system the most important factor is the rate of blood flow; reduced flow rates increase susceptibility to thrombus formation. Vasculitis or inflammation of the vessel wall also causes thrombosis (see Ch. 11).

Micrograph (c) shows venous thrombosis **T** completely occluding the lumen of a vein in a neurovascular bundle from the muscle of the calf. This is known as *deep vein thrombosis (DVT)* and is most frequently seen in postoperative patients who are confined to bed.

BASIC PATHOLOGICAL PROCESSES

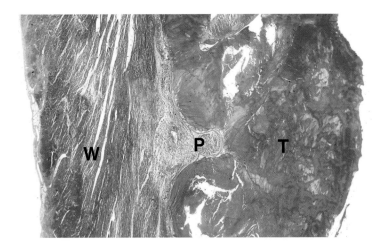

Fig. 9.3 Left ventricular mural thrombus (LP)

Thrombus within the heart chambers most commonly occurs upon endocardium damaged by myocardial infarction (see Fig. 10.2). This micrograph illustrates infarcted ventricular wall **W** with mural thrombus **T** laid down on the luminal surface; the thrombus surrounds a papillary muscle **P**.

The left ventricle is the most common site of mural thrombosis after myocardial infarction.

Consequences of thrombosis

There are two main consequences of thrombosis, namely vascular obstruction and embolisation.

- **Vascular obstruction**. Thrombus may partially or completely occlude a vessel lumen. This is particularly common in the deep veins of the legs in immobilised, debilitated patients, and results in obstruction of venous return from the feet and lower legs causing oedema (Fig. 9.2c). Thrombus forming on the surface of atheroma in an artery may occlude the vessel causing ischaemic damage to tissues distal to the obstruction. This may lead to tissue death (*infarction*), as discussed in Chapter 10.
- **Embolisation**. Embolism is the process in which any abnormal mass forming in, or entering, the bloodstream passes with the circulation to lodge in a more distal vessel with resulting pathological consequences; the abnormal mass is known as an *embolus*. Emboli are most commonly caused by detachment of all or part of a thrombus from its site of formation and this form of embolism, often called *thromboembolism*, is of the greatest clinical importance. Stasis of blood resulting from occlusion or partial obstruction of blood flow by thrombus may lead to propagation of the thrombus in the static blood. As previously outlined, thrombus formed in such conditions contains many blood cells and relatively less fibrin and is thereby much more prone to become detached to form a *thromboembolus*. For example, following deep venous thrombosis in the leg, the thrombus may propagate as far as the common iliac vein or even the inferior vena cava; part of such a huge thrombus may readily become detached and pass via the right side of the heart to the pulmonary arterial tree as a *pulmonary embolus* which is often fatal (see Fig. 9.4).

  Systemic arterial thromboemboli most commonly arise from the heart or major arteries; in such cases, the thrombus often covers only part of the luminal wall as a plaque-like structure and is known as *mural thrombus*. For example, mural thrombus may form on the ventricular endocardium following a myocardial infarct (Fig. 9.3) or in an aneurysmal dilatation or on an atheromatous lesion in the aorta (Fig. 8.5). Emboli which arise in the arterial system impact in peripheral arterial vessels where the most dramatic outcome is necrosis of the tissue supplied (infarction); this is described in detail in the next chapter.

  Whilst thrombotic emboli are the most common, emboli may also arise from other sources. These include atheromatous debris, clumps of tumour cells, bacterial vegetations from infected heart valves, fat and bone marrow after bone fracture, air entering the circulation, and rarely, amniotic fluid in cases of complicated pregnancy.

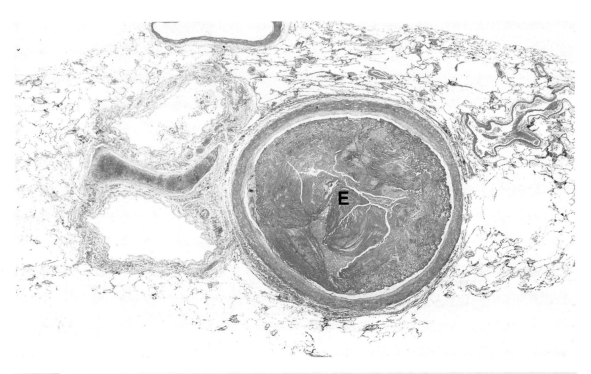

Fig. 9.4 Thromboembolism: pulmonary embolus (LP)

When fragments of thrombus become detached from their site of formation, they travel in the circulation (venous or arterial, according to site of origin) as thromboemboli. On reaching vessels of small enough calibre to prevent further passage, the thromboemboli impact producing sudden vascular occlusion. Depending on the size of the thromboembolus, the tissue or organ involved and the extent of alternative vascular supply, the result may be either inadequate blood flow for normal sustenance of the tissue (ischaemia) or frank tissue necrosis (infarction); these phenomena are described in the next chapter.

This micrograph illustrates lung tissue in which the pulmonary artery branch is occluded by an embolus **E** originating from thrombus in the deep veins of the leg.

This condition, known as *pulmonary embolism*, is an important cause of sudden death, especially in debilitated or immobilised patients predisposed to deep venous thrombosis.

Fate of vascular thrombosis

Whether a thrombus arises in situ or by embolisation from elsewhere, it may be dealt with in one of two ways:

- **Resolution**. This involves the normal physiological phenomenon of fibrinolysis as well as autolytic disintegration of the cellular elements of the thrombus; the end result is complete dissolution with restoration of blood flow.
- **Organisation**. Ingrowth of granulation tissue from the vessel wall and subsequent fibrous repair occur when fibrinolysis is ineffective in removing the thrombus. By an extraordinary mechanism, the organised thrombus may undergo recanalisation, a process whereby new vascular channels are formed to reestablish a patent lumen. The processes of organisation and recanalisation are illustrated in Figure 9.5.

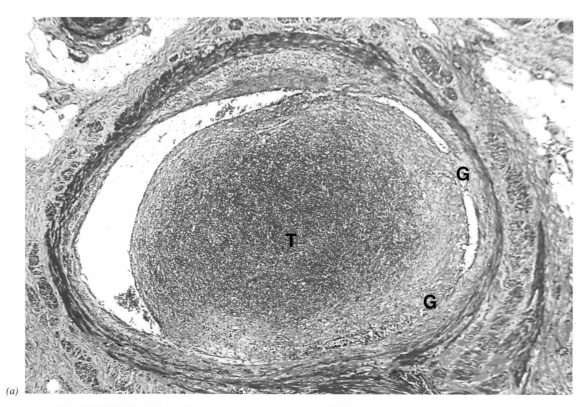
(a)

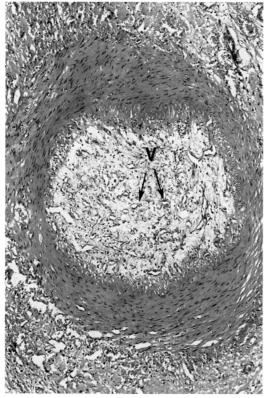
(b)

Fig. 9.5 Fate of thrombi
(a) Organisation (LP)
(b) Recanalisation (MP)

Following occlusion of a vessel by thrombus, there is an
initial inflammatory response in the vessel wall. Within a
few days, the thrombus becomes ***organised*** by ingrowth
of granulation tissue from the intima of the vessel wall.
Micrograph (a) shows a vein occluded by thrombus **T**. At
various points, granulation tissue **G** extends from the
vessel wall into the thrombus. This eventually results in
replacement of the thrombus by fibrovascular granulation
tissue. In some cases, larger vessels develop within the
fibrovascular granulation tissue of the organising
thrombus and may permit passage of blood through the
damaged, previously occluded area. This occurs most
commonly in arteries and is termed ***recanalisation***.

Micrograph (b) illustrates this process in an artery
which has been occluded by thrombus and is at a later
stage of organisation than in micrograph (a). Note that the
granulation tissue in the lumen contains numerous small
blood vessels **V**. These vessels may conduct blood across
the thrombosed area and some will enlarge with time and
acquire smooth muscle walls.

10. Infarction

Introduction

Infarction occurs in any tissue when there is interruption of blood supply sufficient to cause tissue necrosis; the area of tissue involved is described as an ***infarct***. Disturbance of blood supply may not always be sufficient to cause frank tissue necrosis but may instead cause temporary or permanent damage to the tissue or some of its functional elements; this situation is known as ***ischaemia*** and may in due course, though not necessarily, lead to infarction.

Causes of infarction

Infarction may result either from obstruction of arterial supply or, much less commonly, from obstruction of venous drainage.

- **Arterial infarction** is usually due to complete blockage of an artery by thrombosis or embolism. Arterial thrombosis is generally a complication of pre-existing atheroma (Fig. 8.8). Embolisation in the arterial system is most commonly from the heart, either mural thrombus (Fig. 9.3) or from thrombus occurring on heart valves (vegetations: see Fig. 11.6), or from thrombosis and/or atheroma of arteries; examples of infarcts from the kidney and myocardium are shown in Figures 10.1 and 10.2 respectively.

- **Venous infarction** is most commonly due to mechanical compression of the vascular supply, particularly in organs which receive their blood supply via a vascular pedicle. Such organs may become infarcted if the pedicle becomes twisted, for example torsion of the testis (Fig. 19.2), or constricted by becoming entrapped in a narrow space, for example bowel infarction caused by hernial strangulation (Fig. 10.5). In such cases, venous obstruction occurs as extrinsic pressure affects the thin-walled, low pressure veins without initially compromising the arteries; tissues become massively suffused with red cells, and prolonged venous obstruction eventually causes the tissue to become ischaemic owing to stasis of blood. The resulting cessation in tissue perfusion results in overt infarction. Venous infarction may also occur in the brain as a result of thrombosis of the dural venous sinuses.

Macroscopic appearance of infarcts

When infarction is due to simple cessation of arterial supply, the shape of the infarct reflects the geographical distribution of the artery involved. In most organs (e.g. kidney, spleen or brain), the infarct appears wedge-shaped on section, with the broad part of the wedge at the periphery. In contrast, infarcts in the heart are not wedge-shaped but rather involve part or full thickness of the myocardium and its overlying endocardium and/or visceral pericardium.

Like most forms of tissue damage, infarction excites an acute inflammatory response followed by replacement of necrotic tissue by granulation tissue which then undergoes fibrous repair and scarring (see Ch. 2). The naked eye and histological appearances of infarcts thus depend on how far this sequence has progressed. One important exception to this process is the brain, which does not normally show the usual processes of granulation tissue formation and fibrous repair. Cerebral infarcts undergo central liquefaction known as colliquative necrosis (see Ch. 1) with reactive gliosis at the margins of the lesion, and old infarcts are usually marked by a cystic area surrounded by a zone of gliosis; brain infarction is illustrated in Figures 1.7 and 23.2.

Organs in which there are extensive capillary, sinusoidal or arteriovenous anastomoses often have infarcts which in their earliest stages are dark red in colour because of congestion with blood and haemorrhage (from the Latin, *infarcire*: to stuff); important examples are the lung (Fig. 10.4) and spleen.

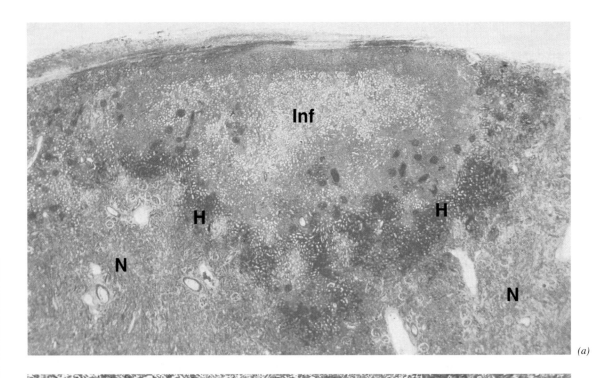

(a)

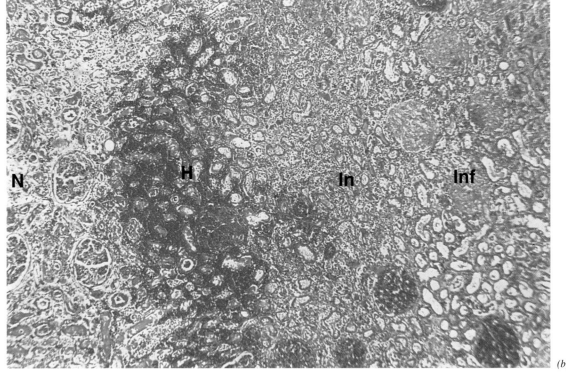

(b)

Fig. 10.1 Renal infarction *(illustrations a and b opposite)*

(a) Early infarct (LP)
(b) Margin of infarct (MP)
(c) Old renal infarct (MP)

The general features of infarction induced by thromboembolism are well illustrated by renal infarcts which usually result from emboli originating from thrombus in the left ventricle (e.g. mural thrombus after myocardial infarction) or the left atrial appendage (e.g. in atrial fibrillation).

In the very early stages (i.e. within 12 hours of infarction), gross examination shows the infarcted area to be ill-defined and dark, but progressively the lesion becomes paler until its wedge-shaped margins may be clearly distinguishable.

Micrograph (a) shows the histological appearance of a typical early renal infarct. The recently infarcted necrotic area **Inf** stains less intensely than the normal cortex **N**, but the general architecture of the infarct remains intact with still discernible 'ghosts' of glomeruli and renal tubules. The infarcted area has become demarcated from normal cortex by a narrow hyperaemic zone **H** representing the earliest vascular stages of a typical acute inflammatory response. Between this hyperaemic zone and the necrotic tissue is a purple-staining band containing the neutrophils of an early cellular acute inflammatory exudate.

Micrograph (b) shows, at higher magnification, the edge of the infarct in micrograph (a). Note that the normal cortical tissue **N** with its well-defined glomeruli and tubules gives way to a zone of hyperaemia **H**; next to this is a purplish band of acute inflammation **In** at the margin of the infarcted area **Inf** where marked necrotic changes are evident in both glomeruli and tubules (see Fig. 1.6). The acute inflammatory zone exhibits typically dilated and congested capillaries and an influx of small, dark-staining neutrophil polymorphs.

The necrotic tissue is progressively removed by neutrophils and macrophages and replaced by granulation tissue which eventually undergoes fibrous repair to form a small fibrous scar. This is shown in micrograph (c) which illustrates the end result of a renal infarct occurring 2 months previously; the infarct was of a similar size to that shown in (a). All that now remains is a small, narrow, pink-staining, wedge-shaped scar **S** with its broad aspect at the capsular surface. Note that the capsular surface at the site of the scar is depressed as a result of contraction of the collagen fibres within the scar (a process known as cicatrisation; see Fig. 2.10).

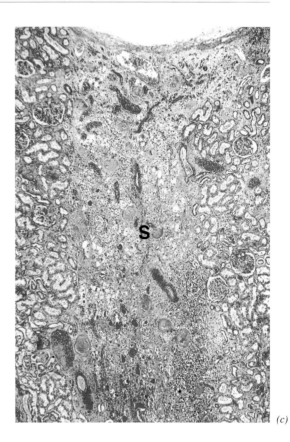

(c)

Ischaemic heart disease

Disease of cardiac muscle as a result of impaired blood supply is a major cause of death in all industrialised countries. Atherosclerosis of coronary arteries accounts for the vast majority of cases and gives rise to four main clinical syndromes: angina pectoris (chest pain on exertion), acute myocardial infarction ('heart attack' or 'coronary occlusion'), chronic ischaemic heart disease, and sudden cardiac death (immediately fatal myocardial infarct or dysrhythmia).

Acute myocardial infarction takes two main pathological forms:

- **Transmural infarction**. This involves the full thickness of a segment of the ventricular wall and is associated with complete blockage of a main coronary artery by thrombosis superimposed on an area of arteriosclerotic narrowing. As mentioned in Chapter 8, fissure or ulceration of an atheromatous plaque is the usual cause of thrombus formation.
- **Subendocardial myocardial infarction**. In this case, myocardial necrosis is limited to cells in the inner third of the ventricular wall and tends to be associated with severe arteriosclerotic narrowing of both right and left coronary arteries. The pathogenesis of infarction is limitation of flow to the end arteries supplying the inner part of the ventricular wall rather than complete occlusion of the main arterial trunks.

The histological changes following infarction are illustrated in Figures 10.2 and 10.3.

Fig. 10.2 **Myocardial infarction** (*illustrations opposite*)
(a) **24-hour infarct (HP)** (b) **3-day infarct (HP)** (c) **10-day infarct (HP)** (d) **14-day infarct (HP)**

The most common clinical example of infarction is that of the myocardium following occlusion of a coronary artery.

Using routine staining methods, the earliest histological evidence of infarction is visible some 12 to 24 hours after the onset of acute ischaemia as illustrated in micrograph (a). The infarcted cardiac muscle fibres **In** exhibit patchy loss or blurring of cross striations and tend to become more intensely stained by eosin when compared to normal myocardial fibres **M**; there may also at this stage be some degree of early capillary engorgement and interstitial oedema, representing the earliest stages of the acute inflammatory response.

By about 2 or 3 days, as shown in micrograph (b), the infarcted fibres are intensely eosinophilic and most have lost their nuclei; there is marked infiltration by neutrophils **N** into the oedematous interstitium. The acute inflammatory process evolves during the succeeding days, during which time the necrotic myocardium undergoes autolysis and fragmentation, and the neutrophil infiltration becomes more intense.

By about the 10th day, as illustrated in micrograph (c), most of the necrotic muscle has disappeared as a result of the combined phagocytic activity of neutrophils and macrophages (see Fig. 2.8). The infarcted area is now largely occupied by residual macrophages, some

lymphocytes and plasma cells, in a loose oedematous mesh in which a few capillaries and fibroblasts herald the earliest signs of granulation tissue formation.

By about the 14th day, the infarct is almost wholly replaced by fibrovascular granulation tissue **G**, as illustrated in micrograph (d), and the necrotic myocardium has been almost completely removed by the phagocytic activity of macrophages and neutrophils (Fig. 2.8).

Over succeeding weeks, the fibrovascular granulation tissue becomes progressively more fibrous and less vascular, leading to the formation of a highly collagenous and relatively acellular scar by about the end of the second month following infarction; examples of myocardial scars are shown in Figure 10.3.

The infarcted myocardium offers the least resistance to pressure around days 5 to 10, and at this time the patient is most vulnerable to myocardial rupture. This not uncommon complication is almost invariably fatal, the ruptured ventricle wall spilling blood into the pericardial cavity (***haemopericardium***). If the interventricular septum is involved in the infarct, there may be rupture of the septum with the sudden appearance of a systolic murmur. Similarly, rupture of an infarcted papillary muscle may lead to mitral valve incompetence with the sudden appearance of a characteristic systolic murmur.

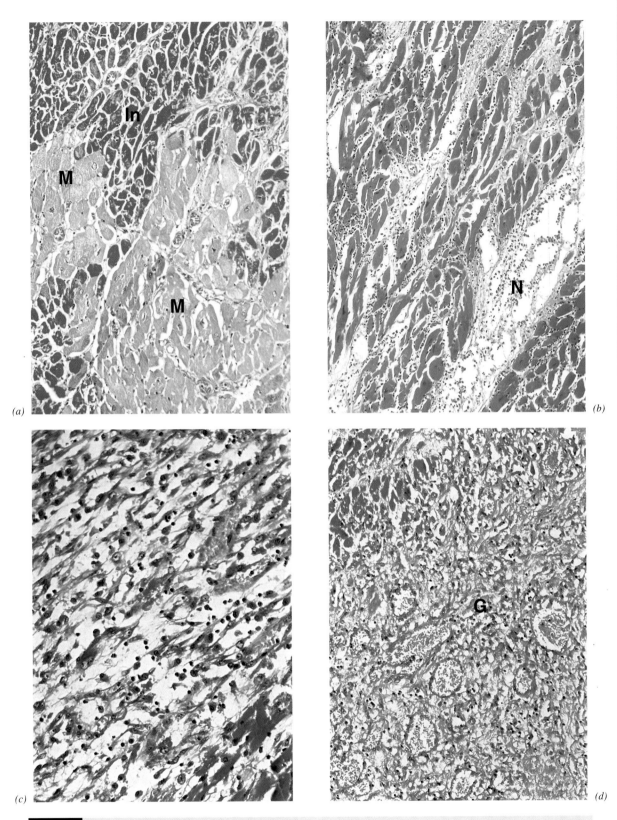

Fig. 10.2 Myocardial infarction *(caption opposite)*

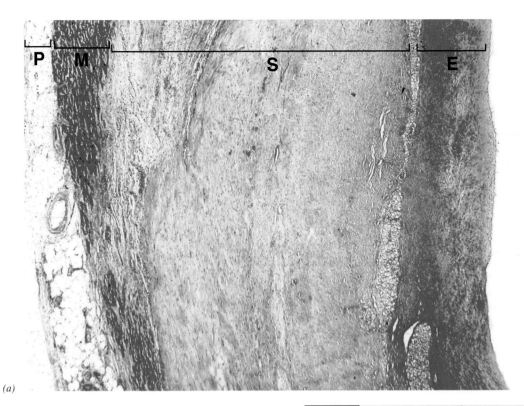

(a)

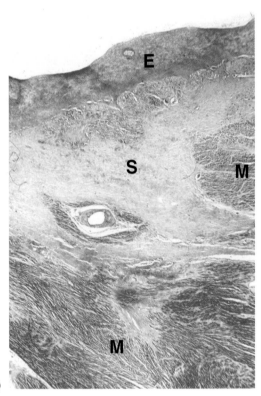

(b)

Fig. 10.3 Old myocardial infarcts
(a) Full thickness scar (LP)
(b) Partial thickness scar (LP)

These two micrographs show examples of myocardial scars several months after infarction. The sites of infarction are marked by densely collagenous pale pink-staining scar **S**, contrasting with the more eosinophilic surviving myocardial muscle **M**. Continuing contraction (cicatrisation) of the fibrous scar over succeeding months leads to thinning of the infarcted area of the ventricular wall. If the scar is inadequate to withstand ventricular pressures (most likely after a full thickness infarct), a ventricular aneurysm may develop by ballooning of the ventricular wall. With or without aneurysm formation, stasis in the region of the non-contractile scar predisposes to formation of a ventricular mural thrombus.

If the original infarct involves the endocardium **E** or visceral pericardium **P**, or both as in some full thickness infarcts, these normally delicate layers become markedly thickened as a result of their involvement in the inflammatory process and subsequent organisation and repair.

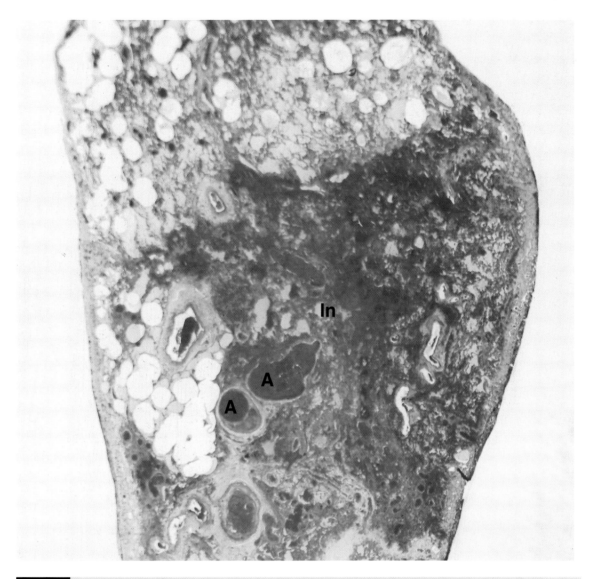

Fig. 10.4 Lung infarct (LP)

Infarcts of the lung usually result from small pulmonary emboli arising from fragments of thrombus within the veins of the legs (see Fig. 9.2c). In their early stages, lung infarcts are firm, dark red, wedge-shaped areas at the lung periphery; their firmness and colour derive from the fact that the alveolar spaces are filled with erythrocytes, partly owing to leakage from damaged capillary walls and partly to blood carried by the unobstructed bronchial arterial circulation. The pleura becomes involved in the resulting acute inflammatory response; in this case, the fibrinous pleurisy results in characteristic sharp pleuritic pain and a pleural friction rub. Larger emboli which obstruct the main pulmonary arteries tend to result in sudden death.

This micrograph illustrates the edge of a lung with a small congested infarct **In**. Note the obstructed branches of the pulmonary artery **A** and the clearly defined margins of the infarct demarcating the area supplied by this vessel.

BASIC PATHOLOGICAL PROCESSES

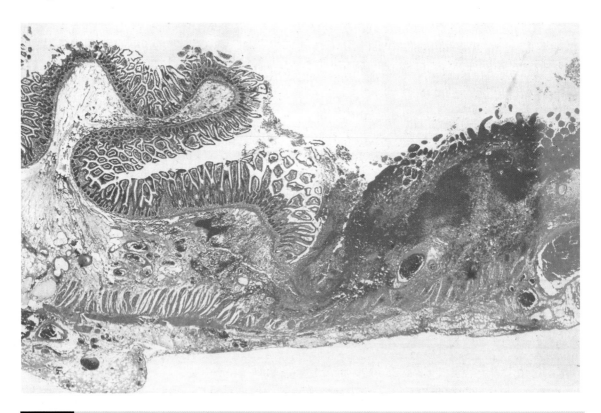

Fig. 10.5 Venous infarction of bowel following volvulus (LP)

Bowel infarction may occur either as a result of arterial occlusion (e.g. mesenteric thrombosis or embolism) or, more commonly, as a result of venous obstruction. Venous obstruction may occur through *torsion* (twisting) of a free loop of bowel around its vascular pedicle (*volvulus*), entrapment in a tight hernial orifice (e.g. *incarcerated indirect inguinal hernia*) or obstruction by fibrous *peritoneal adhesions* (e.g. following previous surgery).

Venous obstruction initially causes the bowel to become intensely congested with blood, giving it a plum-coloured appearance on gross examination; as the dammed-back blood prevents arterial inflow, the bowel becomes progressively hypoxic. Frank necrosis follows unless the venous obstruction is relieved.

In this micrograph of a small bowel volvulus, the necrotic bowel at the right-hand side of the picture is stained bright red because of massive suffusion with blood; the outline of the necrotic mucosal villi is still apparent. Note the sharp demarcation between normal and necrotic bowel, and the marked engorgement of all vessels.

BASIC SYSTEMS PATHOLOGY

11. Cardiovascular system

Introduction

Diseases of the cardiovascular system are the commonest cause of death and serious illness in developed countries. The most common underlying cause is *atherosclerosis* which is the exclusive topic of Chapter 8. Also important are *thrombosis* and *embolism*, which are the subject of Chapter 9, and their frequent sequel, *infarction*, which is described in Chapter 10.

Ischaemic heart disease

Of the diseases involving the heart, ischaemic heart disease is the most important in developed countries. In almost all cases, the cause of ischaemic heart disease is atherosclerosis of the coronary arteries with or without accompanying thrombosis; coronary artery atheroma and thrombosis are illustrated in Figures 8.4 and 8.5, and the stages of myocardial infarction are shown in Figure 10.2.

Inflammation of the heart

Inflammation may affect the pericardium, myocardium or endocardium, either separately or concurrently. The causes are numerous but the most common are ischaemia and infection. Most infections of the pericardium (*pericarditis*) and myocardium (*myocarditis*) are viral, whilst those of the endocardium (*endocarditis*) and valves (*valvulitis*) are bacterial or fungal (Figs 11.6 to 11.8).

The main causes of pericarditis are summarised in Figure 11.1. The histological features of most forms of acute pericarditis are virtually identical whatever the cause and are illustrated and discussed in Figure 2.6. In tuberculous pericarditis, there is a chronic granulomatous response as described in Chapter 4. In malignant pericarditis, clumps of tumour cells are often mixed with the inflammatory exudate.

The term myocarditis implies inflammatory damage to the myocardium and by common usage usually excludes the acute inflammatory reaction to necrotic muscle fibres seen in myocardial infarction (Fig. 10.2). Primary myocarditis can be associated with viral infections, rheumatic fever, and exposure to certain toxins and drugs. In some cases, no causative factor can be identified (*idiopathic myocarditis*).

Endocarditis and valvulitis (see later) involve not only inflammation but also thrombus deposition upon the endocardium and/or valves. These are important diseases and have a high mortality rate, their clinical manifestations often resulting from embolic phenomena or from dysfunction of the valves.

Fig. 11.1 Important causes of pericarditis		
Myocardial infarction	After transmural myocardial infarction	Common
Cardiac surgery	After surgical opening of pericardial sac	Common
Viral infections	Usually young adults. Coxsackie B most common	Common
Malignancy	Local invasion or metastatic tumour desposits	Uncommon
Uraemia	Renal failure	Now uncommon
Bacterial infections	Secondary to lung infection including TB	Uncommon
Rheumatic fever	Part of rheumatic pancarditis	Now rare

Cardiomyopathy

The *cardiomyopathies* are disorders in which there is abnormal myocardial structure and function not resulting from ischaemia or hypertension; a classification is shown in Figure 11.2. The abnormalities usually cause progressive cardiac failure, but sudden cardiac death caused by acute dysrhythmia may be the first manifestation.

The term *secondary cardiomyopathy* is sometimes used to describe cases in which the cause of the myocardial disorder is recognised, for example amyloid infiltration, viral myocarditis, alcohol and certain drugs, or rarely muscular dystrophies.

Fig. 11.2 Classification and causes of cardiomyopathy

Classification	Pathology	Aetiology
Hypertrophic (obstructive) cardiomyopathy	Gross hypertrophy of left ventricular wall (particularly interventricular septum) causing outflow obstruction	Autosomal dominant (some), unknown (majority)
Dilated (congestive) cardiomyopathy	Defective myocardial contractility leading to atrophy and ventricular dilation and cardiac failure	Postviral myocarditis (some), unknown (majority)
Restrictive cardiomyopathy	Abnormal rigidity of myocardium restricts filling and contraction	Infiltration by amyloid (some), unknown (majority)

Rheumatic fever

Rheumatic fever is a systemic inflammatory disease which, in susceptible individuals, appears to follow infection by *group A beta haemolytic streptococci*; such infections commonly occur in the throat and are themselves relatively innocuous. The systemic manifestations represent a disordered immunological response resulting in inflammation of connective tissues. Connective tissues in all parts of the body may be involved, for example the joints and skin, with painful short-term consequences. Involvement of the heart is of great clinical importance because of potentially fatal acute myocarditis and endocarditis and the long-term consequences of chronic scarring of the heart valves.

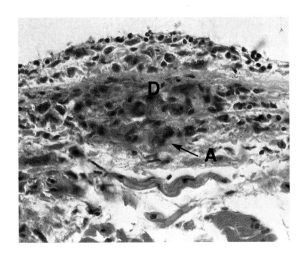

Fig. 11.3 Rheumatic carditis (HP)

The characteristic acute myocardial rheumatic lesion is the *Aschoff body* as shown in this micrograph. The fully developed Aschoff body has a central, ill-defined area of degenerate material **D** surrounded by a mixture of inflammatory leucocytes. Amongst these cells can often be seen a so-called *Anitschow myocyte* **A**, recognised by its irregular, ribbon-like nucleus and extensive eosinophilic cytoplasm. Despite the name, these cells are considered to represent large modified histiocytic cells. Aschoff bodies are found in the interstitial connective tissue of the myocardium, particularly near vessels in the subepicardial fibrous tissue, and (as in this micrograph) in the subendocardial connective tissue.

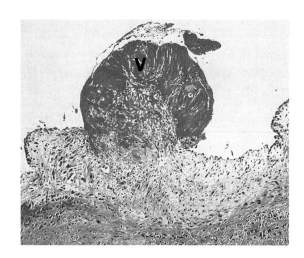

Fig. 11.4 Acute rheumatic endocarditis (MP)

The importance of acute rheumatic endocarditis relates to involvement of the heart valves where endocardial roughening induces formation of fibrin and platelet thrombi. This micrograph illustrates part of a mitral valve leaflet affected by acute rheumatic endocarditis. A small thrombotic vegetation **V** has formed on the upper (atrial) surface of the valve leaflet at the site of the remnants of a large Aschoff body.

Chronic rheumatic valvular disease is the result of organisation and fibrous scarring of affected valves. This continues over many years with eventual thickening and distortion of the valve leaflets as well as the chordae tendinae. Such distortion commonly renders affected valves stenotic or incompetent.

Valvulitis (endocarditis of valves)

The heart valves may become subject to a variety of vegetative lesions which have traditionally been described as forms of **endocarditis**. The primary phenomenon underlying all these conditions is the formation of thrombus on the valve leaflets or cusps.

As in the arterial system, roughening of the endocardial surface predisposes to thrombus formation (Ch. 9). This may occur when valve leaflets or cusps have been previously damaged by rheumatic fever or are congenitally abnormal. Thrombus formation may also follow autoimmune valve damage in systemic lupus erythematosus (**Libman–Sacks endocarditis**) and in the acute phase of rheumatic fever (Fig. 11.4). The most frequent type of valve thrombi, however, occurs in so-called **marantic endocarditis** (Fig. 11.5) in which warty thrombotic vegetations develop on mitral and aortic valves. This phenomenon occurs in seriously ill patients, often those with widely disseminated malignancy, and is usually associated with a state of hyper-coagulability of the blood. Despite use of the term endocarditis in these conditions, inflammation is usually not a feature of the valve at the time of thrombus formation.

True valvular inflammation may arise, however, if these thrombotic vegetations on the valves then become infected with bacteria, fungi or other organisms, conditions collectively referred to as **infective endocarditis**. Bacterial endocarditis tends to be divided into two clinicopathological patterns. In the first, traditionally known as **subacute bacterial endocarditis** (Fig. 11.6), the thrombotic vegetations develop on previously damaged valves, and then become colonised by bacteria of low virulence such as *Streptococcus viridans*; such organisms tend to reach the valves via a transient bacteraemia, for example following dental extraction. The major clinical consequences are those resulting from detachment of small thrombotic emboli, often infected, into the systemic circulation.

In the second type of bacterial endocarditis, known traditionally as **acute bacterial endocarditis** (Figs 11.7 and 11.8), thrombi form on previously normal valves and become infected by virulent organisms such as *Staphylococcus aureus*. In this case, the patient is usually already severely debilitated and septicaemic, for example from an infected urinary catheter, and the infecting organism is that which is responsible for the septicaemia. In contrast with the subacute pattern, in the acute form the fulminating infection extends into the substance of the valve causing tissue necrosis. Rapid destruction of the valve leaflet leads to valvular incompetence with acute cardiac failure as the usual clinical outcome.

Fungal endocarditis (Fig. 4.19), formerly rare, is now appearing more commonly as a complication of immunosuppressive therapy, intravenous drug abuse, or AIDS; *Candida albicans* is the most common organism.

The incidence of the types of endocarditis just described has changed over the past few decades; reasons include the widespread use of broad-spectrum antibiotics and decreasing incidence of rheumatic fever. Furthermore, understanding of the nature of these conditions has changed markedly in recent years, leaving behind a somewhat inappropriate terminology.

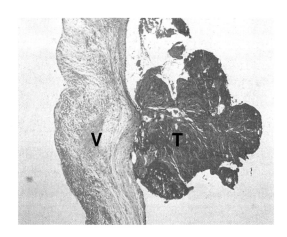

Fig. 11.5 Marantic endocarditis (LP)

This micrograph illustrates a mitral valve lesion of marantic (thrombotic, non-bacterial) endocarditis; masses of thrombus **T** have developed on the superior surface of the valve leaflet **V**. Such thrombotic masses are only loosely attached to the underlying non-inflamed valve and are therefore readily detached leading to major embolic consequences such as cerebral, renal and splenic infarction. In practice, this type of endocarditis is rarely diagnosed in life but is a common necropsy finding.

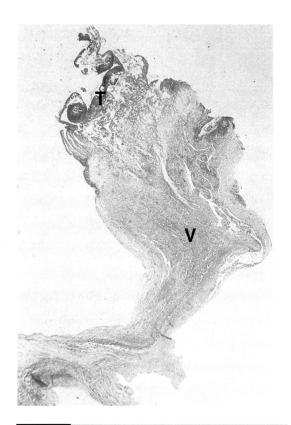

Fig. 11.6 Subacute bacterial endocarditis (LP)

This micrograph shows the subacute form of bacterial endocarditis affecting a mitral valve. The valve leaflet **V** is covered at its tip by pink-staining thrombus **T** containing small colonies of blue-purple-staining bacteria. There is no evidence of bacterial destruction and the organisms are present in relatively small numbers. The underlying valve is thickened as a result of previous rheumatic fever.

Fragments of such vegetations become detached giving rise to multiple small emboli: these may be manifest by splinter haemorrhages of nails and microscopic haematuria.

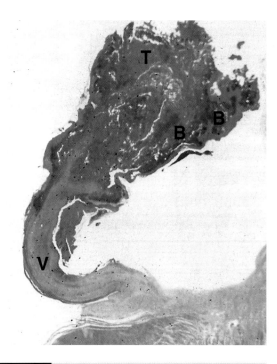

Fig. 11.7 Acute bacterial endocarditis (LP)

This micrograph shows an example of the acute form of bacterial endocarditis involving an aortic valve. The patient was bacteraemic following a fulminant local infection, in this case involving the kidney. The highly virulent bacteria **B** have settled on the heart valves probably colonising small pre-existing thrombi; bacterial proliferation has then stimulated further formation of thrombus **T** forming large vegetations which have eroded and destroyed the previously normal valve **V**. Compare the huge mass of bacteria and thrombus in this case with that of the subacute form shown in Figure 11.6. Since valve destruction is so rapid, the clinical picture is usually of rapidly developing cardiac failure due to valve incompetence rather than embolic episodes.

BASIC SYSTEMS PATHOLOGY

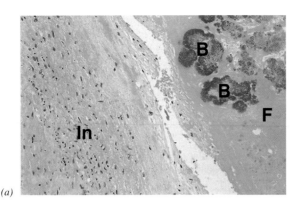

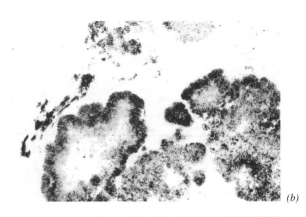

(a)

(b)

Fig. 11.8 **Acute bacterial endocarditis (HP)**
(a) H&E (b) Gram stain

This example of *acute bacterial endocarditis* is taken from a patient who presented with acute heart failure following bacterial destruction of his aortic valve. In micrograph (a), the fibrous tissue comprising the valve is seen at the lower left and is infiltrated by sparse inflammatory cells **In**. In the upper right, there is a mass of eosinophilic fibrin **F** containing large colonies of purple-staining bacteria **B**, in this case *Streptococcus bovis*.

Micrograph (b) is from the same specimen and stained with the Gram stain; this demonstrates large quantities of the Gram-positive, purple-staining streptococci embedded in the fibrin. This patient underwent an emergency aortic valve replacement and with intravenous antibiotic treatment made an excellent recovery.

Diseases of the arterial system

The most common pathological abnormality of the arterial tree is thickening and hardening of the walls, a condition known as arteriosclerosis. Atheroma (atherosclerosis) is the most frequent cause of arteriosclerosis and is discussed in Chapter 8.

The other important causes of arteriosclerosis are hypertension and diabetes mellitus; in both cases, the specific vascular changes are often superimposed upon features of atherosclerosis. Some of the important arterial wall changes associated with hypertension are illustrated in this chapter in Figures 11.9 and 11.10, and in relation to the kidney in Figure 15.12. Diabetic vascular changes are illustrated in relation to the kidney in Figure 15.9. Inflammatory disorders of arterial vessels are of considerable histological importance and are discussed later in the chapter.

Aneurysms
Abnormal dilatations of arterial vessels are known as *aneurysms* and may be divided into five main types as shown in Figure 11.11. One type, the *berry aneurysm*, is shown in Figure 11.12. The main complications of an aneurysm are rupture leading to haemorrhage, and more rarely thrombus formation leading to occlusive or embolic phenomena.

Dissecting aneurysms (Fig. 11.13) arise acutely as a result of idiopathic degeneration of the tunica media; they are not true aneurysms since they do not result in chronic arterial dilatation.

Tumours of blood vessel origin
Benign and malignant tumours may arise from the blood or lymph vascular tissues. The most common are *haemangiomas* (Fig. 11.14), many of which are regarded as hamartomas (see Ch. 7) rather than neoplasms. *Angiosarcoma*, a rare malignant tumour of endothelium, is illustrated in Figure 11.15.

Kaposi's sarcoma is a malignant tumour of vascular tissues which particularly occurs in patients who are immunosuppressed, particularly those with AIDS; this is illustrated in Figure 11.16.

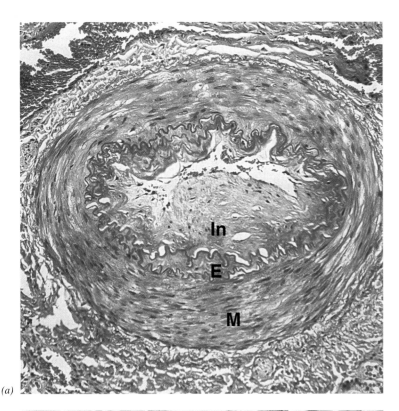

(a)

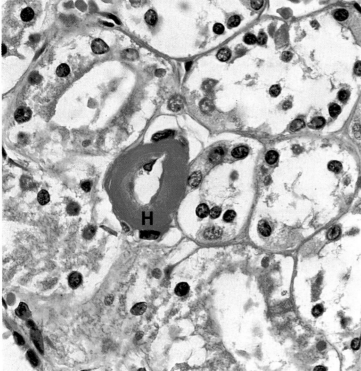

(b)

Fig. 11.9 Essential
hypertension: kidney

(a) **Medium-sized artery (MP)**
(b) **Renal arteriole (HP)**

Hypertension, whether idiopathic
(primary) or secondary, is associated
with changes in peripheral arterial
vessels; whether such changes are part
of the primary causative process,
secondary, or contributory, remains
unresolved.

When the increase in blood
pressure is moderate and gradual in
onset (*essential* or *benign
hypertension*), muscular arteries
undergo progressive thickening of
their walls. Three features are
characteristically seen and are shown
in micrograph (a): symmetrical
hypertrophy of the muscular media **M**,
extensive reduplication of the internal
elastic lamina **E** and fibrotic
thickening of the intima **In**. All these
changes lead to reduction of luminal
diameter.

Arterioles show a different type of
wall thickening sometimes referred to
as *hyaline arteriolosclerosis* and
shown in micrograph (b). The normal
layers of the wall become ill-defined
and replaced by homogeneous
eosinophilic (pink-stained) material
called *hyaline* **H**, thought to consist of
basement membrane-like material.
This results in reduction in size of
arteriolar lumina and may contribute
to further hypertension.

BASIC SYSTEMS PATHOLOGY

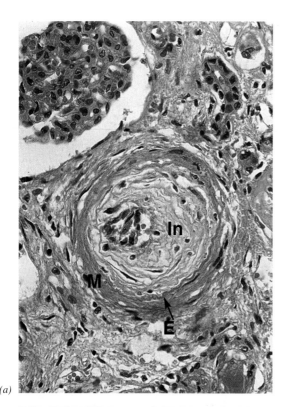

(a)

Fig. 11.10 Accelerated hypertension: kidney
(a) Medium-sized artery (HP)
(b) Arteriole (HP)

When the increase in blood pressure is of marked degree and rapid onset (*accelerated* or *malignant hypertension*), muscular arteries develop severe thickening of the tunica intima **In** by proliferation of intimal cells; this gives the appearance of concentric lamellae which encroach upon the arterial lumen as seen in micrograph (a). In contrast to the findings in moderate hypertension, the tunica media **M** and internal elastic lamina **E** remain largely unchanged.

The impact of sudden and severe hypertension on arterioles is even more dramatic, as shown in micrograph (b). The intimal cells undergo rapid proliferation (as in the muscular arteries) which is often complicated by disruption of the vessel wall, with leakage of plasma proteins, including fibrinogen, into and beyond the arteriolar wall. This change, known inaccurately as *fibrinoid necrosis*, is characterised by obliteration of the wall by intensely eosinophilic amorphous proteinaceous material **P**; the lumen is often completely occluded. Damage to the vessel wall may lead to thrombosis within the lumen.

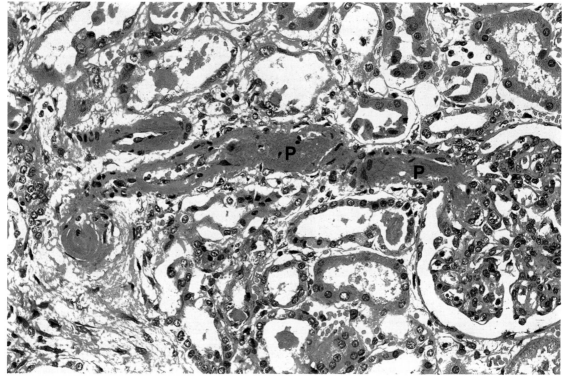

(b)

Fig. 11.11 Classification of aneurysms

Type	Common sites	Aetiology	Common effects of rupture
Atherosclerotic aneursyms	Abdominal aorta	Weakening of tunica media owing to atheroma	Massive haemorrhage into retroperitoneum and peritoneal cavity
Berry aneurysms (Fig. 11.12)	Cerebral arteries	Developmental defects in tunica media and elastic laminae	Subarachnoid haemorrhage
Syphilitic (Fig 4.13)	Ascending thoracic aorta	Damaged tunica media owing to syphilitic arteritis	Massive haemorrhage into mediastinum and thoracic cavity
Mycotic (infective) aneurysms	Any arterial vessels	Destruction of tunica media by infected thrombus	Haemorrhage from affected vessel
Microaneurysms	Brain, retina	Hypertensive and diabetic small vessel disease	Brain and retinal haemorrhages

Note: Dissecting aneurysms (Fig. 11.13) are not true aneurysms, since they do not represent permanent dilations of arteries.

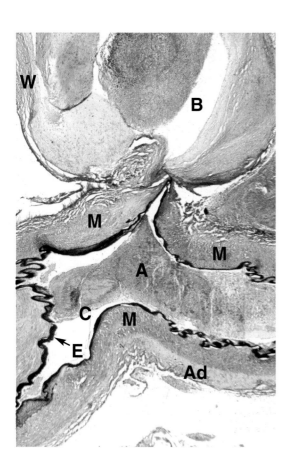

Fig. 11.12 Berry aneurysm (Elastic van Gieson – LP)

Berry aneurysms are a characteristic type of aneurysm found in the cerebral circulation, particularly at junctions in the circle of Willis or at bifurcations of the major cerebral arteries (especially the middle cerebral). Berry aneurysms most often become manifest in middle age by rupturing to cause subarachnoid haemorrhage. These aneurysms are, however, an occasional incidental finding at all ages and are often multiple.

This micrograph illustrates a berry aneurysm **B** arising from the anterior cerebral artery **A** just proximal to the point where it gives rise to its anterior communicating branch **C**. The vessel has a normal tunica media **M**, adventitia **Ad** and internal elastic lamina **E** (elastin stains black with this staining method). Note that at the point of origin of the aneurysm, the tunica media is deficient. The wall of the aneurysm **W** is composed of loose fibrous intimal tissue and the lumen contains blood. There is no medial muscle or elastin in the aneurysm wall.

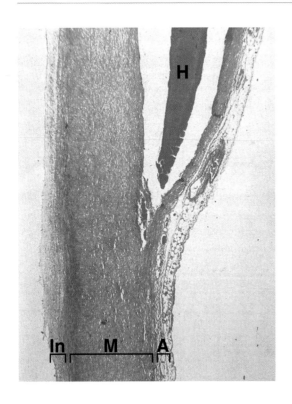

Fig. 11.13 Dissecting aneurysms of the aorta (LP)

Dissecting aneurysms most commonly affect the thoracic aorta. A laceration of the tunica intima **In** leads to tracking of blood into the tunica media **M**. The plane of cleavage (dissection) is usually between the middle and outer thirds of the media, as in this example; note that the site of intimal laceration is not included in this photographic field. The medial haematoma **H** then frequently bursts through the tunica adventitia **A** with rapidly fatal consequences.

The pathogenesis of dissecting aneurysms is poorly understood but almost all cases exhibit a peculiar type of non-inflammatory degeneration of the smooth muscle and elastic tissue of the tunica media known as *medial myxoid degeneration* or *cystic medionecrosis*. In this condition, areas of the tunica media become replaced by irregular masses of acellular polysaccharide material. Dissecting aneurysms may occur in adults at any age though they are most common in middle age, with males outnumbering females.

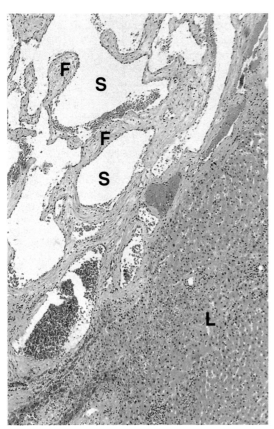

Fig. 11.14 Haemangioma (MP)

Benign tumours of vascular tissues most commonly occur in the skin and liver but may occur in any tissue. Many are present at birth or soon after and may be considered as hamartomas or developmental disorders. Haemangiomas are usually divided into *capillary* and *cavernous* types, the former composed of small capillary-sized spaces, the latter mainly of large dilated vascular spaces.

This micrograph shows a typical *cavernous haemangioma* of the liver at low power. In the bottom right-hand corner of the micrograph is normal liver parenchyma **L**. The upper left half shows the haemangioma consisting of large vascular spaces **S**, some of which contain blood. These are lined by essentially normal endothelial cells, in contrast to angiosarcoma (see Fig. 11.15), and separated by a fibrous stroma **F**. These tumours are common in the liver and are often found incidentally at autopsy or laparotomy.

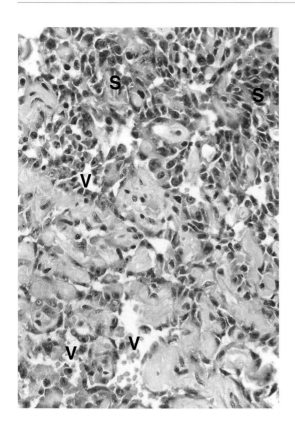

Fig. 11.15 Angiosarcoma (HP)

Angiosarcomas are rare, occurring most commonly in the skin (as shown here), soft tissues, breast and liver. Those in the liver are associated with known carcinogens including arsenic, Thorotrast and polyvinyl chloride. These tumours are formed by malignant endothelial cells which show pleomorphism, increased mitotic figures and hyperchromicity.

This example is from the arm of a woman who underwent a radical mastectomy with axillary clearance years previously; the malignant endothelial cells can be seen forming irregular branching vascular spaces **V** in some areas and solid sheets of cells **S** in other areas. Mitotic figures are common. The difference between these malignant endothelial cells and the benign endothelium lining vascular spaces in the haemangioma of the liver (Fig. 11.14) can be readily appreciated. Malignant tumours arising from the endothelium of the lymphatic system, *lymphangiosarcomas*, are usually similar in appearance except for the absence of blood in the vascular spaces.

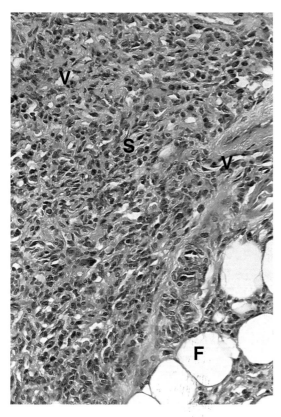

Fig. 11.16 Kaposi's sarcoma (HP)

Until recently, Kaposi's sarcoma was a rare tumour in developed countries, affecting elderly men of Eastern European origin and transplant recipients. A similar tumour was known to be common in children and young men in equatorial regions of Africa. Since the advent of AIDS, Kaposi's sarcoma has become a common tumour in developed countries. It commonly occurs in the skin in the former groups but also spreads widely in the viscera in AIDS patients.

A typical lesion, illustrated here, consists of sheets of plump stromal cells **S** interspersed with irregular slit-like vascular spaces **V**. The tumour is seen here infiltrating subcutaneous fat **F**. Extravasation of red blood cells, not seen here, is common. *Bacillary angiomatosis*, caused by infection with *Rickettsiae quintana*, may appear very similar except for the presence of numerous neutrophils and nuclear dust. This condition also occurs in AIDS patients but can be cured by the antibiotic erythromycin.

BASIC SYSTEMS PATHOLOGY

Inflammation of vessels (vasculitis)

Inflammation of the walls of blood vessels may occur in arteries (*arteritis*), capillaries (*capillaritis*) or veins (*phlebitis, venulitis*); the collective term is *vasculitis*. The classification of this group of disorders has recently changed in line with an increasing understanding of the underlying pathogenic mechanisms. Some cases of vasculitis arise from direct infection of the blood vessel wall, for example *syphilitic aortitis* (Fig. 4.13) and *Aspergillus* infection. Vascular injury and resulting inflammation may also be caused by direct damage to vessels such as mechanical trauma and radiation injury.

The most common types of vasculitis are caused by immunologic mechanisms:

- The deposition of circulating immune complexes in the walls of blood vessels, as in *Henoch–Schönlein purpura* and *hepatitis B-related microscopic polyarteritis*.
- Direct damage to vessel walls by antibodies which react with endothelial cells (*Kawasaki's syndrome, systemic lupus erythematosus*) or glomerular basement membrane (*Goodpasture's syndrome*).
- Vasculitides associated with *anti-neutrophil cytoplasmic antibody (ANCA)* such as *Wegener's granulomatosis* and *microscopic polyarteritis* (Fig. 11.19).
- *Giant cell arteritis* (Fig. 11.17) and *Takayasu's arteritis* may be related to cell-mediated immunity.

Another major type of vasculitis, *classic* or *macroscopic polyarteritis nodosa* (Fig. 11.18), probably belongs to the immunological group but its aetiology is not yet clear.

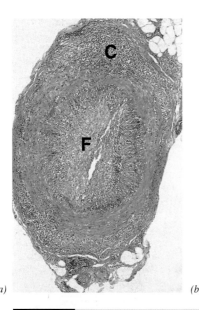
(a)

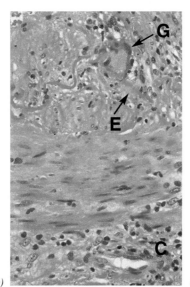
(b)

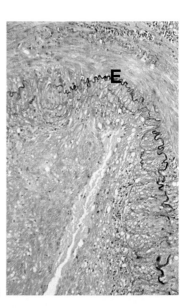
(c)

Fig. 11.17 Giant cell (cranial or temporal) arteritis
(a) LP   (b) HP   (c) Elastic stain HP

Giant cell arteritis is a systemic disease of blood vessels which particularly involves medium-sized arteries of the head. It may be mediated by type IV hypersensitivity to an as yet unknown antigen.

Histologically, the walls of involved vessels exhibit features of a cell-mediated immune response (Type IV hypersensitivity reaction). Multinucleate giant cells **G** are characteristic and tend to be arranged circumferentially, apparently in relation to degenerate fragments of the internal elastic lamina **E**; this is illustrated in micrographs (b) and (c). There is also an infiltrate of lymphocytes and plasma cells **C** in the vessel wall. Marked fibrous thickening **F** of the intimal layer, shown in micrograph (a), may be complicated by thrombosis,

which may produce acute blindness if the ophthalmic artery is affected.

Giant cell arteritis is mainly seen in those over the age of 50. In addition to debilitating constitutional symptoms, the condition often presents as localised throbbing pain or tenderness over the temporal artery. Alternatively, it presents as more generalised pain involving the muscles of the pelvic and shoulder girdles in the condition known as *polymyalgia rheumatica*. Diagnosis of temporal arteritis is confirmed by temporal artery biopsy although results will be negative unless a specific giant cell lesion is included in the biopsy specimen.

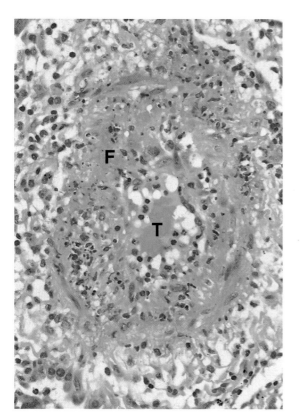

Fig. 11.18 Polyarteritis nodosa (MP)

The *classic type* of *polyarteritis nodosa* (PAN), also known as *macroscopic PAN*, affects mainly medium and small muscular arteries. The most common vessels affected are the arteries supplying the kidneys, gut, heart, liver, peripheral nerves and brain. The typical features of an early lesion are shown in this high power micrograph, where a segment of the vessel wall shows a necrotic area known as *fibrinoid necrosis* F associated with infiltration of the vessel wall with neutrophils. The lumen of the vessel contains fibrin thrombus T giving rise to one of the common effects of vasculitis, namely ischaemia of the tissue supplied by the affected artery. In addition, the necrotic area of vessel wall may rupture during the healing phase when it is replaced by fibrous tissue, and a small aneurysm may form. These small aneurysms appear as nodules on the affected vessels, hence the term *nodosum*.

Apart from systemic symptoms such as fever, malaise, weakness and weight loss, the clinical presentation of this disease is extremely variable depending on which tissues become ischaemic or infarcted as a result of the arterial lesions. For example, kidney involvement may be manifest by pain, haematuria or proteinuria, heart involvement by angina, myocardial infarction or pericarditis, and skin involvement by tender subcutaneous nodules. Clinical diagnosis must usually be substantiated by tissue biopsy.

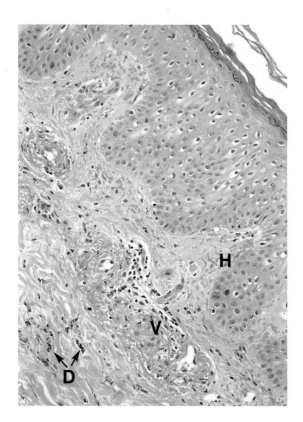

Fig. 11.19 Microscopic polyarteritis (MP)

Microscopic polyarteritis, also known as *leucocytoclastic vasculitis* or *hypersensitivity vasculitis*, occurs in association with a wide range of conditions including drug reactions, serum sickness and immune responses to certain organisms. The smaller vessels are affected including arterioles, capillaries and venules. The condition affects the skin (where it causes palpable purpura), mucous membranes, kidneys, lungs and gastrointestinal tract. In contrast to PAN, microscopic polyarteritis causes haematuria, haemoptysis and bloody diarrhoea rather than frank infarction or major haemorrhage.

This micrograph of the skin shows the classic features of microscopic polyarteritis. Neutrophils infiltrate the vessel walls V, which also show fibrinoid necrosis, and nuclear dust D (fragmented neutrophil nuclei) is commonly seen – hence the term leucocytoclastic. Neutrophils, nuclear dust and haemorrhage H are seen in the surrounding dermis in this micrograph. As in any type of vasculitis, thrombosis of the affected vessels is common although it is not seen in this example.

In the serum of approximately 70% of patients with microscopic polyarteritis, an autoantibody which reacts with cytoplasmic components of neutrophils can be detected. This autoantibody, called *anti-neutrophil cytoplasmic antibody (ANCA)*, is also found in most patients with a rare form of vasculitis called *Wegener's granulomatosis* and may somehow directly cause the damage to blood vessel walls.

BASIC SYSTEMS PATHOLOGY

12. Respiratory system

Diseases of the nose, nasopharynx and larynx

Although viral infections (coryza – the common cold) and allergic inflammation (hay fever – allergic rhinitis) commonly affect the nose, nasal sinuses and nasopharynx, there are only a few conditions of general histopathological interest in the upper respiratory tract. *Nasal polyps* (Fig. 12.1) are a common sequel of prolonged or recurrent inflammation, particularly allergic inflammation. Malignant tumours of the nasal passages and sinuses are rare but *nasopharyngeal carcinoma* (Fig. 12.2) is of special interest because of its association with *Epstein–Barr (EB) virus* infection.

The stratified squamous epithelium of the larynx may undergo hyperplastic or dysplastic change to form benign squamous papillomata or invasive carcinoma (Fig. 12.3). Cigarette smoking and alcohol consumption predispose to the development of carcinoma of the larynx.

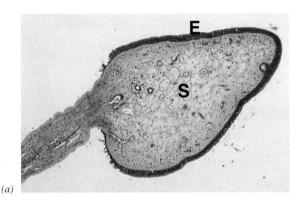
(a)

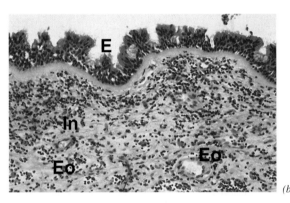
(b)

Fig. 12.1 Nasal polyp
(a) LP (b) HP

Nasal polyps are a consequence of chronic inflammation of the nasal mucosa, commonly infective or allergic in nature. There is marked oedema and engorgement of mucosal connective tissue and infiltration by chronic inflammatory cells; eosinophils are prominent in allergic rhinitis.

In the low power view of a nasal polyp in micrograph (a), note the grossly oedematous stroma **S** and stretched but otherwise relatively normal covering epithelium **E**. As seen in micrograph (b), the mucosal connective tissue contains a marked inflammatory cell infiltrate **In** in which plasma cells and eosinophils **Eo** predominate. Note the thick basement membrane typical of respiratory epithelium.

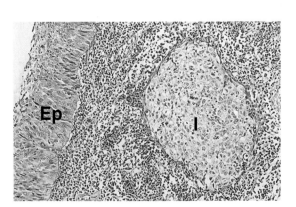

Fig. 12.2 Nasopharyngeal carcinoma (MP)

In the nasal cavities and nasopharynx, malignant tumours take the form of transitional cell, squamous cell or adenocarcinomas, although anaplastic carcinomas also occur, particularly in the nasopharynx. In this micrograph, an invasive transitional cell carcinoma of the nasal cavity is shown. A possible viral aetiology (EB virus) has been postulated for some nasopharyngeal carcinomas. Note the island **I** of invasive carcinoma beneath the dysplastic surface transitional epithelium **Ep**.

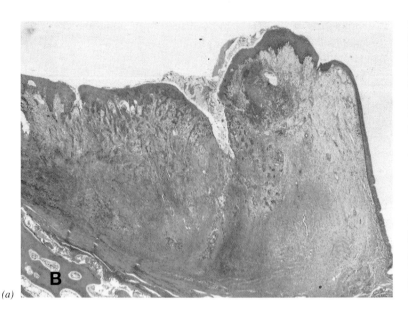
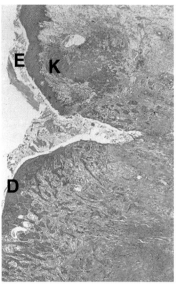

(a) *(b)*

Fig. 12.3 Carcinoma of the larynx
(a) LP (b) MP

Squamous cell carcinomas form the vast majority of malignant tumours of the larynx, most commonly originating in the vocal cords (intrinsic), but also occasionally arising in epiglottis, aryepiglottic folds and pyriform fossae (extrinsic carcinoma of larynx). Squamous carcinomas of the larynx are usually well differentiated and exhibit keratin pearl formation.

Micrograph (a) shows a low power view of squamous carcinoma arising from a vocal cord. The section also includes part of the normal laryngeal wall including bone **B**.

At higher power in micrograph (b), it is possible to see occasional keratin pearls **K**. Normal stratified squamous epithelium **E** is seen at one edge but dysplastic epithelium **D** overlies the main part of the tumour.

Inflammatory diseases of the airways and lungs

The trachea and bronchi may become acutely inflamed as a result of infections by viruses or pyogenic bacteria to cause *acute tracheobronchitis* (Fig. 12.4). Bacterial infections of airways are frequently complicated by extension of inflammation into the surrounding lung parenchyma to cause a pattern of lung infection known as *bronchopneumonia* (Fig. 12.5), a common cause of illness and death in the debilitated and elderly. Another common pattern of bacterial lung infection is *lobar pneumonia* which involves a whole segment or lobe; usually a more virulent bacterium such as the pneumococcus is involved and fit young people may be almost as susceptible as the elderly and debilitated. Lobar pneumonia illustrates many important principles of acute inflammation and the phenomenon of resolution, and is discussed in Chapter 2 (Figs 2.4 and 2.8). In contrast, tuberculosis and sarcoidosis are classical examples of specific chronic inflammations and are discussed fully in Chapters 3 and 4.

Recurrent or persistent suppurative bacterial infections of bronchi may lead to irreversible dilatation of airways with marked thickening and chronic inflammation of the walls, a condition known as *bronchiectasis* (see Fig. 3.3).

Abscess formation in the lungs is a serious complication of certain pneumonias, particularly staphylococcal and *Klebsiella* pneumonias. Lung abscesses may also result from septic emboli causing infarction of the lung, bronchiectasis, bronchial obstruction by tumour, or as a complication of pulmonary tuberculosis.

The term *chronic obstructive airways disease* refers to conditions characterised by chronic or recurrent obstruction of air flow and includes chronic bronchitis and emphysema. Recurrent episodes of acute bronchitis or persistent non-infective irritation of bronchial mucosa (e.g. as a result of cigarette smoking) may produce *chronic bronchitis* (Fig. 12.7), which is frequently associated with persistent dilatation of air spaces and destruction of their walls, a condition known as *emphysema* (Fig. 12.6).

BASIC SYSTEMS PATHOLOGY

Asthma (Fig. 12.8) is a disorder of the airways characterised by reversible bronchoconstriction, often provoked by allergens in susceptible individuals, but also triggered by physical agents or infection. There is also increased secretion of bronchial mucus, leading to plugging of the bronchial lumina.

The massive capillary bed of the lungs makes them vulnerable to a variety of haemodynamic and other vascular disorders. Left ventricular failure results in engorgement of pulmonary capillaries and fluid transudation into the alveolar spaces causing *pulmonary congestion* and *oedema* (Fig. 12.9). Two other common vascular disorders of great clinical importance are *pulmonary embolism* and its sequel *pulmonary infarction* illustrated in Figures 9.4 and 10.4 respectively.

Acute inflammation of the pleura (*pleurisy*) is a frequent accompaniment of lung infections and infarcts, and is characterised by a marked fibrinous exudate typical of serosal surfaces (Fig. 2.6).

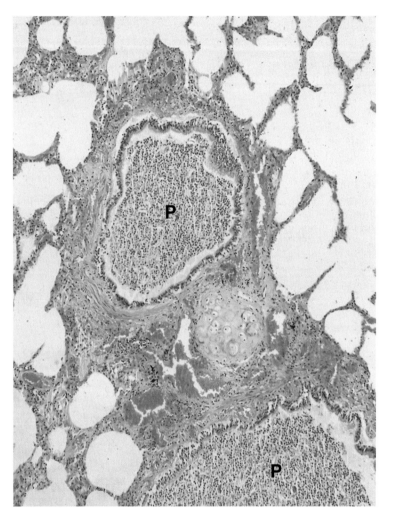

Fig. 12.4 Acute purulent bronchitis (MP)

Bacterial infections of the upper respiratory tract (often following a transient viral infection) tend to spread down the respiratory tract where they may produce an *acute purulent tracheobronchitis* and *bronchiolitis*. The mucosa of the airways becomes acutely inflamed and congested, and the smaller lobular bronchi and bronchioles become filled with purulent exudate **P** composed of protein-rich fluid and numerous neutrophils; strips of necrotic epithelium are often shed into the pus. The inflammatory process inhibits ciliary activity but promotes secretion of mucus which, with the dead and dying neutrophils, pools in the airways and is coughed up as yellow-green sputum. In the early stages, the lung parenchyma is usually unaffected but the alveolar spaces adjacent to the affected bronchioles often become filled with oedema fluid. In susceptible patients, this may then proceed to the development of bronchopneumonia (Fig. 12.5).

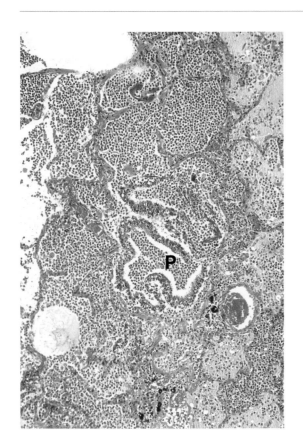

Fig. 12.5 Bronchopneumonia (MP)

Extension of bacterial infection from bronchioles into the surrounding lung parenchyma leads to a patchy pattern of purulent pneumonic consolidation known as bronchopneumonia; this is in marked contrast to the involvement from the outset of a whole lobe or lobule as occurs in lobar pneumonia (Fig. 2.4).

Each peribronchial focus of pneumonic consolidation has within it a small bronchus or bronchiole exhibiting the features of acute purulent bronchitis **P**, as demonstrated in Figure 12.4. As each focus of bronchopneumonia expands, it tends to merge with adjacent foci until the consolidation becomes confluent.

Bronchopneumonia is a threat to the very young, elderly or those debilitated by pre-existing illness such as congestive cardiac failure or carcinomatosis, and is a very common terminal event. No single organism is responsible, but *Streptococcus pneumoniae* and *Haemophilus influenzae* are the most common.

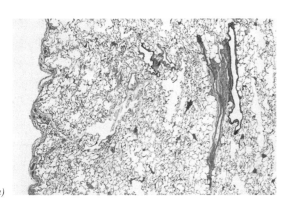

(a)

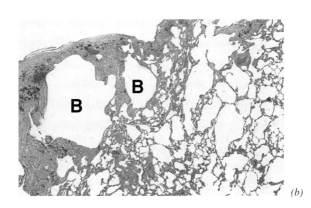

(b)

Fig. 12.6 Pulmonary emphysema
(a) Normal lung (LP) (b) Emphysematous lung (LP)

Emphysema is a condition characterised by permanent enlargement of the respiratory spaces distal to the terminal bronchioles, accompanied by destruction of their walls. Comparison of emphysematous and normal lungs (shown here at the same magnification) demonstrates the marked increase in alveolar volume and consequent marked reduction in area of alveolar wall available for gaseous exchange in emphysema. This problem is compounded by the loss of elastic 'guy rope'

support which alveolar walls normally provide to the airways; thus, in emphysema, the airways tend to collapse during expiration. Emphysema is often associated with recurrent or chronic infection of the airways (chronic bronchitis) and some degree of reversible airways obstruction caused by bronchospasm. In micrograph (b), two small subpleural bullae **B** are present. These are common in emphysema and may rupture into the pleural space causing a pneumothorax.

BASIC SYSTEMS PATHOLOGY

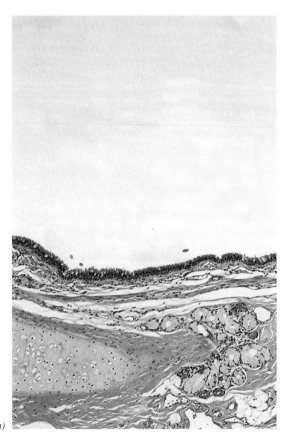

(a)

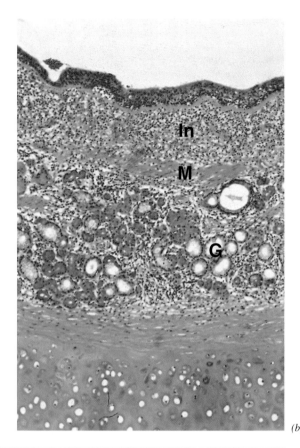

(b)

Fig. 12.7 Chronic bronchitis
(a) Normal bronchial wall (MP) (b) Bronchial wall in chronic bronchitis (MP)

The term chronic bronchitis is used clinically to describe the situation where excess sputum is produced by a patient on most days for at least 3 months of the year for at least 2 consecutive years.

Although well defined as a clinical term, pathological changes in chronic bronchitis are variable and relatively non-specific. Chronic irritation of the bronchial mucosa, either by tobacco smoke, atmospheric pollution or by repeated episodes of infection, induces chronic inflammatory and hyperplastic changes resulting in marked thickening of the bronchial wall. This feature is the main abnormality in cases of chronic bronchitis and is well illustrated in micrograph (b) when compared to the normal bronchial wall shown in micrograph (a) at the same magnification.

Three factors contribute to the increased thickness of the bronchial wall: infiltration of the submucosa by chronic inflammatory cells **In**, marked hypertrophy of mucosal smooth muscle **M** and marked hyperplasia of the mucous glands **G** with the production of copious mucus.

In addition, the surface epithelium undergoes hyperplasia and often squamous metaplasia (not shown here). The consequent loss of ciliary activity then compounds the problem of excessive mucus production by destroying the 'mucociliary escalator' and provides an ideal environment for superimposed bacterial infection.

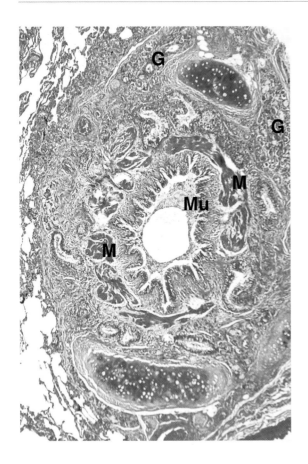

Fig. 12.8 Chronic asthma (MP)

Asthma is a common respiratory disorder characterised by instability of the smooth muscle of bronchiolar walls leading to paroxysmal bronchoconstriction. This results in diminution of airway diameter causing marked resistance to air flow, particularly on expiration. Clinically there is shortness of breath, wheezing and cough. There are several aetiological and trigger factors for bronchospasm including IgE-mediated hypersensitivity reactions to allergens, bacterial or viral infections, exertion, changes in air temperature, and non-allergic sensitivity to specific environmental agents (often through occupational exposure). In severe asthma, reduction in bronchial diameter has three components: bronchospasm, mucosal oedema and luminal occlusion by excessive mucus production.

Single acute asthmatic attacks resolve with therapy leaving no apparent structural disorder. In chronic asthmatics, as in this example, the bronchial walls become thickened because of hypertrophy of smooth muscle **M**, hyperplasia of submucosal mucous glands **G**, protracted oedema of submucosa and marked infiltration by eosinophils. The bronchial lumen becomes obstructed by mucus **Mu** containing numerous eosinophils.

Eosinophils characteristically accumulate in a variety of allergic states and may be involved in deactivation of some of the chemical mediators.

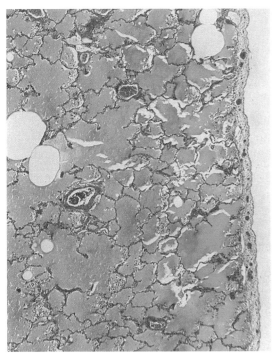

Fig. 12.9 Pulmonary oedema (LP)

Any condition in which the left ventricle or atrium fails to empty adequately increases pressure in the affected chamber which is transmitted back to the pulmonary venous system and pulmonary capillaries. The pulmonary capillaries become *dilated* and *congested* with erythrocytes and the increased hydrostatic pressure results in *transudation* of plasma fluid into the alveolar spaces causing *pulmonary oedema*.

As progressive cardiac failure is a terminal event in many diseases, pulmonary congestion and oedema are common post-mortem findings. This condition also provides an ideal environment for the growth of pathogens of relatively low virulence, so superimposed bronchopneumonia is a common sequel (see Fig. 12.5). Chronic pulmonary congestion, for example owing to mitral stenosis, may result in numerous small intra-alveolar haemorrhages followed by red cell lysis; phagocytosis of released iron pigments, mainly haemosiderin, leads to the gross appearance known as *brown induration*.

BASIC SYSTEMS PATHOLOGY

Interstitial diseases of the lung

A wide range of pathogenic stimuli may cause interstitial lung inflammation, i.e. inflammation primarily involving the alveolar walls; this contrasts with the pneumonic or intra-alveolar inflammation seen in pneumonia.

Acute interstitial inflammation is often called *pneumonitis*. The clinical picture may be of catastrophic acute respiratory distress as seen in *adult respiratory distress syndrome (ARDS)* which has a wide range of causes including viral and atypical pneumonias, shock, drug and hypersensitivity reactions. *Respiratory distress syndrome* of premature infants *(IRDS)* is a similar phenomenon and both the adult and infant forms are characterised by the formation of hyaline membranes upon the alveolar walls (Fig. 12.10).

At the chronic end of the spectrum, interstitial lung disease usually presents as insidious onset of breathlessness secondary to *pulmonary fibrosis* (Fig. 12.11). The development of pulmonary fibrosis again may be due to a wide range of agents and may be preceded by an acute phase. The common causative factors are inorganic dusts such as silica, coal dust and asbestos, organic dusts such as mouldy hay in 'farmer's lung', and disorders of unknown cause such as sarcoidosis and *idiopathic pulmonary fibrosis* (see Fig. 3.6).

The disorders caused by inhalation of inorganic dusts are known as *pneumoconioses* and follow inhalation of mineral dusts (e.g. silica and asbestos), usually over a long period of industrial exposure, leading to fibrotic reactions in the lung. Inhalation of organic dusts (e.g. fungal spores and plant dusts) usually cause pulmonary fibrosis by the development of chronic allergic responses termed *extrinsic allergic alveolitis*. The end result of these diseases is the development of interstitial fibrosis in the lungs. Pulmonary fibrosis of this type results in thickening of the barrier between blood and air causing reduced gas transfer. As the disease progresses, these may cause pulmonary hypertension and respiratory failure may develop. In most of these diseases, there are few clues to the causative agent when the fibrosis is well developed. Exceptions to this rule include silicosis (Fig. 12.12) which has a distinctive pattern of fibrosis, asbestosis (Fig. 12.13) where the presence of plentiful asbestos bodies is diagnostic, and sarcoidosis where characteristic granulomas may be seen (Fig. 3.9).

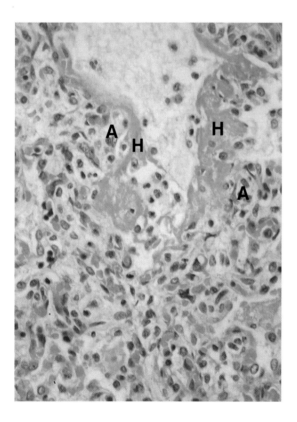

Fig. 12.10 Hyaline membrane disease (HP)

At the very acute end of the spectrum of interstitial lung diseases, the histological appearances of the lung are characterised by the formation of 'hyaline membranes' **H** which represent accretions of protein and necrotic cell debris upon the alveolar surface of the alveolar walls **A**. The other name sometimes used for this condition is *diffuse alveolar damage (DAD)*. Characteristically, the alveolar walls are thickened owing to a mixed inflammatory infiltrate, oedema, congestion of capillaries and haemorrhage. In combination with the hyaline membranes, this greatly inhibits gaseous exchange and results in respiratory failure. Occasionally, there are characteristic histological features of a particular aetiologic agent such as caseating granulomas in miliary TB (Fig. 4.5) or nuclear inclusion bodies in cytomegalovirus infection (Fig. 4.16).

In most cases, the histological appearance is non-specific and a careful history is important in defining the cause. In premature infants (IRDS), the cause is a deficiency of pulmonary surfactant. In adults, there is a wide variety of causes but the common factor is widespread damage to capillary endothelial cells and/or alveolar lining cells. This condition is often fatal but may resolve completely with appropriate treatment, or may progress to pulmonary fibrosis.

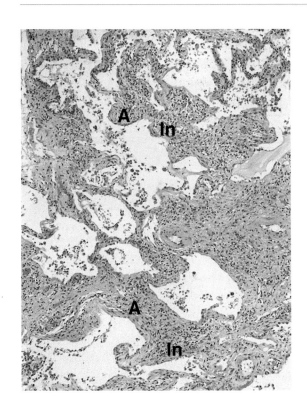

Fig. 12.11 Pulmonary fibrosis (MP)

This condition may represent the end stage of acute diffuse alveolar damage or of subacute disease as in extrinsic allergic alveolitis. Often, however, the condition presents with insidious breathlessness and lung biopsy shows established pulmonary fibrosis. As seen in this micrograph, the alveolar walls **A** are markedly thickened because of the deposition of collagen. There is a variable chronic inflammatory infiltrate **In** consisting mainly of lymphocytes. In addition, the alveolar epithelium consists mainly of type II pneumocytes. When no aetiological factors can be established from the biopsy and careful recording of the clinical history, the condition is called *cryptogenic fibrosing alveolitis* or *usual interstitial pneumonitis* as in this case. In other cases, there are distinctive histological features such as granulomas in late stage tuberculosis and sarcoidosis, and asbestos bodies in asbestosis. Some cases are associated with a significant clinical history such as exposure to particular drugs, for example bleomycin-induced pulmonary fibrosis. In the late stages, the normal lung parenchyma may be densely fibrotic with macroscopically visible spaces; in this situation, it is known as *honeycomb lung*.

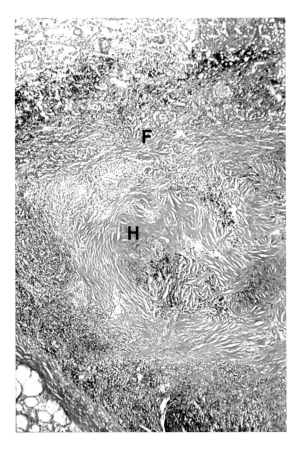

Fig. 12.12 Silicosis (MP)

Silicosis is a form of pneumoconiosis which tends to occur in miners and others with industrial exposure to silica dusts. Initially, the inhaled silica particles are phagocytosed by macrophages which accumulate in clumps, very occasionally forming granuloma-like masses. The presence of silica-laden macrophages excites a vigorous focal fibrotic reaction resulting in the formation of nodules of collagenous tissue. The centre of each focus becomes progressively acellular and hyaline **H** and is surrounded by a variable zone of more cellular fibrous tissue **F**, exhibiting a relatively sparse chronic inflammatory cell infiltrate in which black carbon-laden macrophages abound. Usual histological methods do not reveal the presence of silica which can, however, be demonstrated as refractile particles by polarised light microscopy.

As the process continues, the fibrotic nodules may coalesce, resulting in widespread pulmonary fibrosis. Silicosis is the most common of the pneumoconioses; other examples are asbestosis (Fig. 12.13), and berylliosis in which the inhaled particles excite a giant cell granulomatous reaction similar to that seen in sarcoidosis (Fig. 3.9).

All the clinically significant inorganic dust diseases of the lung lead to progressive fibrosis, with ventilatory failure and diminished gaseous exchange. Disruption of the pulmonary microvasculature may lead to pulmonary hypertension.

The large amounts of black carbon indicate that this case is from a coal miner.

BASIC SYSTEMS PATHOLOGY

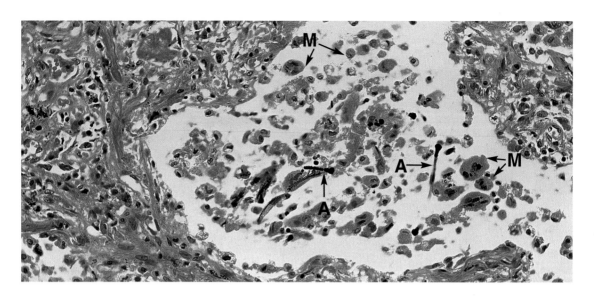

Fig. 12.13 Asbestosis (HP)

Asbestos, a complex silicate, occurs in the form of long needle-like fibres which when inhaled into the lung parenchyma become coated with proteinaceous material to form segmented *asbestos bodies*. The presence of asbestos fibres excites a macrophage and giant cell response which ultimately leads to fibrosis in a similar manner to that of silicosis (Fig. 12.12). The major fibrotic lesions occur initially in the subpleural zone of the lower lobes.

This micrograph shows an alveolar space containing alveolar macrophages **M** and typical asbestos bodies **A**;

the brownish colour of the asbestos bodies derives from the incorporation of haemosiderin in the proteinaceous coat.

Apart from its tendency to produce lung fibrosis, exposure to asbestos predisposes to neoplastic change. Mesotheliomas of the pleura and less often the peritoneum (Fig. 12.19) may follow exposure to a form of asbestos known as 'blue asbestos', whilst common asbestos exposure greatly increases the risk of lung carcinomas, especially in cigarette smokers.

Tumours of the lung and pleura

Genuinely benign lung tumours are rare. Most 'bronchial adenomas' are in fact carcinoid tumours arising from lung neuroendocrine cells; these may be locally invasive and occasionally metastasise. Their histological appearance is similar to carcinoid tumours in the gastrointestinal tract (Fig. 13.17).

The great majority of primary malignant tumours of the lung are carcinomas which arise in the bronchi and are thus often called *bronchogenic carcinomas*; carcinogens in cigarette smoke are the major aetiological agents. Other less important factors include exposure to radiation, asbestos (especially when combined with smoking) as well as other minerals such as nickel and chromium. Air pollution and genetic predisposition are other possible factors. Occasionally tumours arise in a pre-existing lung scar.

Bronchopulmonary carcinomas are of four main types:

- *Differentiated squamous cell carcinoma* (Fig. 12.14)
- *Differentiated adenocarcinoma* (including bronchioloalveolar pattern) (Figs 12.16 and 12.17)
- *Undifferentiated squamous/adenocarcinoma* (large cell undifferentiated) (Fig. 12.18)
- *Malignant neuroendocrine carcinoma* (small cell carcinoma or oat cell carcinoma) (Fig. 12.15)

The current vogue is to call the last type *small cell carcinoma*, and to group all other types together as *non-small cell carcinoma*. This unsatisfactory grouping system is based on the likely response of the tumour to the present limited therapeutic options. Metastatic tumours, usually blood-borne from distant organs, are also very common in the lungs (Fig. 7.9).

The pleura is the site of uncommon but fatal tumours known as *mesotheliomas* (Fig. 12.19). These occur almost exclusively in those exposed to asbestos.

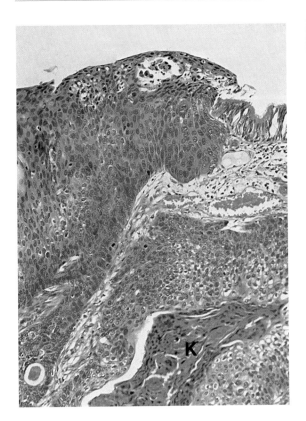

Fig. 12.14 Squamous cell carcinoma of bronchus: well differentiated (MP)

Squamous cell carcinoma, the commonest primary malignancy of the lung, usually arises in the main bronchi or their larger branches close to the lung hilum and often in an area of epithelium which has previously undergone squamous metaplasia, for example as a result of cigarette smoking. Such tumours invade the local parenchyma and tend to obstruct the involved airway as well as spreading via local lymphatics to regional lymph nodes.

These tumours have the typical features of squamous cell carcinoma but tend to vary widely in degree of differentiation. At one end of the spectrum is the well-differentiated keratinising type as in this micrograph where the likeness to stratified squamous epithelium is evident and there is formation of keratin **K** in some areas. Towards the other end of the spectrum are poorly differentiated tumours in which squamous characteristics such as intercellular bridges are only visible at high magnification (see Fig. 7.14). Some tumours are so poorly differentiated that squamous features cannot be seen by light microscopy; such tumours are classified as large cell undifferentiated carcinomas (Fig. 12.18).

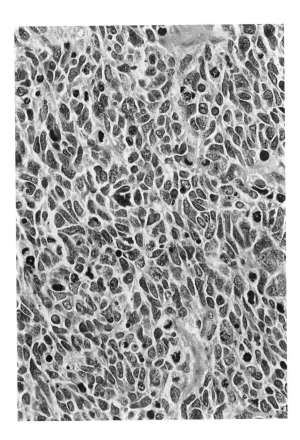

Fig. 12.15 Small cell carcinoma (HP)

In addition to squamous carcinoma, the proximal bronchi may also give rise to another important carcinoma known as small cell or oat cell carcinoma. As seen at high magnification in this micrograph, the name derives from the supposed resemblance of the small, tightly packed, darkly stained, ovoid tumour cells to oat grains. These tumours rapidly and extensively invade the bronchial wall and surrounding parenchyma and may compress and invade nearby pulmonary veins. Early lymphatic and blood-borne spread is a feature of these tumours. Small cell tumours have the worst prognosis of all bronchogenic carcinomas because, although they are the most responsive to chemotherapy, they almost always relapse early.

Apart from their local and metastatic effects, these tumours may also secrete peptide hormones, such as ADH and ACTH (*ectopic hormone secretion*) giving rise to various *tumour-related endocrine syndromes*.

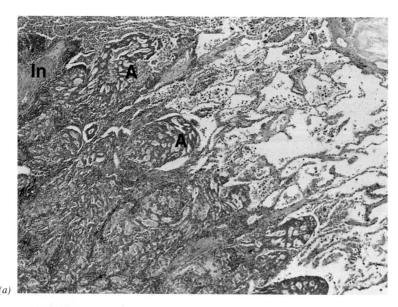

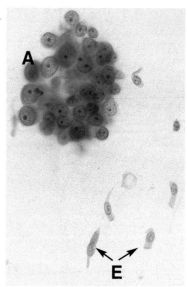

(a)　　　　　　　　　　　　　　　　　　　　　　　　　　　　　*(b)*

Fig. 12.16 Adenocarcinoma of the lung
(a) LP　(b) Cytology; Giemsa (HP)

Adenocarcinomas tend to arise more peripherally in small bronchi and bronchioles; they have a particular predilection for old areas of scar tissue, for example healed tuberculosis. Adenocarcinoma of the lung is not as closely linked with cigarette smoking as other primary lung tumours.

The main histological feature of this type of tumour is the formation of the tumour cells into a glandular acinar pattern **A**, the acini often being filled with mucus. The tumour (in common with many others) excites a local inflammatory response **In** and the alveoli in the adjacent lung parenchyma contain numerous alveolar macrophages. Very poorly differentiated variants of adenocarcinoma are included in the category of ***large cell undifferentiated carcinoma*** (Fig. 12.18); here also, only electron microscopy can demonstrate the glandular origin of such tumours.

All lung tumours may be diagnosed by cytological examination of sputum, bronchial washings or brushings, and by fine needle aspiration biopsy. In micrograph (b), note the cluster of large adenocarcinoma cells **A** with prominent nucleoli; these contrast with occasional normal bronchial epithelial cells **E**.

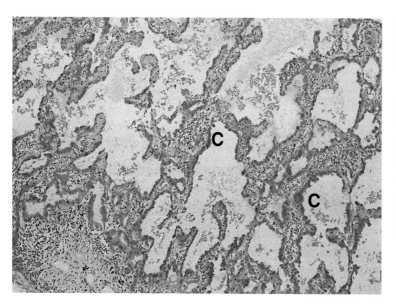

Fig. 12.17 Bronchioloalveolar cell carcinoma (MP)

This is an uncommon subtype of adenocarcinoma which may appear as a solitary well-defined mass in the lung periphery on X-ray or, more commonly, as a diffuse infiltrate. The characteristic feature of this tumour is that the malignant cells grow along the alveolar walls as shown in this micrograph. The alveolar epithelium is replaced by crowded columnar cells **C** with enlarged hyperchromatic nuclei. The alveolar walls are somewhat fibrotic and inflamed.

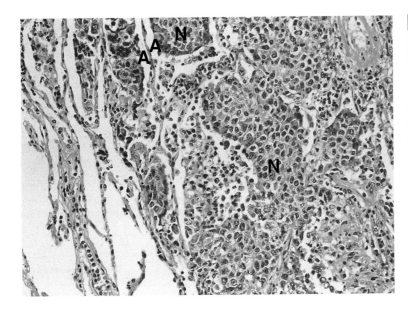

Fig. 12.18 Large cell undifferentiated carcinoma (MP)

This micrograph shows the advancing edge of a large cell undifferentiated carcinoma of the lung. As mentioned earlier, large cell undifferentiated carcinomas include extremely poorly differentiated squamous cell carcinomas and adenocarcinomas with no discernible features of squamous or adenocarcinoma by light microscopy, although such features can be seen on electron microscopy. These tumours consist of large anaplastic epithelial cells growing in nests **N** and sheets. No evidence of keratinisation, intercellular bridges or intracytoplasmic mucin is seen. Invasion of adjacent alveolar spaces **A** can be clearly seen in this micrograph.

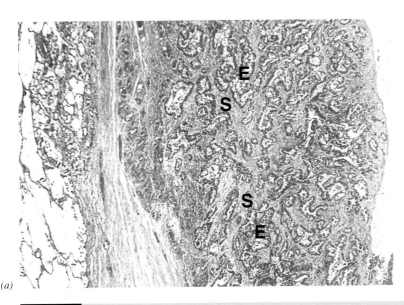

(a)

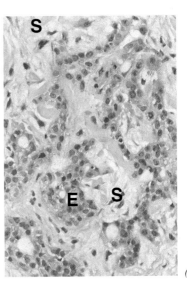

(b)

Fig. 12.19 Mesothelioma of pleura
(a) LP   (b) HP

The pleura is frequently involved in secondary spread of bronchial and breast carcinoma. Primary malignant tumours of the pleura, known as *mesotheliomas* because of their origin from mesothelial cells, are rare but of great interest since they are related to exposure to asbestos dust; exposure is often trivial and in the distant past. Even more rarely, mesotheliomas arise from the peritoneum and are also often associated with a history of asbestos exposure.

Pleural mesotheliomas form a dense sheet of tumour extending over the pleural surface as in micrograph (a),
often encasing the lung in a hard white shell; the tumour extends only a little distance into the lung parenchyma and metastatic spread is uncommon.

At low magnification, the tumour can be seen to have both a glandular epithelial component **E** and a fibrous stromal component **S**. At high magnification as in micrograph (b), both epithelial **E** and spindle-celled stromal components **S** exhibit the pleomorphism characteristic of malignancy. Most mesotheliomas contain both spindle cell and glandular components but occasionally one pattern predominates.

13. Alimentary system

Introduction

The alimentary system includes the mouth and its associated salivary glands, the oesophagus, stomach, small and large bowels, appendix and anus. The function of the alimentary tract is the ingestion, digestion and absorption of nutrients along with the storage and expulsion of waste products. A wide range of congenital and acquired diseases may affect all parts of the tract.

Diseases of the oral tissues and salivary glands

The mouth and associated structures may be involved in a wide variety of disease states that may be loosely divided into three categories. First, many systemic diseases, particularly dermatological conditions, exhibit oral manifestations (e.g. *lichen planus*, *syphilis*). Second, all oral tissues may be subject to acute or chronic inflammatory states, the most common being dental caries and its sequel periapical abscess formation, and periodontal disease (i.e. inflammation of the gums). Of more general histopathological interest is inflammation of the salivary glands leading to *chronic sialadenitis* (Fig. 13.2). Third, many benign and malignant tumours may arise in the oral tissues, the most common being squamous cell carcinomas of the lips, oral mucosa and tongue (Fig. 13.1). Salivary tumours, both benign (Figs 13.3 and 13.4) and malignant (Fig. 13.5), can arise in both major and minor salivary glands.

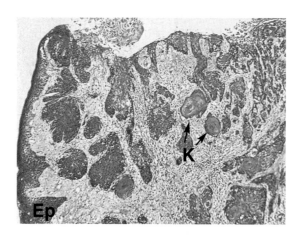

Fig. 13.1 Carcinoma of the tongue (LP)

Malignant tumours of the mucosa of the lips, tongue, cheeks and gums are almost invariably squamous cell carcinomas; they tend to be well differentiated and metastasize to regional lymph nodes.

This micrograph illustrates a squamous carcinoma involving the tongue. The tumour has arisen from adjacent normal stratified squamous epithelium **Ep**, and has deeply infiltrated the tongue. It exhibits keratin pearl formation **K**. Although these tumours may arise in normal epithelium, squamous dysplasia similar to that seen in the skin and cervix (Fig. 17.6) is a common premalignant lesion, and may be identifiable clinically as an abnormality of the mucosa.

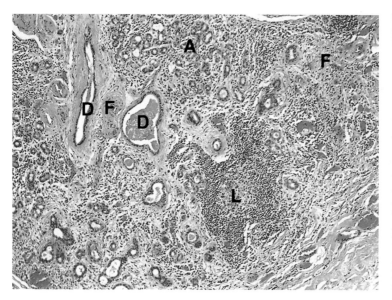

Fig. 13.2 Chronic sialadenitis (LP)

Prolonged obstruction of a large salivary gland duct by a calculus (*sialolith*) results in chronic inflammation and acinar atrophy in the gland, termed *chronic sialadenitis*.

This micrograph is from the submandibular gland, the gland most frequently involved. Two salivary duct branches **D** are dilated, with periductal fibrosis **F** and infiltration by lymphocytes with the formation of lymphoid follicles **L**. The surrounding secretory acini **A** are markedly atrophic and the interstitial spaces have become expanded by fibrous tissue **F**.

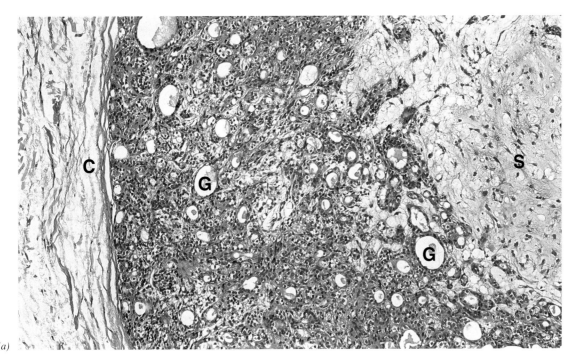

(a)

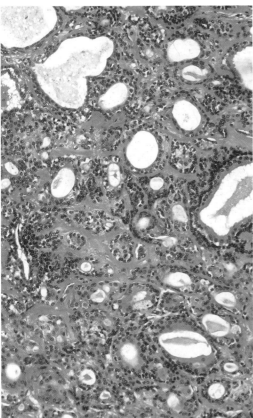

(b)

Fig. 13.3 Pleomorphic adenoma of the salivary glands

(a) Typical pleomorphic form (MP)
(b) Monomorphic variant (HP)

The most common salivary gland tumour is the *pleomorphic adenoma*, formerly known as *mixed salivary tumour*. The latter term was acquired from the histological appearance of columns and islands of benign epithelial cells separated by loose myxomatous connective tissue stroma in which areas resembling cartilage may be found.

Pleomorphic adenomas occur most commonly in the parotid gland. They are usually encapsulated but irregular in shape; in the parotid gland, this leads to difficulty in achieving total excision (bearing in mind the facial nerve) and local recurrence may become a problem. Almost all pleomorphic adenomas are benign but, vary rarely, malignant change may supervene after many years.

Micrograph (a) demonstrates the typical features of benign pleomorphic adenomas, namely a strongly staining neoplastic epithelial element with glands **G** and a pale blue-stained, loose connective tissue stroma **S**, somewhat resembling cartilage. Note that the tumour is circumscribed by a thin fibrous capsule **C**.

Much less commonly, salivary adenomas are entirely composed of the glandular epithelial component and contain none of the myxomatous stromal component which often dominates the picture in the typical pleomorphic salivary adenoma; this variant is described as a *monomorphic salivary adenoma* and an example is shown in micrograph (b).

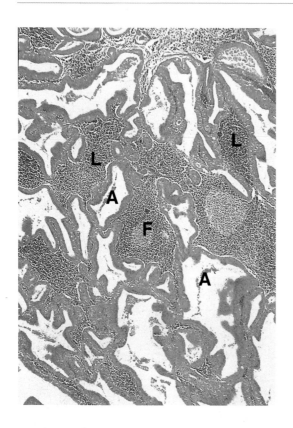

Fig. 13.4 Adenolymphoma (MP)

This unusual benign tumour occurs almost exclusively in and around the parotid gland; it commonly arises in middle-aged and older men.

The tumour, which is often cystic, is composed of large glandular acini **A** embedded in dense lymphoid tissue **L** in which typical lymphoid follicles **F** are often seen. The glandular element consists of tall columnar epithelium rather resembling that of large salivary ducts.

The histogenesis of this tumour is not understood but the glandular element may represent hamartomatous salivary duct tissue within lymph nodes in and around the parotid gland. Adenolymphomas are also known by the eponym *Warthin's tumour*, a term which is preferable as it avoids the erroneous impression of malignancy implied by the term adenolymphoma.

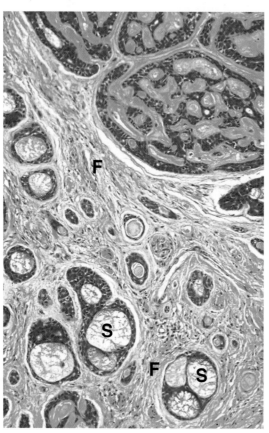

Fig. 13.5 Adenocystic carcinoma (MP)

The most common malignant tumour of salivary tissue is the *adenocystic* or *adenoid cystic carcinoma*. This tumour is uncommon in the parotid glands but is seen in the other major glands and in the minor salivary glands. Histologically, it has a characteristic cribriform (sieve-like) appearance owing to the presence of small spaces **S** in a mass of tightly packed tumour cells. The tumour cells are arranged in clumps and cords separated by a fibrous stroma **F** which may exhibit a marked degree of hyalinisation.

As well as occurring in the major salivary glands, adenocystic carcinomas can arise in the minor or accessory salivary glands of the palate. These tumours are locally invasive and prone to recurrence following surgical excision. Spread to regional lymph nodes is frequent and wide local spread is common, although the rate of growth is often slow. Perineural invasion, which is often extremely painful, is a common feature of this tumour.

Oesophageal diseases

Infections of the oesophagus are rare in healthy individuals but in debilitated or immunosuppressed patients, infection with *Herpes simplex virus* or *Candida albicans* can occur (see Ch. 4). The lower oesophagus frequently becomes inflamed as a result of gastric acid reflux, producing either *oesophagitis* or sometimes *chronic peptic ulceration* analogous to that seen in the stomach and duodenum (Figs. 3.2 and 13.8). In response to reflux of acid-pepsin, the squamous mucosa of the lower oesophagus may undergo metaplastic transformation into a form of glandular epithelium similar to that seen in the stomach or small intestine. This metaplastic condition is termed *Barrett's oesophagus* (Fig. 13.6).

The most common oesophageal neoplasm is *squamous cell carcinoma*, which is similar to squamous cell carcinomas at other sites, although *adenocarcinomas* may arise in Barrett's oesophagus at the lower end of the oesophagus. The lower oesophagus may also be involved by local spread of adenocarcinoma of the upper stomach.

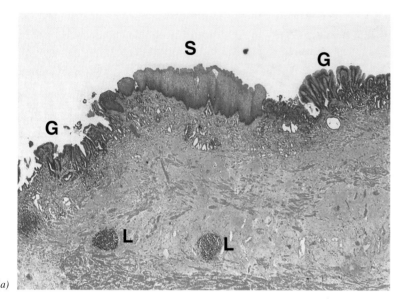

(a)

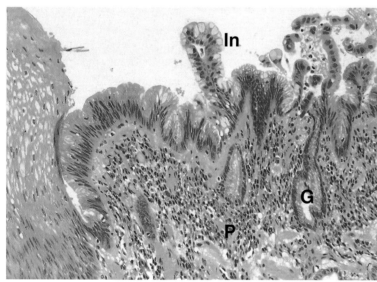

(b)

Fig. 13.6 Barrett's oesophagus
(a) LP   (b) HP

At the lower end of the oesophagus, long-standing acid reflux from the stomach may give rise to metaplastic change in which the epithelium may exhibit a gastric or intestinal type pattern or a mixture of both; this is known as *Barrett's oesophagus*.

Micrograph (a) shows a longitudinal section of the lower oesophagus in which there is abrupt transition from squamous epithelium **S** to metaplastic gastric epithelium **G**. An infiltrate of lymphocytes and plasma cells with occasional lymphoid aggregates **L** is indicative of chronic inflammation.

At high magnification in micrograph (b), both gastric **G** and intestinal **In** epithelial patterns are seen as well as a dense infiltrate of plasma cells **P** in the lamina propria. In addition, the epithelial cells exhibit changes of low grade dysplasia with enlargement, crowding and disorganisation of the nuclei of the epithelial cells. High grade dysplasia of gastric epithelium is shown in Figure 13.9. Patients with Barrett's oesophagus have a greatly increased risk of adenocarcinoma, especially if there is superimposed dysplasia. Thus this condition is usually endoscopically monitored and biopsied regularly. Both adenocarcinoma and squamous cell carcinoma of the oesophagus have a very poor prognosis.

BASIC SYSTEMS PATHOLOGY

Diseases of the stomach

Gastritis

Inflammation of the stomach is termed *gastritis* and may be divided into acute and chronic forms.

- **Acute gastritis** may be associated with the use of aspirin and other anti-inflammatory drugs, excessive alcohol and severe stress.
- **Chronic gastritis** can be divided into distinct subtypes, each of which has particular histological features (Fig. 13.7):
  — *Chronic infection* – *Helicobacter pylori* is the usual infective agent.
  — *Chronic autoimmune gastritis* is associated with autoantibodies to gastric parietal cells and with pernicious anaemia.
  — *Chronic chemical gastritis* (also known as *reactive gastritis*) is associated with reflux of bile into the stomach, especially following surgical procedures, and with chronic alcohol consumption.
  — Less common causes include *Crohn's disease*, *graft-versus-host disease* and *gastric outlet obstruction*.

Chronic gastritis is often associated with the later development of peptic ulceration and, less commonly, gastric carcinoma, which is usually preceded by intestinal metaplasia and dysplasia (Fig. 13.9).

Peptic ulceration

The histological details of chronic peptic ulceration in the stomach are described in Chapter 3 (Fig. 3.2). Acid-induced necrosis of the gastric wall, the acute inflammatory response, organisation and granulation tissue formation, and fibrous scarring occur concurrently. *H. pylori* infection is almost always present in chronic duodenal ulceration and most cases of chronic gastric ulceration, and must be eradicated for permanent healing. The outcome of this dynamic process depends on which is the dominant element, i.e. the damaging stimulus or the attempts of the body to heal the damage.

There are three main complications of chronic peptic ulceration:

- **Perforation** – if tissue destruction outstrips attempts to confine or repair it, the process may extend rapidly through the wall, leading to perforation (Fig. 13.8a).
- **Haemorrhage** – tissue necrosis may extend deeply enough to involve the wall of a large artery. This is most common in long-standing chronic gastric ulcers on the posterior wall in the region of the left gastro-epiploic artery. This vessel tends to become incorporated in the fibrous scar on the serosal aspect of a chronic gastric ulcer, and may then be eroded during a subsequent acute exacerbation of ulceration (Fig. 13.8b). This may produce torrential haemorrhage, presenting as *haematemesis* and/or *melaena,* which may be fatal.
- **Obstruction** – persistent attempts at repair lead to progressive fibrous scarring which undergoes shrinkage and ultimately causes distortion and thickening of the wall of the viscus, commonly at the lower end of the oesophagus or in the pyloric region of the stomach. The narrowing may cause *stricture* formation with partial or even complete obstruction of the lumen. When the ulcerative process is still active, obstruction may be compounded by inflammatory oedema of the mucosa surrounding the ulcer.

Neoplasia

By far the most common malignant tumours of the stomach are *adenocarcinomas*. These may asume a variety of gross morphological forms including *malignant ulcers* with heaped-up edges, *fungating polypoid tumours* or *diffuse infiltration* of the wall *(linitis plastica)* giving rise to the so-called 'leather bottle stomach'. Gastric adenocarcinomas are classified histologically as *intestinal type* (Fig. 13.10) or *diffuse type* (Fig. 13.11). *Gastric lymphoma* (Fig. 13.12) and *carcinoid tumours* (Fig. 13.17) make up a small percentage of stomach malignancies. Both adenocarcinoma and gastric lymphoma are associated with *H. pylori* infection. Of the benign tumours, gastric adenomas comprise only a small proportion of gastric polyps, most of which are inflammatory or regenerative. Mesenchymal tumours occur in the stomach and other parts of the gastrointestinal tract. Previously these tumours were considered to be leiomyomas. However, although all these lesions appear similar histologically, it is now apparent that some are derived from smooth muscle cells (leiomyomas), some from neural cells and others from dendritic or histiocytic cells. This group of tumours is now known as *gastrointestinal stromal tumours (GIST)*. They may be benign or malignant and occur at any age. *Lipomas* may also occur in several parts of the gastrointestinal tract and often form a submucosal mass that may become polypoid.

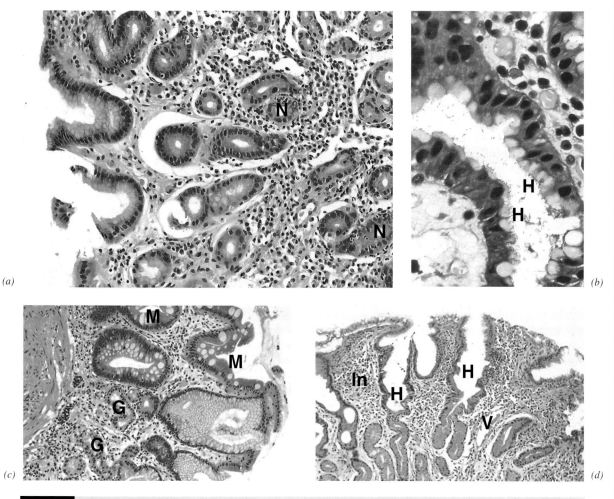

Fig. 13.7 Chronic gastritis

(a) *H. pylori* infection (MP)   (b) *H. pylori* infection (Giemsa – HP)   (c) Autoimmune gastritis (MP)
(d) Chemical gastritis (MP)

Helicobacter pylori is now thought to be the most common cause of chronic gastritis characteristically affecting the mucosa of the gastric antrum but extending to the body of the stomach in severe cases. The histological features, as shown in micrograph (a), include a mixed inflammatory infiltrate in the lamina propria including neutrophils, plasma cells, lymphocytes and eosinophils. Typically, neutrophils **N** are seen infiltrating the epithelium of the gastric glands; *H. pylori* organisms can sometimes be seen in routine H&E preparations. Intestinal metaplasia and dysplasia are commonly seen in association with this type of gastritis. The Giemsa stain shown in micrograph (b) at high power demonstrates the organisms **H** at the surface of the epithelium. Bacterial invasion of the mucosa is not a feature.

In contrast, autoimmune-type chronic gastritis affects primarily the body of the stomach. As seen in micrograph

(c), which is taken from the gastric body, the histological features include atrophy of the gastric glands with loss of parietal cells. The glands **G** are small and the mucosa is thinned. The lamina propria is infiltrated primarily with lymphocytes and plasma cells, and intestinal metaplasia **M** is a prominent feature. In intestinal metaplasia, the gastric epithelial cells are replaced with goblet cells and columnar absorptive cells typical of the small intestine. Chronic autoimmune gastritis in its late stages is often termed ***chronic atrophic gastritis***.

Chemical or reactive gastritis, as shown in micrograph (d), is characterised by inflammation of the superficial mucosa with a scanty infiltrate of inflammatory cells **In** (lymphocytes and plasma cells). The necks of the gastric glands show hyperplasia **H** and characteristically the lamina propria is oedematous with marked vasodilatation **V**.

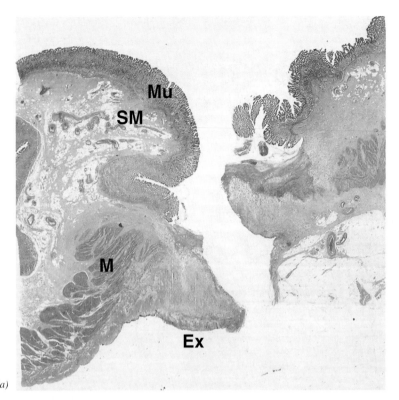

(a)

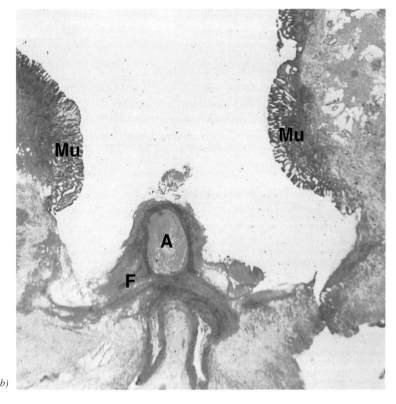

(b)

Fig. 13.8 **Complications of peptic ulceration**
(a) Perforated gastric ulcer (LP)
(b) Bleeding gastric ulcer (LP)

Perforation of peptic ulcers has become less common with the advent of effective medical treatment for gastritis and peptic ulcer. It results in discharge of gastric contents into the peritoneal cavity with resulting *acute peritonitis*. In the perforated gastric ulcer shown in micrograph (a), tissue necrosis has extended through the full thickness of the wall, with complete destruction of the mucosa **Mu,** submucosa **SM** and muscle layers **M**. Peritonitis is manifest by an acute inflammatory exudate **Ex** on the serosal surface of the stomach. The margins of the perforated ulcer are lined by necrotic tissue, beneath which is a zone of acute inflammation similar to that found in the floor of a more chronic ulcer (Fig. 3.2). There is no evidence of fibrous granulation tissue or fibrous scar since the destructive process has been too acute. Perforations such as this occur most commonly in peptic ulcers in the first part of the duodenum, but also occur in the stomach as in this example.

Haemorrhage from erosion of a large artery in the base of an ulcer may occur in untreated chronic gastric ulcers as shown in micrograph (b). Note the eroded artery **A** trapped in the fibrous scar tissue **F** forming the floor of the ulcer. Part of the arterial wall is undergoing necrosis as a result of acid attack and massive haemorrhage will follow.

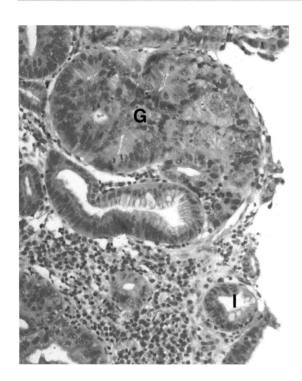

Fig. 13.9 Gastric dysplasia (LP)

Dysplasia of the gastric epithelium may arise in association with longstanding chronic gastritis of any of the three common types described. This micrograph shows *high grade dysplasia* **G** of the gastric mucosa. There is marked irregularity of the glands with nuclear enlargement, hyperchromicity and crowding of the epithelial cells. There is little evidence of mucus production by epithelial cells and cellular polarity (basal alignment of nuclei) is completely lost. The adjacent epithelium shows *intestinal metaplasia* **I** (see also Fig. 13.7c). Note in this micrograph that the surface epithelium has been partly stripped off. This feature is commonly found in dysplastic epithelium at many sites and is a result of the loss of cohesiveness of dysplastic cells compared with normal.

In this example, the dysplasia is high grade in contrast to that in Figure 13.6(b), which shows *low grade dysplasia* in Barrett's oesophagus. Dysplasia is almost always seen in association with intestinal metaplasia. Both of these conditions imply an increased risk of gastric carcinoma.

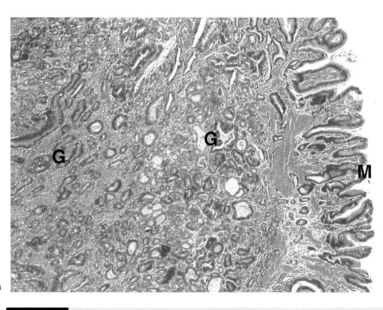

(a)

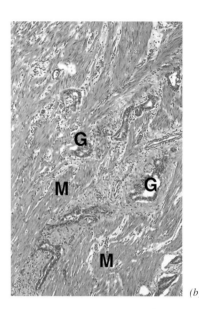

(b)

Fig. 13.10 Gastric carcinoma: intestinal type
(a) LP (b) MP

Gastric adenocarcinomas of the *intestinal type* are well or moderately differentiated and usually form a polypoid tumour mass or an ulcer with heaped-up edges. They are usually found in association with intestinal metaplasia (Fig. 13.7c) and dysplasia of the adjacent mucosa (Fig. 13.9). The low power view in micrograph (a) shows irregular malignant glands **G** infiltrating the gastric wall beneath a dysplastic mucosa with focal intestinal metaplasia **M**. Deeper in the gastric wall in micrograph (b), abnormal glands **G** can be seen infiltrating the muscularis propria **M**.

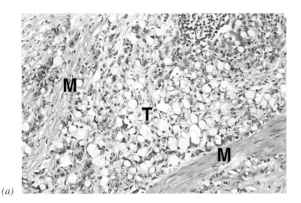

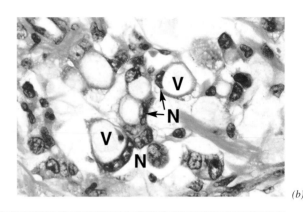

(a)   *(b)*

Fig. 13.11 Gastric carcinoma: diffuse type
(a) MP   (b) HP

Diffuse type gastric carcinomas are poorly differentiated adenocarcinomas with little or no discernible gland formation. This pattern tends to take the form of a diffuse infiltration of the stomach wall as in ***linitis plastica***. In micrograph (a), the tumour cells **T** can be seen forming a diffuse sheet infiltrating between bundles of smooth muscle **M**. At high power in micrograph (b), the tumour is seen to consist of ***signet ring cells***, so named because the cytoplasm is occupied by a mucin-filled vacuole **V** pushing the nucleus **N** to the periphery of the cell. Note the great degree of cellular pleomorphism in this poorly differentiated adenocarcinoma in contrast to that of the well-differentiated intestinal type in Figure 13.10(b). Some gastric carcinomas produce large amounts of extracellular mucin giving rise to '***mucinous adenocarcinomas***' (Fig. 7.16).

Carcinoma of the stomach may be staged histologically as ***early*** or ***late*** with early carcinomas infiltrating into the submucosa but not into the muscularis propria. Early gastric carcinomas have an excellent prognosis in contrast to late gastric carcinomas.

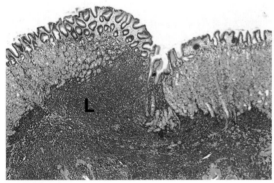

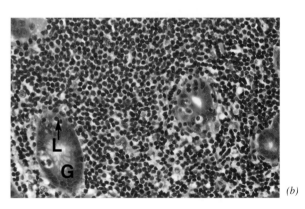

(a)   *(b)*

Fig. 13.12 Gastrointestinal lymphoma
(a) MP   (b) HP

Lymphoma is the second most common malignant tumour of the stomach (comprising about 5% of the total) and the third most common malignant tumour of the small intestine; lymphomas are rare in the colon and oesophagus. The typical gastrointestinal lymphoma is often termed a ***MALToma*** as it is derived from ***M***ucosal ***A***ssociated ***L***ymphoid ***T***issue. In the stomach, lymphomas may be macroscopically indistinguishable from adenocarcinomas but in the small intestine they often cause a diffuse thickening of the intestinal wall. As mentioned above, gastric lymphoma is often associated with *H. pylori* infection and eradication of *H. pylori* may bring about regression of the tumour.

Micrograph (a) shows a gastric lymphoma (MALToma) at low magnification. A diffuse sheet of small, densely staining atypical lymphocytes **L** has replaced the gastric mucosa at the centre-left of the field and elsewhere is infiltrating between the gastric glands. At high magnification in micrograph (b), the relative uniformity of the malignant lymphocytes can be seen. There are also typical ***lymphoepithelial lesions***, in which malignant lymphocytes **L** can be seen infiltrating the epithelium of two gastric glands **G**. The malignant lymphocytes of MALTomas are typically of small size and resemble ***centrocytes***. High grade lymphomas composed of large atypical lymphocytes may arise from transformation of a MALToma or occur de novo. High grade gastric lymphomas have the same histological appearance as diffuse large cell lymphoma occurring in lymph nodes (see Ch. 16).

Diseases of the small intestine and appendix

Primary inflammatory disorders of the small intestine are relatively uncommon with the exception of *coeliac disease* (Fig. 13.13) and *Crohn's disease* (Fig. 13.16). *Appendicitis* (Fig. 13.15) is extremely common and is a classical example of acute inflammation. *Giardiasis* (Fig. 13.14) is a common infective cause of inflammation in some countries.

Primary tumours of the small intestine and appendix are very rare with the exception of *neuroendocrine (carcinoid) tumours* (Fig. 13.17) and *lymphomas*, which resemble gastric lymphomas (Fig. 13.12). Neuroendocrine tumours occur in the appendix as well as rare adenomas, which are similar to colonic adenomas. However, the anatomy of the appendix means that mucin-producing adenomas may produce enough mucin to distend the appendix and form a *mucocoele* or *mucinous cystadenoma*. Very rarely these tumours may become malignant.

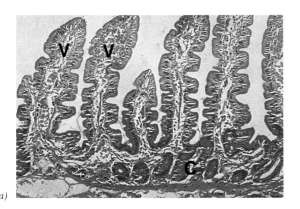

(a)

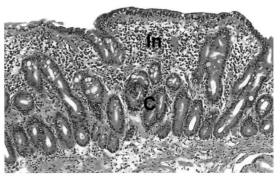

(b)

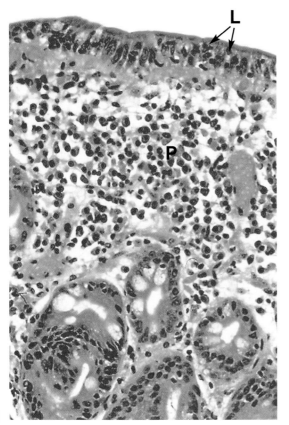

(c)

Fig. 13.13 Coeliac disease (gluten enteropathy)
(a) Normal jejunal mucosa (MP)
(b) Atrophic jejunal mucosa (MP)
(c) Atrophic jejunal mucosa (HP)

Hypersensitivity to gluten (a constituent of wheat, rye and barley) gives rise to *coeliac disease (gluten enteropathy)*, a condition in which the villi of the small bowel mucosa undergo total or subtotal atrophy leaving a flat mucosal surface with greatly diminished absorptive capacity. Clinically, this results in a malabsorption syndrome characterised by weight loss and *steatorrhoea* (diarrhoea containing unabsorbed lipid).

The diagnosis is usually confirmed by duodenal or jejunal biopsy. Micrograph (a) shows normal mucosa with villi **V** and short crypts **C**. In coeliac disease, as shown in micrograph (b), there is infiltration of the duodenal mucosa by inflammatory lymphocytes and plasma cells **In**, loss of villi (villous atrophy), and hyperplasia (elongation) of crypts **C**. The result is a flat small bowel mucosa. At high power, micrograph (c) shows the preponderance of plasma cells **P** in the lamina propria with the typical increase in *intraepithelial lymphocytes* **L**. These lymphocytes are mainly T cells and represent a cell-mediated immune reaction to gluten. Change to a gluten-free diet results in eventual restoration of the normal villous mucosal pattern. This restitution of normal mucosa is important to confirm the diagnosis as several other causes of inflammation or infection (see Fig. 13.14) can bring about a similar histological appearance.

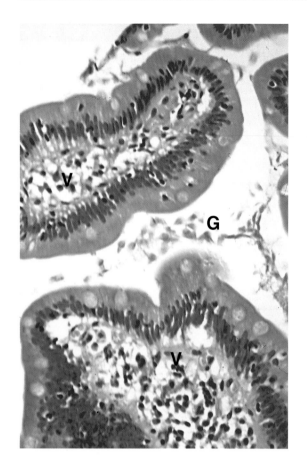

Fig. 13.14 Giardiasis (HP)

Giardia lamblia is a common protozoal cause of infective diarrhoea. The organism is spread via contaminated water supplies and the condition is particularly prevalent in institutionalised patients and those with immunodeficiency states. The diagnosis is often made by small intestinal biopsy.

As shown in this high power micrograph, the *Giardia* **G** are seen on the surface of and between the small intestinal villi **V**. The organisms are binucleate and flagellate although these features are not discernible at this magnification. The intestinal mucosa may appear virtually normal or there may be inflammation of the lamina propria with clubbing or even flattening of villi similar to that seen in coeliac disease (Fig. 13.13).

Fig. 13.15 Acute appendicitis (*illustrations opposite*)
(a) Early acute appendicitis (MP)   **(b) Later acute appendicitis (MP)**
(c) Established acute appendicitis (HP)   **(d) Gangrenous appendicitis (MP)**

Acute inflammation of the appendix is one of the most common surgical emergencies. The earliest change, shown in micrograph (a), is ulceration of the mucosa **U** with an overlying acute fibrinopurulent inflammatory exudate **Ex** and a purulent exudate **P** within the lumen. At this stage, the patient may experience vague central abdominal pain.

As the condition progresses, the inflammation spreads throughout all layers of the wall of the appendix and the mucosal ulceration becomes more extensive. This is illustrated in micrograph (b). Few of the original mucosal glands **G** now remain intact and large numbers of neutrophils have infiltrated through the submucosa **SM** and muscle layer **M** to the serosa **S**, where at one point a fibrinous exudate **F** is beginning to form on the peritoneal surface. This ***peritonitis***, involving the parietal peritoneum in the right iliac fossa, is responsible for the classical clinical features of acute appendicitis with localisation of the pain to the right iliac fossa. The peritoneal exudate often spreads to cover most of the serosal surface of the appendix and the mesoappendix

even though the point at which the inflammation spreads through the appendix wall may remain well localised. At high power, micrograph (c) shows the acute inflammatory infiltrate in the muscular layer of the wall of the appendix; the inflammatory infiltrate consists mainly of neutrophils **N**. The smooth muscle fibres **M** are separated by inflammatory oedema. Severe continuing inflammation of the appendix wall often leads to extensive necrosis of the muscle layer (***gangrenous appendicitis***) which predisposes to perforation of the appendix with more widespread peritonitis. This feature can be seen in micrograph (d) where the muscle layer **M** is identifiable up to a point where it has undergone necrosis **N**. Perforation of the appendix is imminent and will almost certainly take place at this site. The pus **P** that fills the lumen will then be discharged into the peritoneal cavity, leading to a more severe and extensive peritonitis which is infective. In the absence of appropriate treatment, the complications of perforation, including appendiceal abscess, subdiaphragmatic abscess, septicaemia, shock and death, may ensue.

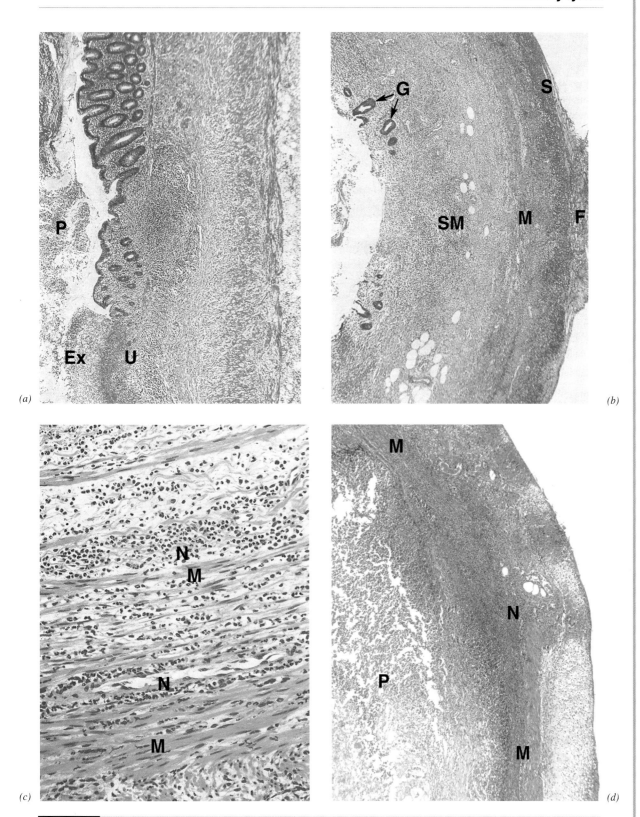

Fig. 13.15 **Acute appendicitis** (*caption opposite*)

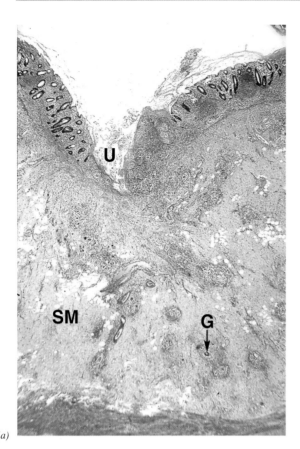

(a)

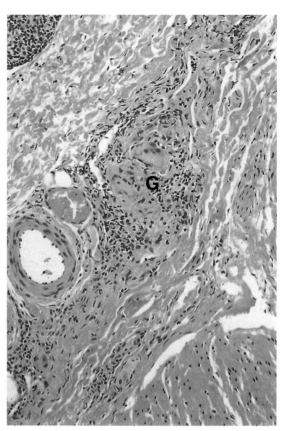

(b)

Fig. 13.16 Crohn's disease
(a) Fissured ulcer (MP)   (b) Crohn's granuloma (HP)

Crohn's disease is a chronic inflammatory disease of unknown aetiology which mainly involves the small intestine, especially the terminal ileum, but which also often affects the large bowel and anus and occasionally the upper gastrointestinal tract. In the colon and anus, it may be confused clinically with ulcerative colitis and anal fissures and fistulae respectively. Crohn's disease is characteristically patchy in distribution, affecting short segments with lengths of normal small intestine in between (*skip lesions*).

As shown in micrograph (a), the affected segments of small intestine show gross thickening of the wall, mainly because of marked oedema and inflammation of the submucosa **SM.** This oedema produces the typical 'cobblestone' macroscopic appearance of the mucosa in which domed areas of swollen mucosa and submucosa are criss-crossed by linear depressions caused by narrow

fissured ulcers. A typical fissured ulcer **U** can be seen here in midfield. Micrograph (a) also demonstrates two other characteristic features of Crohn's disease. First, the chronic inflammatory changes are ***transmural*** (i.e. affect all layers from mucosa to serosa). Second, granulomas **G**, often containing giant cells, may be found in all layers. A granuloma in the submucosa is illustrated at higher magnification in micrograph (b). The granulomas in Crohn's disease are often loose aggregates of epithelioid macrophages and giant cells rather than the well-circumscribed granulomas found in tuberculosis or sarcoidosis. Granulomas such as these may also be found in lymph nodes draining the affected segment of bowel. The result of longstanding transmural inflammation is widespread fibrosis, which may cause bowel obstruction; the deep-fissured ulceration predisposes to the formation of fistulae, a common complication of Crohn's disease.

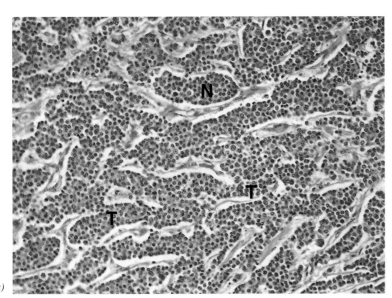
(a)

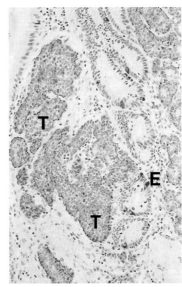
(b)

Fig. 13.17 Gastrointestinal neuroendocrine tumour (carcinoid)
(a) H&E (MP)   (b) Chromogranin (HP)

These tumours are found in the stomach, small intestine, appendix, pancreas and lung and, more rarely, the oesophagus, colon and biliary tract. Most are locally invasive but all may metastasise. They are derived from neuroendocrine cells and may secrete a variety of hormone products such as *serotonin*, which may cause *carcinoid syndrome*; insulin or glucagon are the usual secretory products of pancreatic lesions.

Whatever the location and secretory product, the histological appearance is very similar with tumour cells forming nests **N** and trabeculae **T** as in micrograph (a),

glandular structures or diffuse sheets of cells. The cells characteristically are small and uniform with round nuclei, stippled chromatin and pinkish granular cytoplasm. Immunoperoxidase staining will often reveal the hormone products within the cells. Similarly, in micrograph (b) of duodenal mucosa, tumour cells **T** have been stained for *chromogranin A*, a protein found in the secretory granules. Note also the positive staining of normal neuroendocrine cells scattered in the adjacent normal duodenal epithelium **E**.

Diseases of the large intestine

The colon and rectum are subject to various viral, bacterial and parasitic infections that are usually short-lived and readily diagnosed by microbiological methods; an important exception is *amoebic colitis* (Fig. 4.25), which is often diagnosed only after histological examination of biopsy specimens. Of great importance is the chronic relapsing inflammatory disease of the large intestine known as *ulcerative colitis* (Fig. 13.19). More recently discovered causes of chronic diarrhoea include *collagenous colitis* and *lymphocytic (microscopic) colitis* (Fig. 13.18).

Raised intraluminal pressure in the colon, probably as a result of a low residue diet, commonly leads to saccular herniation of mucosa through the muscle layers of the bowel wall; the diverticula so formed may become inflamed giving rise to *diverticulitis* (Fig. 13.23) which may have serious sequelae.

The large intestine may undergo infarction either as a result of mesenteric artery occlusion by thrombus or embolus, or more commonly by venous infarction following hernial strangulation or *volvulus*; this is shown in Fig. 10.5.

Colonic polyps are exceedingly common. By far the most common is the *hyperplastic polyp* (Fig. 13.20), a reactive rather than neoplastic lesion. Less common non-neoplastic polyps include *inflammatory pseudopolyps* as seen in ulcerative colitis (Fig. 13.19a) and polypoid hamartomas such as *Peutz–Jeghers' polyps*. Neoplastic benign polyps include *tubular adenomas, villous adenomas* and *tubulovillous adenomas* (Fig. 13.21), all of which have a definite risk of malignant transformation.

Malignant tumours of the colon and rectum are very common, and almost all are *adenocarcinomas* (Fig. 13.22); most appear histologically moderately differentiated with a clearly defined glandular pattern. The anal canal, being lined by squamous epithelium, is occasionally the site of *squamous carcinoma* (Fig. 7.14), although local invasion of the anal canal by adenocarcinoma of the lower rectum also occurs.

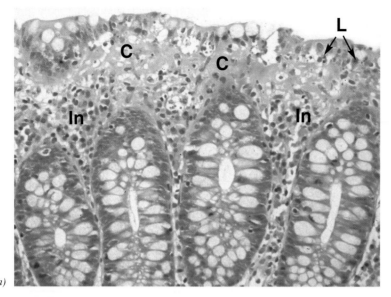
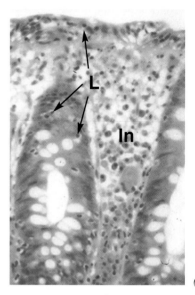

(a)   *(b)*

Fig. 13.18 Collagenous and lymphocytic colitis
(a) Collagenous colitis (HP)   (b) Lymphocytic colitis (HP)

Both of these recently identified conditions cause chronic watery non-bloody diarrhoea with a normal appearing bowel at colonoscopy. The two conditions have many similarities but their exact relationship is as yet unknown. The aetiology of these conditions is also unknown but an immunological cause seems most likely. ***Collagenous colitis***, which is a disorder found mainly in middle-aged and elderly women, is shown in micrograph (a). It is characterised by a band of collagen **C** deposited immediately below the epithelial basement membrane. There is also inflammation **In** of the lamina propria with inflammatory cells and erythrocytes trapped within the collagen band. The surface epithelium contains increased

numbers of intra-epithelial lymphocytes **L**. The changes may be patchy throughout the colon and are generally least prominent in the distal colon and rectum. ***Lymphocytic*** or ***microscopic colitis***, shown in micrograph (b), occurs in both men and women and generally affects the whole colon. Typically, there is a marked increase in intraepithelial lymphocytes **L** in both the surface epithelium and glands with degenerative changes in the surface epithelium. There is also an inflammatory infiltrate **In** in the lamina propria. The changes are in fact similar to collagenous colitis but without the collagen band.

Fig. 13.19 Ulcerative colitis *(illustrations opposite)*
(a) Active disease with pseudopolyp formation (LP)   (b) Acute disease (HP)   (c) Quiescent phase disease (HP)

Ulcerative colitis is a chronic relapsing inflammatory disease of unknown cause affecting the large bowel. The disease always involves the rectum but often extends proximally to involve the whole colon. It is sometimes accompanied by systemic features such as anaemia, arthritis and uveitis.

In active disease, there is acute inflammation of the mucosa with neutrophils accumulating in the lamina propria and in the lumina of the colonic glands to form ***crypt abscesses***; ulceration of the mucosa occurs, but the ulcers are superficial rather than fissured as in Crohn's disease (Fig. 13.16).

In severe cases, ulceration may develop extensively throughout the length of the colon as shown in micrograph (a). Note that the ulcerative process has destroyed much of the mucosa and submucosa in this field, leaving an isolated island of non-ulcerated mucosa which is swollen by acute and chronic inflammatory changes; some of the colonic glands **G** remain. Non-ulcerated areas such as this project above the surrounding ulcerated areas to produce so-called ***inflammatory pseudopolyps***. Despite the severity and extent of the inflammation and ulceration, the changes are mainly confined to the mucosa and submucosa, and the muscularis **M** is not involved. The inflammatory changes are rarely transmural, a useful distinguishing feature from Crohn's disease. In micrograph (a),

a peritoneal exudate **Ex** is present but this resulted from peritonitis owing to surgical instrumentation causing perforation and does not represent true transmural inflammation.

Micrograph (b) illustrates features indicative of acute-on-chronic inflammatory activity, namely the presence of crypt abscesses **A** in the glands, depletion of mucus-containing goblet cells and the presence of neutrophils as well as chronic inflammatory cells in the lamina propria.

During quiescent periods between acute exacerbations, the mucosa damaged by earlier severe inflammation or ulceration shows mixed features of chronic inflammation and attempts at restitution. Micrograph (c) shows a mucosal biopsy taken during a quiescent phase. The lamina propria **LP** is infiltrated by lymphocytes and plasma cells. The colonic glands usually show reduction in the numbers of mucin-secreting goblet cells although that is not a major feature in this example, and there is mild reactive change in the epithelial cells. The crypts are shortened and often branched **B**.

Repeated episodes of inflammation, ulceration and epithelial regeneration may lead to dysplastic change in the constantly irritated epithelium. This factor may contribute to the high incidence of colonic adenocarcinoma arising in patients with a long history of ulcerative colitis.

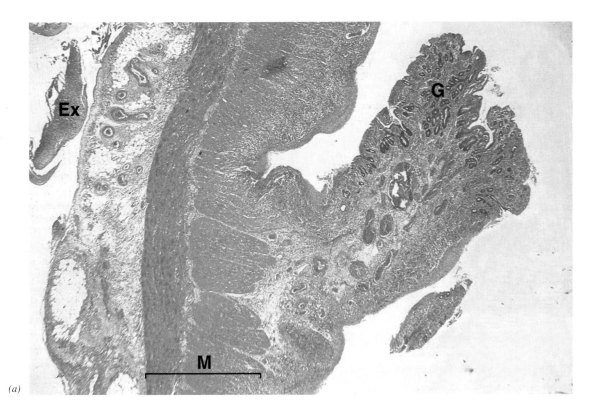

(a)

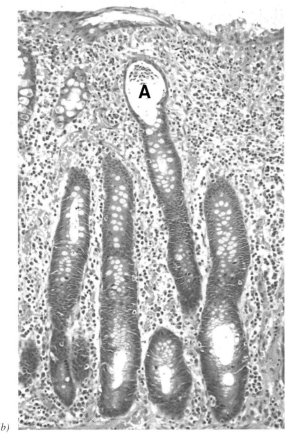

(b)

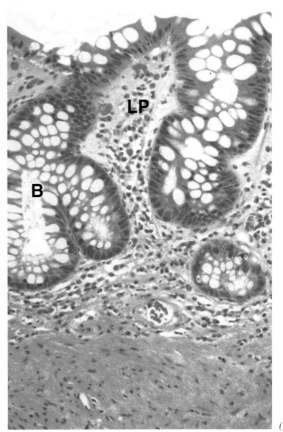

(c)

Fig. 13.19 Ulcerative colitis *(caption opposite)*

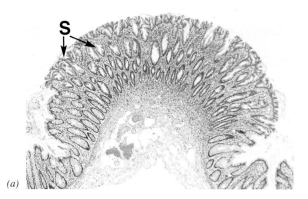

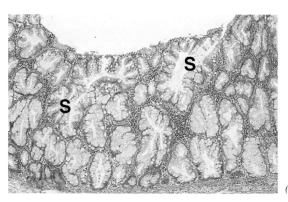

(a) *(b)*

Fig. 13.20 Hyperplastic polyp
(a) LP   (b) HP

Hyperplastic polyps far outnumber neoplastic polyps (Fig. 13.21) in the large bowel. They are usually small, often multiple and occasionally bleed. They may coexist with neoplastic polyps and malignant tumours but do not themselves have malignant potential.

At low magnification, micrograph (a) shows a typical hyperplastic polyp composed of crypts with a characteristic 'sawtooth' outline **S**; this is also seen at medium power in micrograph (b). Apart from mild crowding, i.e. hyperplasia, the epithelial cells lining the crypts are very similar in appearance to normal colonic epithelium and exhibit no evidence of dysplasia in contrast to the epithelial cells of neoplastic polyps.

Fig. 13.21 Colonic adenomatous polyps *(illustrations opposite)*
(a) Tubular adenomas: polyposis coli (LP)   (b) Villous adenoma (LP)
(c) Tubulovillous adenoma (LP) (d) Villous adenoma (HP)

Benign neoplastic polyps of the colonic mucosa are of three main histological patterns: *tubular adenoma, villous adenoma* and *tubulovillous adenoma*.

Tubular adenomas are usually pedunculated polypoid lesions, the adenoma proper being connected to the mucosa by a narrow stalk of normal tissue. The adenoma consists of dysplastic colonic epithelium arranged in straight tubular glands. When seen with the naked eye, these tumours have a smooth or slightly bosselated surface. Tubular adenomas may be either solitary or multiple. In one heritable condition, known as *familial polyposis coli*, numerous tubular adenomas develop throughout the colon and there is a strong predisposition for the transformation of benign lesions into adenocarcinoma.

Micrograph (a) shows two tubular adenomas **T** in a segment of colon from a patient with polyposis coli. Note the darkly stained adenomatous masses connected to the underlying mucosa by stalks, which merely represent extensions of the normal mucosa and submucosa.

Villous adenomas are sessile, rather than pedunculated, lesions, arising from a broad base; they are composed of narrow, frond-like outgrowths of epithelial cells supported by a delicate connective tissue stroma giving a papillary appearance both histologically and with the naked eye. A typical sessile villous adenoma is illustrated in micrograph (b).

Many longstanding tubular adenomas acquire a partially villous histological pattern, particularly at the surface, although the general configuration of the lesion (pedunculated and non-sessile) resembles that of a pure tubular adenoma. Such adenomas are called tubulovillous adenomas. In the example shown in micrograph (c), note that the stalk is covered by normal colonic-type mucosa that contrasts markedly with the densely staining dysplastic epithelium of the adenoma.

Cytologically, all three types of adenoma show varying degrees of *dysplasia* ranging from mild to severe. Micrograph (d) shows a high power view of dysplasia in a colonic adenoma, in this case a villous adenoma. The cells are enlarged and crowded with large pleomorphic nuclei, increased nuclear to cytoplasmic ratio, palisading of nuclei and increased mitotic figures (see also Fig. 7.1). By definition, adenomas show no evidence of invasion.

All the above types of colonic polyps have the potential for malignant change with the development of invasive adenocarcinoma. This occurs more frequently in villous adenomas than in the other types, and is more likely with increasing severity of dysplasia.

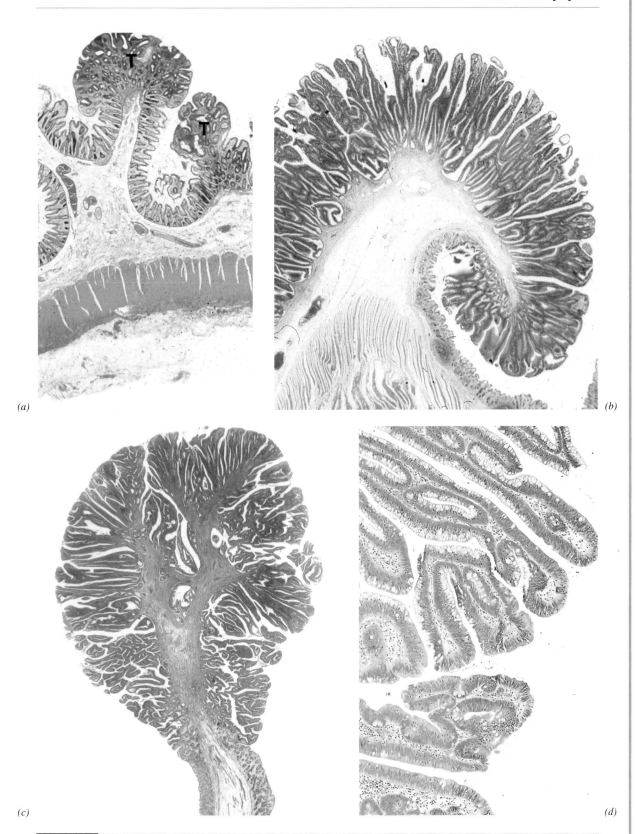

(a)

(b)

(c)

(d)

Fig. 13.21 Colonic adenomatous polyps *(caption opposite)*

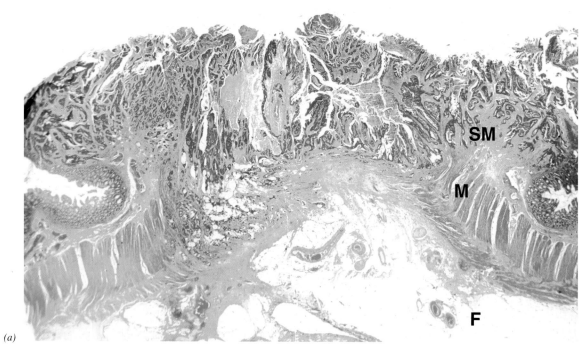

(a)

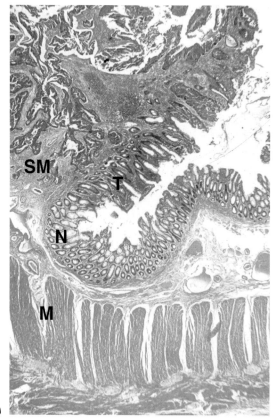

(b)

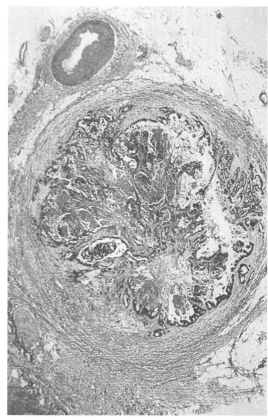

(c)

Fig. 13.22 **Adenocarcinoma of the colon** *(caption opposite above)*

Fig. 13.22 Adenocarcinoma of the colon *(illustrations opposite)*
(a) Invasive tumour (LP) (b) Edge of lesion in (a) (MP) (c) Invasion of vein (MP)

Adenocarcinoma is the most common and important malignant tumour of the large bowel and arises most frequently in the sigmoid colon as well as in the rectum. There are three common macroscopic patterns of growth; tumours may be raised with central ulceration elevated margins, extensive lesions may involve the whole circumference of the bowel forming an annular stricture, or lesions may develop as a protruberant cauliflower-like mass most commonly seen in the caecum and proximal colon.

Micrograph (a) shows an ulcerated adenocarcinoma of the rectum; the tumour has infiltrated deeply through the submucosa **SM**, muscularis **M**, and out into the pericolic fat **F**. Micrograph (b) shows the raised everted edge of this tumour at higher magnification. There is an abrupt transition between normal rectal mucosa **N** and the malignant tumour epithelium **T**. In this area, the tumour has infiltrated into the submucosa **SM**, but not the muscularis propria **M**. Micrograph (c) shows a vein in the serosa of the colon; it is filled with colonic

adenocarcinoma which is growing along it as a solid cord.

The prognosis of colonic and rectal carcinomas depends on a number of factors, the most important being tumour stage as assessed by the depth of invasion of the bowel wall, the presence of lymph node and distant metastases and evidence of tumour invasion into veins and lymphatics.

Dukes' classification (staging) has been in general use since 1932 and despite many modifications and revisions, the initial classification continues in general usage. This system, initially applied to rectal tumours only, divides tumours into three stages designated A to C. In *Dukes' stage A*, the tumour may invade the bowel wall as far as the muscularis propria. If the tumour extends through the muscularis propria into the subserosal fat, it is classified as *Dukes' stage B*. The presence of metastases in lymph nodes automatically classifies it as *Dukes' stage C*. These three stages have approximately 100%, 70% and 35% 5-year survival rates respectively.

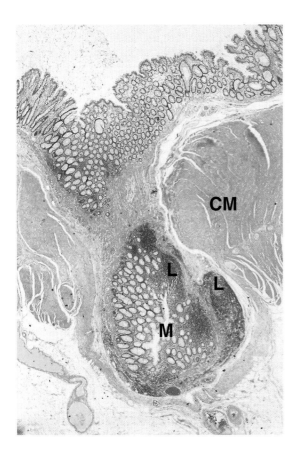

Fig. 13.23 Diverticular disease (LP)

Diverticular disease is a common condition in the elderly; it may involve any part of the colon, although the sigmoid colon is the most frequently and most severely affected part.

The normal muscular wall of the colon consists of an inner circular layer and a discontinuous outer longitudinal layer represented by the *taeniae coli*. Diverticula are formed by herniation of pouches of colonic mucosa **M**, including mucosal lymphoid tissue **L**, through unsupported areas of the circular muscle between the taeniae coli. The diverticula bulge towards the outer surface and often contain faecal material. This probably results from abnormally high intraluminal pressure associated with low residue diets. A characteristic histological feature is marked hypertrophy of the circular muscle layer **CM**.

Acute inflammation, *diverticulitis*, may develop following obstruction of the narrow neck of a diverticulum. Complications include rectal haemorrhage, perforation, peritonitis, paracolic abscess formation and fistula formation with other viscera such as bladder and vagina.

14. Hepatobiliary system and pancreas

Disorders of the liver

The liver is affected by a wide range of disorders, the most important of which are below.

- **Acute hepatic necrosis** has been described in Ch. 1, and usually results from exposure to certain drugs or poison, or as part of a fulminant viral infection.
- **Acute hepatitis** has many causes (see p. 155); it may resolve, or become persistent (chronic hepatitis).
- **Chronic hepatitis** is diagnosed when biochemical manifestations of liver cell damage have persisted for over 6 months, and may eventually progress to cirrhosis.
- **Cirrhosis** is the end stage of several types of liver disease in which there is liver cell loss and architectural distortion over a long period. It is characterised by destruction of normal liver architecture which is replaced by regenerative nodules of liver separated by bands of fibrous tissue. There may be evidence of continuing active damage to liver hepatocytes. Eventually liver function is impaired or fails totally (**chronic liver failure**). The distortion of vascular architecture leads to **portal hypertension**. Various different types of cirrhosis are illustrated and discussed in Figure 14.9.
- **Malignant disease** frequently involves the liver, most commonly as secondary spread, especially from primary lesions in gut, breast and lung (Fig. 7.8); less frequently, the liver becomes diffusely infiltrated in lymphoreticular malignancies such as Hodgkin's disease and other lymphomas.
- **Primary malignancy** of the liver, **hepatocellular carcinoma** (Fig. 14.11), is uncommon and most often arises in pre-existing cirrhosis.
- **Right-sided cardiac failure** involves the liver when raised pressure is transmitted to the central veins resulting in congestion of sinusoids with blood. Hepatocytes in the centrilobular zones then frequently undergo atrophy or even frank necrosis.
- **Inborn errors of metabolism**, in most cases probably reflecting single gene defects, result in the abnormal accumulation of various metabolites within hepatocytes. These are known as **storage diseases** and include **glycogen storage diseases, mucopolysaccharidoses, lipidoses, haemochromatosis** (see Fig. 14.10) and **Wilson's disease**. Liver biopsy may be useful in the diagnosis of such disorders.

Fig. 14.1 Clinical features of hepatobiliary diseases and their pathophysiology

Sign/Symptom	Clinical feature	Mechanism
Jaundice	Yellow coloration of tissues owing to bile	Failure of metabolism or excretion of bile pigments
Bleeding	Easy bruising and prolonged clotting time of blood	Failure of synthesis of clotting factors
Oedema	Swelling of dependent parts owing to extracellular accumulation of water	Failure of synthesis of albumin resulting in reduced plasma oncotic pressure
Ascites	Fluid in peritoneal cavity	Low serum albumin and portal hypertension
Gynaecomastia	Enlarged male breasts	Failure to detoxify endogenous oestrogens
Encephalopathy	Altered consciousness, lack of coordination; may lead to coma	Failure to detoxify ammonia and excitatory amino acids which result from protein breakdown
Haematemesis and/or melaena	Vomiting blood and passing blood per rectum	Bleeding from oesophageal varices owing to portal hypertension

Acute inflammation of the liver

Hepatocytes, with their high degree of metabolic activity, are readily disturbed by toxins and demonstrate the histological cellular responses known as cloudy swelling, fatty change and necrosis as described in Chapter 1. Acute inflammation of the liver parenchyma is usually marked by focal accumulations of inflammatory cells usually in relation to the site of necrotic hepatocytes. The exception to this is in the formation of *hepatic abscesses* which usually develop either as a result of bacterial infections from the biliary tract or from a septic focus in the abdomen drained by the portal venous system to the liver.

Acute hepatitis is a general term for inflammation of the liver parenchyma which can then be further classified according to aetiology. The four most important groups of conditions causing acute hepatitis are:

- **Viral hepatitis** (outlined in Fig. 14.3) – histological appearance shown in Figure 14.2.
- **Toxins** – alcohol is the most common hepatic toxin (Fig. 14.4).
- **Drugs** – hepatitis may be caused by the anaesthetic gas *halothane*, particularly after repeated exposure. *Isoniazid*, a drug commonly used in the treatment of tuberculosis, results in acute hepatitis in a small proportion of cases. Many other drugs occasionally cause acute hepatitis.
- **Systemic infections** – infections caused by *Leptospira* and *Toxoplasma* usually involve the liver as part of disseminated disease. Other systemic infections may cause multiple minute infective lesions as in bacterial septicaemia and miliary tuberculosis.

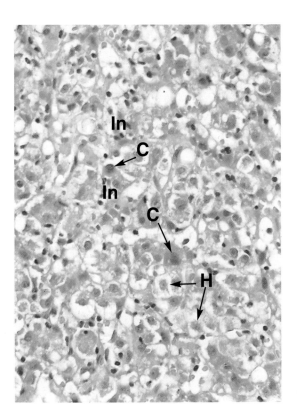

Fig. 14.2 Acute viral hepatitis (HP)

The viral agents causing acute hepatitis all produce a similar histological picture in the acute phase.

There is widespread swelling and ballooning of hepatocytes owing to hydropic degeneration **H** and this progresses to focal or *spotty necrosis* throughout the lobule; the areas of necrosis are identified by aggregates of inflammatory cells **In** surrounding eosinophilic (pink-stained) bodies called *Councilman bodies* **C**, representing the cytoplasm of necrotic liver cells. The Kuppfer cells are very active and within portal tracts there are increased numbers of chronic inflammatory cells (not illustrated here).

In time, regeneration of the dead hepatocytes occurs. In hepatitis A and E, complete resolution is the rule but in hepatitis B, C and D, activity may persist or progress to chronic hepatitis (Fig. 14.7).

Rare cases of viral hepatitis occur in which there is massive liver necrosis instead of the focal type seen here. This is particularly seen with hepatitis E in pregnancy; such fulminant cases are usually fatal.

Fig. 14.3 Viral causes of hepatitis

Virus Type	Mode of transmission	Acute hepatitis	Chronic hepatitis	Chronic carrier	Notes
Hep A	Faeco-oral	Yes	No	No	Mild, self-limiting (rarely fulminant)
Hep B	Blood, saliva, semen	Yes	5-10%	Yes	Transmission – 'needle sharing', sexual, transfusion
Hep C	Blood, saliva, semen	Yes	50%	Yes	Transmission – 'needle sharing' transfusion
Hep D	Blood, saliva, semen	Yes	Yes	Yes	Only in association with hepatitis B
Hep E	Faeco-oral	Yes	No	No	Usually mild, self-limiting (rarely fulminant)

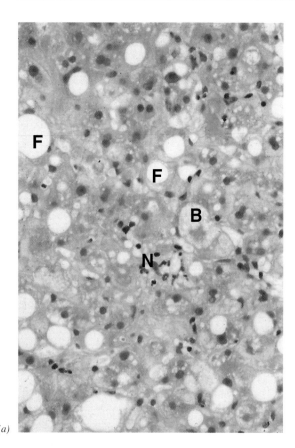

(a)

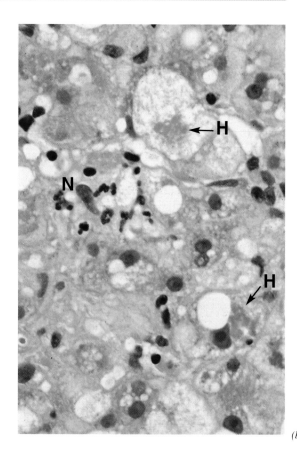

(b)

Fig. 14.4 Alcoholic hepatitis
(a) MP (b) HP

Alcohol is a potent hepatotoxin when taken in large quantities and liver changes occur even after isolated bouts of heavy drinking.

Early evidence of metabolic injury to the hepatocytes is the appearance of fatty change **F** manifest by the accumulation of lipid in the form of large cytoplasmic vacuoles within some hepatocytes, usually displacing the nucleus to one side (see also Fig. 1.5). With more severe metabolic disruption, the hepatocytes undergo hydropic degeneration (Fig. 1.4) and become swollen and vacuolated, an appearance described as ***ballooning degeneration*** **B**. In some cases, the metabolic disruption may be irrecoverable and some hepatocytes undergo necrosis. The location of necrotic hepatocytes **N** is marked by foci of neutrophils and lymphocytes. As seen in micrograph (b), some hepatocytes accumulate an eosinophilic material, derived from cytokeratin intermediate filaments, termed ***Mallory's hyaline*** **H**; this

material forms irregular cytoplasmic globules, usually near the nucleus, and stains a glassy pink colour, slightly darker than the normal cytoplasm. The hepatocytes around the centrilobular veins appear to be most vulnerable to alcohol toxicity and in some individuals delicate fibrosis may be seen around the central veins.

With prolonged alcohol abuse, there is progressive fibrosis because of hepatocyte necrosis and regeneration of liver cells which can develop into ***alcoholic cirrhosis*** (Fig. 14.9a). Fatty change, alcoholic hepatitis and hepatic cirrhosis may all occur in the same individual. Some individuals develop recurrent alcoholic hepatitis and are likely to proceed to cirrhosis; others may develop cirrhosis insidiously with no preceding episodes of acute hepatitis. Reversible fatty change may occur in a healthy individual after a single drinking binge; the presence of fatty change in a known alcoholic is an indicator of continued alcohol intake.

Chronic hepatitis

When inflammation of the liver continues without improvement for 6 months or more, the condition is described as *chronic hepatitis*; this term, however, excludes chronic inflammation of the liver caused by alcohol, bacterial agents and biliary obstruction. There are several causes of chronic hepatitis shown in Fig. 14.5.

Fig. 14. 5 Causes of chronic hepatitis
Viral infection
Hepatitis B Hepatitis C Other hepatitis viruses
Autoimmune disease
Autoimmune hepatitis Primary biliary cirrhosis Primary sclerosing cholangitis
Toxic / metabolic
Wilson's disease α1 Antitrypsin deficiency Drug hepatitis

Histologically, chronic hepatitis is characterised by:

- Necrosis of liver cells (hepatocytes), either concentrated around portal tracts or scattered within the liver lobules, or both.
- The presence of inflammatory cells (mainly lymphocytes) in portal tracts or scattered within the liver lobules, or both.
- The presence of fibrosis, either in the portal tracts, the septa between adjacent lobules, or cutting across the lobular structure, causing architectural distortion.

Assessment of these features can be used to determine how active the disease is (*grade of chronic hepatitis*) and how far the disease has progressed (*stage of disease*). This is shown in Fig. 14.6 (but you do not need to learn it!)

Fig. 14. 6 Staging and grading of chronic hepatitis		
Grade of inflammation or necrosis		
Score	**Portal**	**Lobular**
0	None	None
1	Portal inflammation	Inflammation but no necrosis
2	Mild necrosis of periportal hepatocytes	Focal necrotic cells with Councilman bodies
3	Moderate necrosis of periportal hepatocytes	Severe focal cell damage
4	Severe necrosis of periportal hepatocytes	Necrosis of liver cells bridges between portal tracts
Stages of fibrosis		
Stage score		
0	None	
1	Enlarged portal tracts	
2	Fibrosis of periportal area	
3	Fibrosis in septa but no distortion of liver architecture	
4	Fibrosis with regenerative nodules (cirrhosis)	

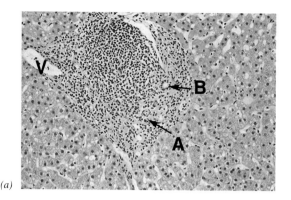

(a)

Fig. 14.7 Chronic hepatitis
(a) MP (b) MP (c) HP (d) HP

Micrograph (a) shows inflammation confined to a portal tract. The periportal hepatocytes (called the limiting plates) show no necrosis. Bile duct **B**, artery **A** and vein **V** are easily seen. This corresponds to low grade disease. In contrast, micrograph (b) shows higher grade disease. Inflammation and necrosis extend out from the portal tract to involve periportal hepatocytes **L** which show necrosis **N**. In addition to changes around the portal tract, individual hepatocytes in the liver lobule are affected, sometimes called spotty necrosis **S**, shown in both micrographs (b) and (c). Reference back to Figure 14.6 shows how these features equate to higher grade disease and reflect active liver cell destruction. Regeneration of liver cells may be seen, reflected in binucleate cells **Bn** or liver cell plates two cells wide.

In more severe cases, liver cell necrosis and inflammation may become confluent to form bands of bridging necrosis extending between adjacent portal tracts.

If disease progresses, there is fibrosis in the liver, with continued liver cell regeneration that ultimately leads to cirrhosis.

In chronic hepatitis caused by hepatitis B virus, the cytoplasm of hepatocytes may assume a ground-glass pale pink appearance **G** seen in micrograph (d), caused by accumulation of viral proteins.

In hepatitis C infection, lymphoid follicles and focal fatty change may be a clue to diagnosis.

Previous classifications have used the terms chronic persistent and chronic aggressive hepatitis. These are no longer used. Current classifications define chronic hepatitis in terms of aetiology and histological grading (see Figs. 14.5 and 14.6).

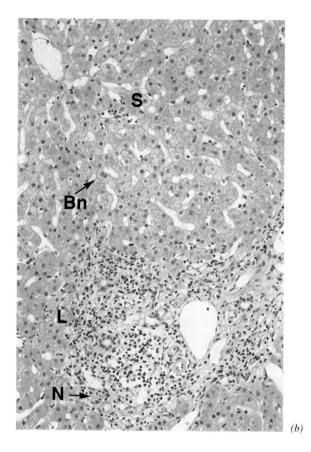

(b)

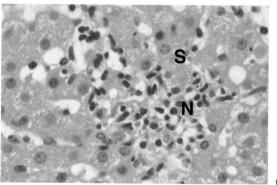

(c)

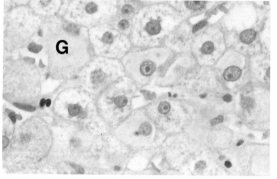

(d)

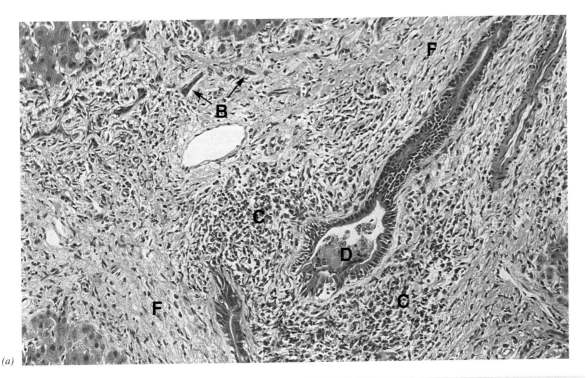

(a)

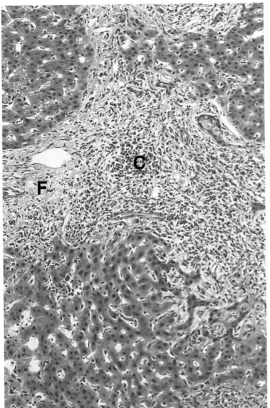

(b)

Fig. 14.8 Primary biliary cirrhosis
(a) Early lesion (HP) (b) Later lesion (HP)

Primary biliary cirrhosis is a chronic inflammatory disease of the liver in which destructive inflammatory changes are centred primarily on bile ducts; hepatocytes are, however, also affected.

The earliest changes are seen in the epithelium of the larger bile ducts **D** as shown in micrograph (a). There is vacuolation of the epithelial cells and infiltration of the wall and surrounding tissues by lymphocytes. A characteristic feature at this stage is the formation of histiocytic granulomas in relation to damaged bile ducts (not shown here). Portal tracts then become progressively expanded by chronic inflammatory cells **C**.

As seen in micrograph (b), the inflammatory cells progressively extend from the portal tracts into the liver parenchyma, with piecemeal necrosis occurring along the limiting plate in a manner similar to chronic hepatitis (Fig. 14.7). As liver cells are destroyed, the portal tracts also become expanded by fibrosis **F**. Large bile ducts are no longer visible, having been destroyed.

At the periphery of the portal tracts, there is proliferation of small bile ducts **B** which do not appear to be canalised; this feature is best seen in micrograph (a).

If primary biliary cirrhosis proceeds unchecked, true cirrhosis develops (Fig. 14.9); note that this disease is referred to as primary biliary cirrhosis even in the early stages when there is no evidence of cirrhotic changes.

BASIC SYSTEMS PATHOLOGY

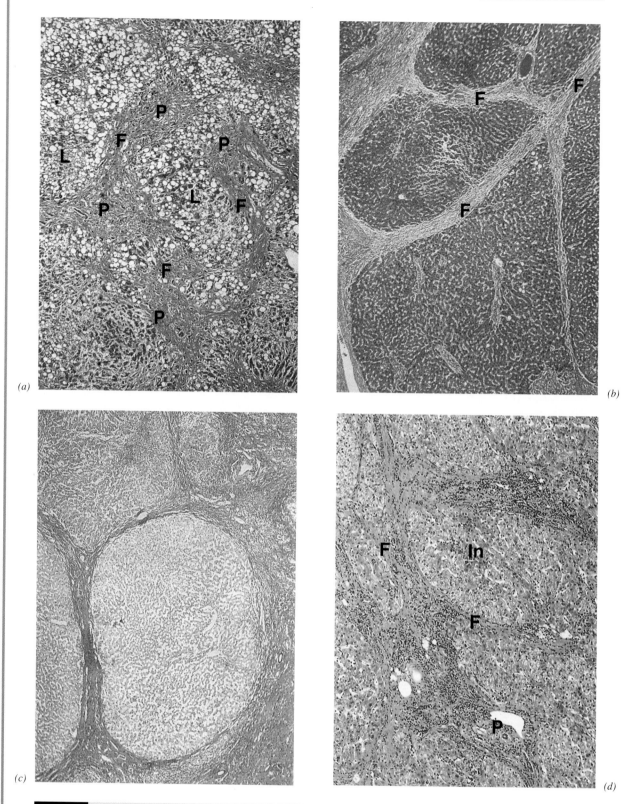

(a)

(b)

(c)

(d)

Fig. 14.9 Cirrhosis *(caption opposite)*

Fig. 14.9 Cirrhosis *(illustrations opposite)*
(a) Alcoholic cirrhosis (MP)   (b) Cryptogenic cirrhosis (MP)
(c) Cryptogenic cirrhosis (van Gieson stain) (MP)   (d) Cirrhosis due to progressive chronic hepatitis (MP)

Cirrhosis is the end result of continued damage to liver cells from a great many causes. It is characterised by wholesale disruption of the liver architecture and the formation of nodules of regenerating liver cells separated by fibrous bands. There are two main effects of this altered liver architecture and cellular damage, namely disordered hepatocyte function (Fig. 14.1) and disturbance of blood flow through the liver from portal vein to hepatic vein.

The effect of vascular obstruction within the liver is an increase in portal venous pressure termed *portal hypertension*. Anastomoses open up between the portal circulation and the systemic venous system resulting in large dilated veins called *varices*. The most important site of varices is in the lower oesophagus but they can occur elsewhere. These dilated thin-walled veins are liable to rupture and this is a common fatal event in patients with cirrhosis.

The classification of cirrhosis is based on the disease which caused the underlying liver damage. The most important causes are chronic alcohol abuse, chronic hepatitis and biliary cirrhosis (primary and secondary to obstruction). In a small percentage of cases no underlying disease can be found; this is known as *cryptogenic cirrhosis*.

The diagnosis of cirrhosis is confirmed by percutaneous liver biopsy. Histological examination is directed towards identifying the nature of any underlying disease process as well as establishing evidence of cirrhosis.

In micrograph (a), the features of cirrhosis are broad fibrous bands **F** connecting portal areas **P**, and intervening nodules of liver cells **L** showing marked fatty change; this is an example of *alcoholic cirrhosis*.

Micrograph (b) shows a typical cirrhotic pattern, with bands of fibrous tissue **F** disrupting the lobular architecture; there is no inflammation, fatty change or specific features. If there are also no clinical pointers to the aetiology, this is classified as cryptogenic cirrhosis. Micrograph (c) is from the same case, this time stained by a method which emphasises the fibrosis (stained red).

Cirrhosis following progressive chronic hepatitis is illustrated in micrograph (d). The portal tracts **P** contain large numbers of chronic inflammatory cells and in some areas these inflammatory cells spill over the limiting plate into nodules of hepatocytes. There are also focal areas of inflammation **In** in the liver parenchyma. The portal tracts show evidence of fibrosis and fibrous bands **F** containing chronic inflammatory cells have formed bridges between adjacent portal areas. These features are all characteristically seen in the more active forms of chronic hepatitis (see Fig. 14.7).

Treatment of cirrhosis is aimed at controlling the underlying liver disease. Once fibrous tissue has been deposited, it is virtually irreversible. Repeated liver biopsy can be used to monitor progress.

Older classifications of cirrhosis grouped the diseases according to the size of the regenerative nodules seen at post-mortem or laparotomy. In *macronodular cirrhosis*, large nodules up to several centimetres in diameter are present. *Micronodular cirrhosis* is characterised by uniform small regenerative nodules up to 1 cm in diameter. While it is useful to describe macroscopic features, this classification does not help in assessing disease type or progress. In active cirrhosis as seen in micrograph (d), there is evidence of continuing damage to liver cells, whereas in inactive cirrhosis there is no evidence of continuing liver damage.

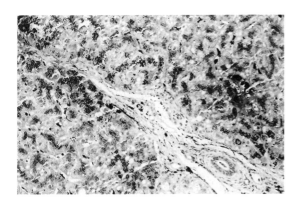

Fig. 14.10 Haemochromatosis (Perls stain) (MP)

Haemochromatosis is a condition characterised by excessive deposition of iron in the tissues. It is due to an inherited defect of iron transport such that excessive iron is absorbed from a normal diet. Pathologically excessive iron is deposited in many tissues, especially myocardium, liver, adrenal glands and pancreas.

Hepatic involvement causes cirrhosis. As seen in this micrograph, liver cells accumulate enormous amounts of iron which are stained blue by Perls stain. Excessive iron may also be stored in the liver owing to dietary excess or frequent blood transfusion. This is termed *secondary haemosiderosis*.

BASIC SYSTEMS PATHOLOGY

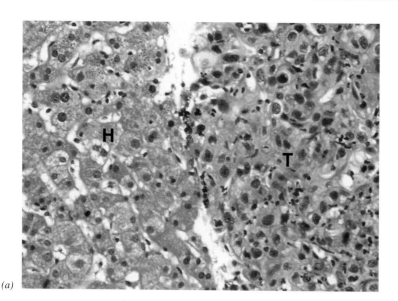

(a)

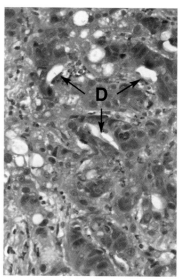

(b)

Fig. 14.11 Hepatocellular carcinoma
(a) HP   (b) MP

Primary carcinoma of the liver is a relatively uncommon condition compared to metastatic tumours from other sites. On a world-wide basis, the incidence of hepatocellular carcinoma, often called *hepatoma*, is closely related to the prevalence of hepatitis B virus infection. In some parts of Africa it accounts for up to 40% of all cancers; however, in Europe and the USA, it only accounts for around 2%. Cirrhosis from any cause also predisposes to the development of hepatocellular carcinoma. These tumours are associated with rapid clinical progression with average survival from diagnosis being around 6 months.

The tumour may form a single massive nodule, multiple small nodules, or exhibit a diffuse infiltrating pattern. Micrograph (a) shows normal hepatocytes **H** on the left and malignant hepatocytes **T** on the right. Sometimes the tumour cells have a ductular pattern **D** as shown in (b).

Alphafetoprotein is secreted by a large proportion of hepatocellular carcinomas and is a useful diagnostic marker.

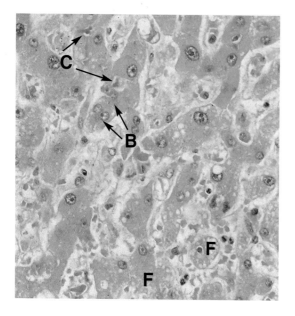

Fig. 14.12 Cholestasis (HP)

Cholestasis, or accumulation of bile within the liver, is a consequence of obstruction to bile flow. This may occur in the extrahepatic biliary tree (most commonly as the result of gallstones), in the intrahepatic biliary tree because of destruction of bile ducts (as in primary biliary cirrhosis), or at the level of the hepatocytes owing to failure to secrete bile; the last is a common feature of liver cell damage from any cause or may be a reaction to certain drugs. In all types of cholestasis, there is accumulation of bile **B** within the hepatic parenchyma. In ductal obstruction, there are also plugs of bile within the canaliculi **C**. Hepatocytes containing bile show *feathery degeneration* **F** where the cytoplasm becomes foamy. Long standing obstruction of the biliary tract may lead to secondary biliary cirrhosis.

Disorders of the biliary system

Gallbladder disease is a common surgical problem in developed countries and is often associated with stone formation and chronic obstruction of the cystic duct leading to *chronic cholecystitis* (Fig. 14.13). Tumours of the biliary system are relatively rare and usually take the form of highly malignant adenocarcinomas (Fig. 14.14). *Cholestasis* is the term applied to accumulation of bile within the liver; this is illustrated in Figure 14.12.

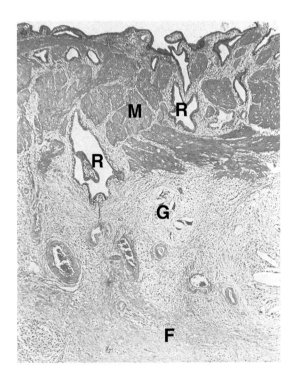

Fig. 14.13 Chronic cholecystitis (LP)

Many gallbladders containing stones are removed surgically because of abdominal pain. On histological examination, there is evidence of low grade chronic inflammation with marked muscle hypertrophy **M** and an infiltrate of lymphocytes and plasma cells in the submucosal layer. Irregular gland-like mucosal pockets extend deep into the thickened muscle layer and are known as *Rokitansky–Aschoff sinuses* **R**.

Outside the muscle layer, aggregates of histiocytes form around inspissated bile, forming *bile granulomas* **G**. There is fibrosis **F** and mild chronic inflammation beneath the serosa.

If bile becomes inspissated and concentrated within the gallbladder, it may cause an acute chemical cholecystitis with a more neutrophilic inflammatory component and often extensive haemorrhage within the gallbladder wall.

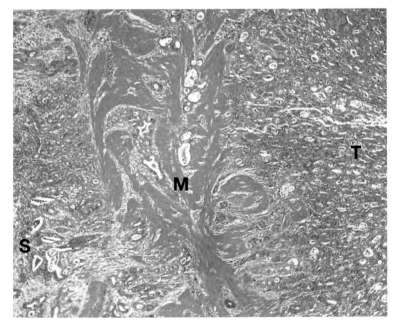

Fig. 14.14 Carcinoma of gallbladder (LP)

Carcinoma of the gallbladder occurs in the elderly. The photomicrograph shows the gallbladder mucosa replaced by adenocarcinoma with a glandular pattern **T**. Invasion has occurred through the submucosa into the muscle layer **M** of the gallbladder and beyond into the outer serosa **S**. On the aspect of the gallbladder where the serosa is loosely attached to the liver, direct tumour invasion into the liver occurs, usually rendering the tumour inoperable.

Similar carcinomas can also occur in the intrahepatic and extrahepatic bile ducts (*intrahepatic* and *extrahepatic cholangiocarcinomas*); these tumours usually cause early obstructive jaundice, but tumours in the gallbladder rarely cause obstruction to the bile flow and therefore usually present late in the disease.

Pancreatic disorders

Inflammation of the pancreas (*pancreatitis*) may present in acute or chronic form. *Acute pancreatitis* has a high mortality partly because of the release of pancreatic enzymes into surrounding tissues causing severe local tissue destruction and is discussed in Figure 14.15. *Chronic pancreatitis* is frequently associated with intractable pain and in some cases causes chronic pancreatic insufficiency.

Malignant disease of the pancreas is now appearing with increasing frequency; these *adenocarcinomas* (Fig. 14.16) are highly malignant and metastases are almost always present by the time of diagnosis.

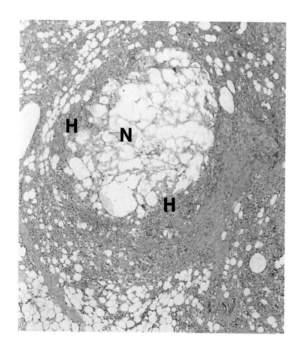

Fig. 14.15 Fat necrosis in acute pancreatitis (MP

Acute pancreatitis is a condition in which there is destruction of the pancreas because of liberation of pancreatic enzymes. Severe cases result in a massive chemical peritonitis causing severe abdominal pain and shock. The two most important predisposing conditions are alcohol abuse and biliary tract disease (usually stones).

Histologically, there is extensive haemorrhagic necrosis of the pancreas and surrounding tissues. Release of pancreatic enzymes gives rise to a characteristic feature termed *fat necrosis*. With the naked eye, numerous chalky-white spots are seen in peripancreatic and omental fat. Histologically, they represent foci of necrotic adipose tissue **N**, surrounded by a rim of foamy histiocytes **H** which contain phagocytosed lipid within their cytoplasm.

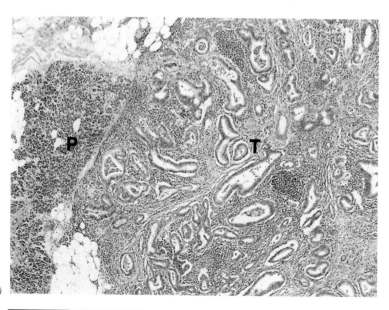

(a)

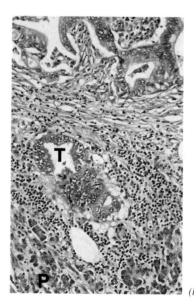

(b)

Fig. 14.16 Adenocarcinoma of the pancreas
(a) LP (b) HP

Pancreatic adenocarcinomas virtually all arise from the pancreatic ductal epithelium and are of great importance because of their insidious manner of growth, often remaining undetected until a very advanced stage. Most arise in the head of the gland where they tend to obstruct the bile duct, thus presenting with painless jaundice. Tumours arising from the islets of Langerhans belong to the neuroendocrine group of tumours (Fig. 13.17) although they are usually named according to their

secretory products, for example insulinoma, glucagonoma.

Macroscopically, pancreatic adenocarcinomas are hard and white. Micrograph (a) shows tumour **T** with normal pancreas **P** on the left. Note the characteristic tortuous, irregular glands in a dense fibrous stroma. At higher magnification in micrograph (b), the tumour is seen to have a ductular pattern, with marked variation in size and shape of neoplastic glands.

15. Urinary system

Introduction

The **urinary tract** comprises the kidneys, pelvicalyceal systems, ureters, bladder and urethra. The kidney is responsible for the excretion of waste products from body metabolic processes, the waste products being excreted in the form of an aqueous solution called **urine**. The urine passes from the kidney into the pelvicalyceal systems and thence via the ureter to the bladder, which acts as a reservoir. Urine is held in the bladder by a series of muscular sphincters until sufficient volume has accumulated. Relaxation of the sphincters and contraction of smooth muscle in the bladder wall allows the urine to be voided to the exterior through the urethra (**micturition**) at a convenient time.

The kidney

Disorders of the kidney arise from a wide range of pathological causes, many of which are common in other organ systems (e.g. infections, tumours, drug reactions, vascular disorders). However, the kidney is unusual in that it is much more prone to immunological disorders than most other organs and is of the greatest importance in the progress of the common metabolic disease, diabetes mellitus. Vascular diseases such as hypertension and vasculitis may also have profound effects on renal function. Disorders of the kidney can be conveniently divided into categories according to which structural component of the kidney is primarily affected:

Glomerulus

- **Glomerulonephritis** of various types, most of which are due to deposition of immunoglobulins and/or complement components (collectively called **immune complexes**) within the glomerulus.
- **Vasculitis** – strictly speaking this is a vascular disorder, but some forms affect the glomerular capillaries giving the clinical and pathological appearances of a glomerulonephritis.
- **Diabetes mellitus** – deposition of abnormal glycosylated proteins causes irreversible structural and functional abnormalities in the glomerulus (see Fig. 15.9).
- **Amyloidosis** – deposition of amyloid proteins in the glomerulus alters the structure and therefore the function of the glomerulus.

Tubules and interstitium

- **Acute tubular necrosis** is usually due to profound hypotension causing ischaemic damage to tubular epithelial cells.
- **Infections** including acute pyelonephritis, renal abscess and TB.
- **Drug toxicity** usually causes tubulo-interstitial nephritis due to a hypersensitivity reaction, but other patterns may occur including direct toxicity to tubular epithelial cells.
- **Mechanical obstruction** of the ureters or bladder may lead to **hydronephrosis**.

Blood vessels

- **Hypertension** causes marked changes to both large and small renal vessels.
- **Vasculitis** may affect larger vessels as well as glomerular capillaries.

Irreversible damage to one component of the kidney inevitably damages the other parts leading eventually to *chronic renal failure*, a condition invariably fatal until the advent of renal dialysis and transplantation. Severe reversible damage to any of the above components of the kidney may lead to *acute renal failure*.

- **Chronic renal failure** – progressive retention of nitrogenous metabolites manifest as a slow rise in serum creatinine levels owing to insufficient glomerular filtration. Concomitant failure of tubular function produces widespread abnormalities in biochemical homeostasis, including salt and water retention, metabolic acidosis, and other electrolyte imbalances, particularly hyperkalaemia.
- **Acute renal failure** – abrupt cessation of activity of the nephrons usually manifest initially as a marked fall in urine production (*oliguria*) which may even be total (*anuria*). This is accompanied by an abrupt rise in urea and potassium. Disturbances of fluid and electrolyte balance soon follow, particularly a rise in the serum potassium level and metabolic acidosis.

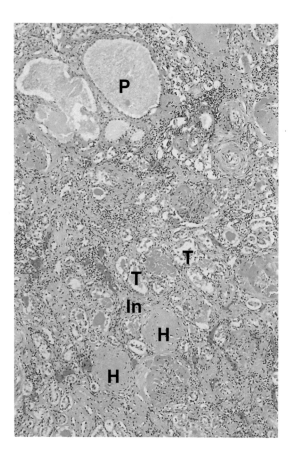

Fig. 15.1 End-stage kidney (MP)

Many progressive renal diseases of greatly differing pathogenesis are followed by progressive nephron destruction paralleled clinically by insidious deterioration of renal function, culminating in chronic renal failure. Macroscopically, the kidneys are usually found to be small and firm with symmetrical atrophic thinning of the cortex and poor demarcation of cortex from medulla. This condition is known as *end-stage kidney*. In both gross and histological appearance, there is often little clue to the original renal pathology.

In the cortex, there is widespread replacement of glomerular tufts by avascular, acellular hyaline material **H** (*hyalinisation*). The cortical tubules **T** also become shrunken and atrophic and the relatively expanded interstitial spaces **In** undergo fibrosis; some atrophic tubules may become cystically dilated with *casts* of inspissated proteinaceous material **P** which is highly eosinophilic (pink-staining) and thus often called *thyroidisation*. The shrunken cortex is sometimes marked by scars, formerly attributed to chronic infection; this is now believed to contribute to only a small proportion of cases and most of the scars are probably ischaemic in origin.

Diseases of the glomerulus

Glomerular disorders are a source of endless fascination for renal pathologists and unbounded confusion to almost everyone else. There are two major causes of glomerular disease: ***immunological*** (including disorders confined to the kidney and systemic diseases) and ***metabolic*** (the most important being diabetes mellitus). It is confusing to many students that there is not a direct one-to-one relationship between a particular mechanism of damage and a particular histological appearance and/or clinical syndrome. In fact, most causes of glomerular damage will give rise to one of five clinical syndromes, namely: nephritic syndrome, nephrotic syndrome, mixed nephritic–nephrotic syndrome, asymptomatic haematuria and asymptomatic proteinuria. Acute and chronic renal failure are described above and may supervene in any of the above conditions. For example, an individual with a very severe nephritic syndrome may progress quickly to acute renal failure or an individual with undiagnosed diabetes, who has had undetected proteinuria for some time, may first be diagnosed in chronic renal failure. These clinical conditions are summarised in Figure 15.2 along with the glomerular diseases with which they are most commonly associated.

Fig. 15.2 Clinical syndromes associated with glomerular diseases

Clinical syndrome	Clinical features	Pathophysiology	Most common examples
Acute nephritis	Haematuria Hypertension Uraemia ($\uparrow$ BUN) Oedema (often periorbital) Oliguria or anuria	Hypercellular glomerulus with obstructed capillary loops, reduced blood flow, reduced urine output. May progress to crescent formation and acute renal failure	Diffuse proliferative glomerulonephritis (GN) (post–streptococcal GN, other infections) Systemic lupus erythematosus (SLE) Vasculitis Goodpasture's syndrome
Nephrotic syndrome	Proteinuria (> 3.5gm/24h) Hypoalbuminaemia Oedema Hyperlipidaemia	Changes to the structure of the glomerular filtration mechanism – most often the glomerular basement membrane	Diabetes mellitus Amyloidosis Minimal change nephropathy Focal segmental glomerulosclerosis (FSGS) Membranous nephropathy SLE
Mixed nephritic–nephrotic syndrome	Features of both nephritic and nephrotic syndromes	Both cellular proliferation and glomerular basement membrane alterations	Mesangiocapillary GN (membranoproliferative GN) SLE
Asymptomatic haematuria	Periodic dark coloured urine or microscopic haematuria Insidious hypertension	Proliferation of glomerular cells or structural abnormalities of basement membrane	IgA nephropathy Thin basement membrane disease SLE
Asymptomatic proteinuria	Proteinuria	Early stages of the changes in the basement membrane	Early phases of all of the conditions which cause nephrotic syndrome

Role of renal biopsy

The introduction of safe and reliable techniques of percutaneous needle biopsy of the kidney has greatly increased knowledge about the natural history of renal diseases, particularly by elucidating the underlying lesion early in the course of glomerular diseases when treatment might be effectively applied. It is of limited value in chronic renal failure when the kidney is shrunken and histological changes are non-specific, i.e. **end-stage kidney** (see Fig. 15.1). Renal biopsy is also frequently used in the assessment of renal transplants to detect the presence of transplant rejection, drug toxicity and a number of other conditions which may cause reduced function of the graft. Maximum information is obtained from a needle biopsy of renal tissue using a combination of the following methods:

- *light microscopy* including special stains to define glomerular structures
- *electron microscopy* to show the presence and precise location of immune complexes, which appear as irregular deposits of electron-dense material (*dense deposits*)
- *immunofluoresence microscopy* to localise and identify the class of immunoglobulins and complement components.

The immunofluoresence and electron microscopic patterns of immune complex deposition can be vital to differentiate between different types of glomerulonephritis which have similar patterns of glomerular damage by light microscopy. Examples include:

- **IgA nephropathy** – granular deposits of IgA in the mesangium
- **Membranous nephropathy** – granular deposits of IgG +/- complement on the epithelial side of the glomerular basement membrane (GBM)
- **Goodpasture's syndrome** – linear deposits of IgG along the GBM
- **Systemic lupus erythematosus** – deposits of most classes of immunoglobulin and many complement components at any site in the glomerulus
- **Mesangiocapillary glomerulonephritis type I** – granular deposits of complement component 3 (C3) on the endothelial side of the GBM.

Glomerulonephritis

Most types of glomerulonephritis (GN) are caused by immune complex deposition in the glomerulus. This applies to **primary glomerulonephritis** where the condition is confined to the kidney (e.g. **membranous nephropathy, mesangiocapillary GN**) and to diseases with a systemic component, for example **Goodpasture's syndrome, systemic lupus erythematosus, Henoch–Schönlein purpura**). The site of immune complex deposition is dependent on the size of the complexes, which is in turn dependent on the type of antigen and on the class of immunoglobulin produced; that is to say the host response. The antigen may be either a normal component of the body (a self antigen as in Goodpasture's) or an external antigen such as a bacterial product (as in **post-streptococcal GN**). Immune complexes may be deposited from the circulating blood or may be formed in situ. In the latter situation, the complexes may involve intrinsic glomerular antigens (basement membrane components in Goodpasture's) or antigens which have been deposited there from the circulation (e.g. DNA in the case of SLE). An important exception to this rule is minimal change nephropathy where the podocytes are thought to be damaged by a cell-mediated immune response rather than by immune complex deposition. Whatever the mechanism of damage to the glomerulus, the various immunological insults alter the structure and therefore the function of the glomerulus and ultimately of the nephron as a whole.

In response to damaging stimuli, the glomerulus appears to react in one or more of the following ways:

- swelling and/or proliferation of the normally flat endothelial cells lining the glomerular capillaries
- proliferation of the epithelial cells investing the outer surface of the glomerular capillary tuft (the podocytes) and the cells lining Bowman's capsule (*crescent formation*)
- thickening of glomerular basement membranes
- proliferation of the cells of the mesangium and excessive production of acellular mesangial material.

These reactions give rise to various histological patterns of glomerulonephritis, which can be identified by light microscopy. This is then put together with the immunofluorescence and electron microscopy findings, clinical history and other investigations to come to a definitive diagnosis. As in many other areas of histopathology, good communications between pathologist and clinician are vital to arrive at an accurate diagnosis, which is essential for appropriate treatment.

Glomerulonephritis is first divided into:

- **Diffuse** – affecting all glomeruli
- **Focal** – affecting some glomeruli
- **Global** – the entire glomerulus is abnormal
- **Segmental** – only part of the glomerulus is abnormal.

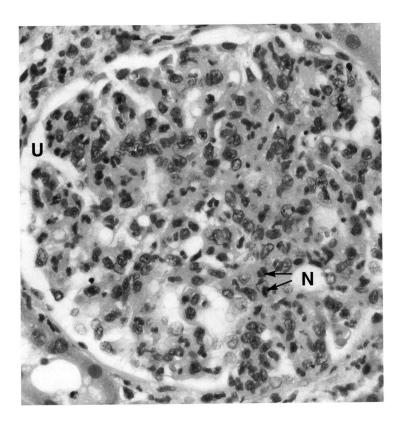

Fig. 15.3 Acute proliferative ('endocapillary') glomerulonephritis (HP)

This form of global diffuse glomerulonephritis most commonly occurs in children and often follows a streptococcal infection, usually of the throat. As seen in this micrograph, the cellularity of the glomerulus is increased owing to swelling and proliferation of endothelial cells which have virtually obliterated the capillary lumina; neutrophils **N** are also present in the glomerular tufts and there is usually also some degree of mesangial cell proliferation. The urinary space **U** remains clear since there has been no proliferation of podocytes. The obstruction of glomerular capillary lumina diminishes glomerular filtration and causes leakage of erythrocytes; hence this condition usually presents with haematuria, transient hypertension and oedema, i.e. the *acute nephritic syndrome*.

A similar pattern of glomerular damage may occur in SLE, Goodpasture's syndrome and rarely in vasculitis. In severe cases, from whatever cause, crescentic glomerulonephritis may be superimposed.

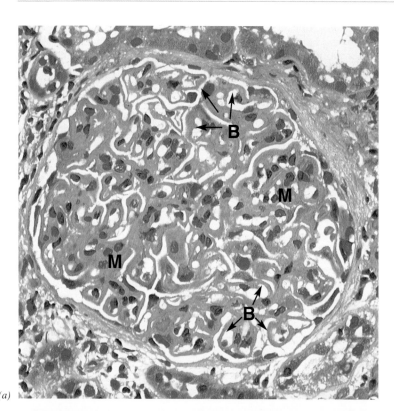

(a)

Fig.15.4 **Membranous nephropathy** (*caption on facing page above*)

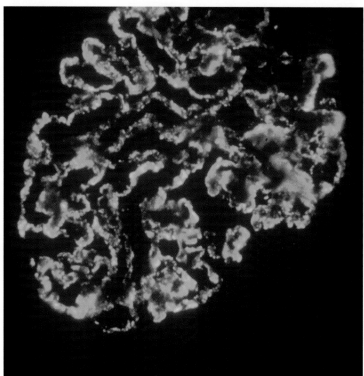

(b)

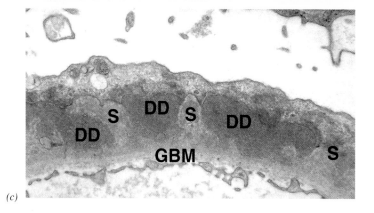

(c)

Membranous nephropathy is a diffuse global pattern of glomerular injury where damage to the glomerular basement membrane leads to proteinuria and often the nephrotic syndrome. This pattern may arise in a variety of situations. *Primary* or *idiopathic membranous nephropathy* accounts for about 85% of cases. The identical pattern of injury, known as *secondary membranous nephropathy*, may arise in individuals with malignant tumours elsewhere in the body (5–10% of cases), individuals taking certain drugs (gold, penicillamine, captopril and non-steroidal anti-inflammatory drugs) and in certain infections (hepatitis B and C, malaria). A third important category is the autoimmune disease SLE which can give rise to almost any pattern of glomerular damage (see Fig. 15.2).

In membranous nephropathy, immune complexes are deposited on the epithelial side of the glomerular basement membrane (sub-epithelial deposits). These deposits induce deposition of additional basement membrane material between the deposits giving rise to the pathognomonic 'spikes' on the outer surface of the basement membrane which can be seen with the silver stain by light microscopy or by electron microscopy (micrograph (c)). By light microscopy (a), the basement membranes **B** appear thick, eosinophilic and sometimes slightly refractile. There is no associated endothelial or epithelial (podocyte) proliferation although there may be a slight increase in mesangial material **M** in severe and longstanding cases. The immune complexes in most cases of membranous nephropathy consist of IgG and complement (C3). Obviously the antigen in the immune complexes will depend on the underlying cause (e.g. DNA in SLE, viral antigens in hepatitis, probably self-antigens in the idiopathic form). Micrograph (b) shows the characteristic immunofluorescence pattern of membranous nephropathy. An antibody specific for IgG and labelled with fluorescein is incubated with a section of kidney. The antibody binds to IgG deposited in the kidney. This micrograph demonstrates IgG as bright green fluorescent granular deposits incorporated on the epithelial surface of the glomerular basement membranes. Micrograph (c) is a high power electron micrograph of a glomerular basement membrane. The glomerular basement membrane **GBM** has additional spikes of basement membrane material **S** on the epithelial side. Between the spikes dense deposits (immune complexes) **DD** are easily identified. The presence of the immune complexes probably activates complement which, by means of the membrane attack complex, damages the glomerular basement membrane allowing leakage of protein.

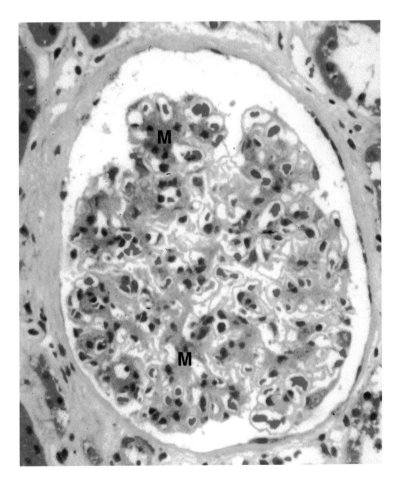

Fig. 15.5 Mesangioproliferative glomerulonephritis

This pattern of glomerular disease is characterised by a diffuse increase in mesangial matrix and variable degrees of increased mesangial cellularity without basement membrane abnormality. This pattern of glomerular damage is characteristic of IgA nephropathy and the related condition Henoch–Schönlein purpura (HSP). Both may present with asymptomatic haematuria or nephritic syndrome. The renal changes of HSP are identical to those in IgA disease, but in HSP there is a typical vasculitic rash plus or minus gastrointestinal symptoms and signs. Immunofluorescence staining reveals deposits of IgA in the mesangium and there are corresponding dense mesangial deposits by electron microscopy. Acute exacerbations of IgA nephropathy may develop segmental necrotising glomerulonephritis (Fig. 15.8) and even occasionally crescentic glomerulonephritis (Fig. 15.7). Healing of these lesions leads to secondary focal segmental glomerulosclerosis (see Fig. 15.8b).

Other conditions which may have a similar light microscopic appearance (but different immunological and electron microscopy findings) are resolving acute proliferative. glomerulonephritis and SLE.

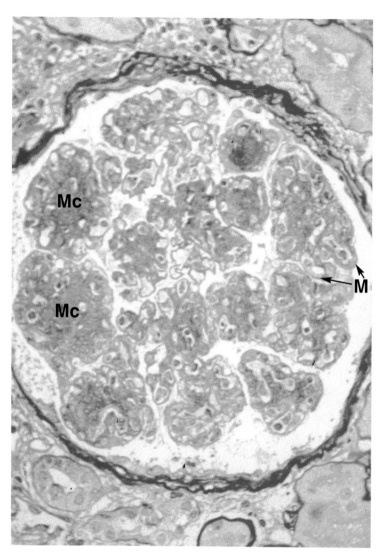

Fig. 15.6 Mesangiocapillary (membranoproliferative) glomerulonephritis – PAS (HP)

This pattern of glomerulonephritis may be either primary or occur in association with SLE. The clinical presentation is either nephrotic syndrome or mixed nephrotic–nephritic syndrome. *Primary mesangiocapillary glomerulonephritis (MCGN)* is divided into *type I* and *type II*, both having a similar appearance by light microscopy. Readily visible, as in this micrograph, is the expansion of each segment of the glomerulus producing an exaggerated lobular appearance. The characteristic feature is reduplication of the glomerular basement membrane **M** with interposition of mesangial cells between the two layers. There is increased mesangial cellularity and matrix *Mc*. White blood cells also infiltrate the glomerulus and there is often mild endothelial cell proliferation. In MCGN type I, dense deposits composed of C3 +/– IgG, are found in the subendothelial position. Type II MCGN is characterised by deposition of a ribbon of dense material of unknown composition in the glomerular basement membrane giving rise to the alternative name of *dense deposit disease*.

This pattern of glomerulonephritis is also commonly seen in SLE where it may have additional features including immunoglobulin deposits in all parts of the glomerular basement membrane and in the mesangium, 'wire-loop lesions', a mixed pattern of immunoglobulins and complement deposition, and superimposed membranous or segmental patterns of glomerulonephritis.

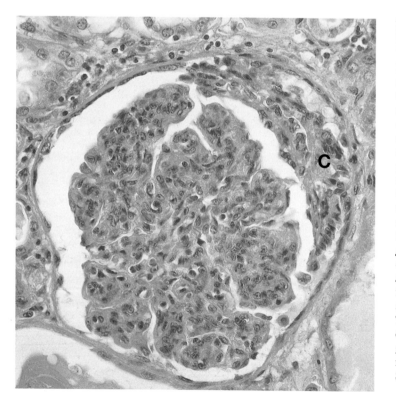

Fig. 15.7 Acute crescentic glomerulonephritis (HP)

In many types of glomerular disease, there is proliferation of podocytes and the epithelial cells lining Bowman's capsule. Proliferation of Bowman's capsule cells around only part of the circumference of the capsule produces a so-called *crescent* **C**. Continued proliferation of the crescent may obliterate the glomerular tuft, leading to irreversible glomerular destruction and subsequent nephron atrophy, with rapidly progressive renal failure. This is known as *rapidly progressive glomerulonephritis* and is characteristic of *Goodpasture's syndrome* where autoantibodies are formed which react with glomerular and alveolar basement membranes. The formation of crescents may also occur in acute proliferative glomerulonephritis, segmental necrotising glomerulonephritis and SLE.

Fig. 15.8 Focal segmental glomerulonephritis

(a) Segmental necrotising glomerulonephritis (HP) (b) Focal segmental glomerulosclerosis (HP)

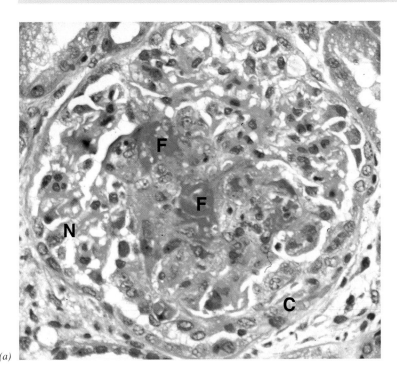

(a)

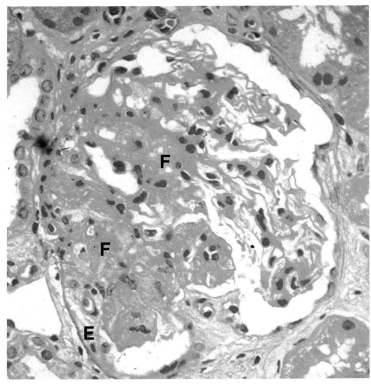

(b)

Focal segmental glomerulonephritis occurs in two related patterns. In contrast to the diffuse and global types of glomerulonephritis mentioned above, these lesions affect only a proportion of the glomeruli (focal) and only part of the glomeruli (segmental).

In segmental necrotising glomerulonephritis (a), a segment of the glomerular tuft becomes necrotic with invasion by neutrophils and deposition of fibrin **F**. Adjacent segments are normal **N** or nearly normal (depending on the underlying disease). Segmental necrosis is often associated with proliferation of epithelial cells of Bowman's capsule, which may progress to frank crescent formation. An early crescent **C** is seen here. Large numbers of crescents are associated with a poor prognosis. This pattern of glomerulonephritis is found in glomerular involvement in IgA disease, systemic vasculitis, SLE and some cases of Goodpasture's syndrome. Segmental necrotising lesions heal by fibrosis, leaving a lesion very similar to focal segmental glomerulosclerosis (FSGS).

FSGS (b) may occur as a primary glomerulonephritis or secondary to other lesions such as those mentioned above. In addition, almost any lesion that causes marked loss of nephrons may induce secondary FSGS. The histological lesion in all these situations is similar. Segments of some glomeruli are replaced by mesangial matrix **F** (*sclerosis*). The sclerotic segment is adherent to a mass of proliferated epithelial cells **E** some of which have foamy cytoplasm. *Hyalinosis*, the deposition of plasma proteins to give a bland eosinophilic mass, is also commonly a feature of these lesions, although not demonstrated in this example.

While focal necrotising glomerulonephritis presents with haematuria or a nephritic syndrome, FSGS is characterised by proteinuria which may progress to nephrotic syndrome. Both of these lesions may be seen in SLE.

BASIC SYSTEMS PATHOLOGY

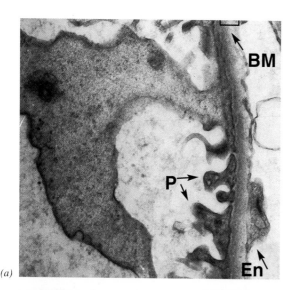

(a)

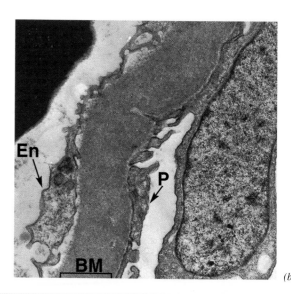

(b)

Fig. 15.9 Diabetic glomerulosclerosis *(illustrations (c) (d) and (e) opposite)*
(a) Normal glomerular basement membrane (EM)   (b) Diabetic basement membrane (EM)
(c) Nodular glomerulosclerosis (HP)   (d) Diffuse glomerulosclerosis (HP)   (e) Capsular drop – PAS (HP)

In diabetes mellitus, renal disease may occur in several ways. Diabetics have an increased predisposition to the development of renal infections such as pyelonephritis (Fig. 15.10) and papillary necrosis (Fig. 15.11), as well as a tendency to severe large vessel atherosclerosis increasing the risk of renal ischaemia and infarction.

Longstanding diabetes mellitus may result in characteristic changes to the glomeruli (*diabetic glomerulosclerosis*). Among the early glomerular changes is a uniform and homogeneous thickening of the glomerular capillary basement membrane. This is best seen by electron microscopy as in micrograph (b), with the normal shown for comparison in micrograph (a). In both micrographs, note the glomerular capillary basement membrane **BM** invested by thin endothelial cell cytoplasm **En** on the inner aspect, and by epithelial cell (podocyte) foot processes **P** externally. In diabetes, the basement membrane may be up to 4 or 5 times normal thickness.

Later, there is an increase in mesangial matrix, the latter often segmental and localised to produce characteristic acellular *Kimmelstiel–Wilson nodules*, often with compressed mesangial cell nuclei pushed to their periphery. This is called *nodular diabetic glomerulosclerosis* and is shown in micrograph (c); note the Kimmelstiel–Wilson nodules **K**.

In another pattern, the mesangial matrix increase is diffuse and global, not segmental and nodular, producing the change called *diffuse diabetic glomerulosclerosis*,

illustrated in micrograph (d). Both patterns may occur in the same kidney, and nodule formation may be superimposed upon the diffuse change within the same glomerulus. In both patterns, there is escape of plasma protein across the thickened but leaky glomerular capillary wall into the urinary space. Occasionally, inspissated protein may be deposited on the outer surface of the glomerular tuft forming *fibrin caps* **FC** as seen in micrograph (d) or on the inner surface of Bowman's capsule forming *capsular drops* **C** as seen in micrograph (e).

A characteristic feature of diabetic renal disease is *hyalinisation* of arterioles similar to that seen in hypertension (Fig. 15.12) but characteristically affecting both afferent and efferent arterioles. This arteriolar hyalinisation **H**, well shown in association with nodular diabetic glomerulosclerosis in micrograph (c), may also extend into the vascular hilum of the glomerulus. The combination of arterial atherosclerosis and arteriolar hyalinisation progressively reduces the blood flow to the glomeruli; thus chronic ischaemic changes, such as hyalinisation of glomeruli and periglomerular fibrosis, are common associated findings in diabetic renal disease.

The initial glomerular basement membrane changes result in proteinuria and even the nephrotic syndrome, but with progressive diabetic glomerulosclerosis and chronic ischaemic nephron atrophy, the features of chronic renal failure supervene. Acute pyelonephritis (Fig. 15.10) or renal papillary necrosis (Fig. 15.11) may precipitate acute renal failure.

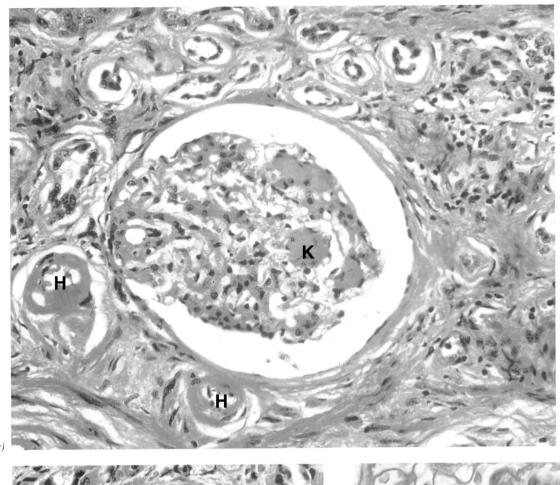

(c)

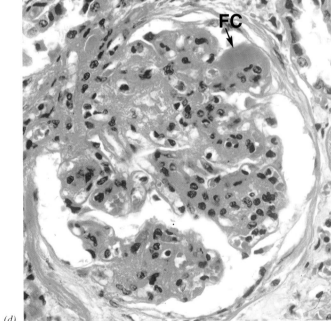

(d)

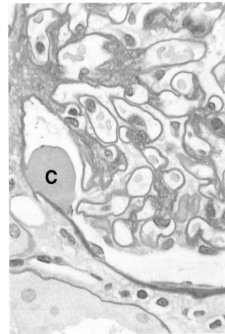

(e)

Fig. 15.9 Diabetic glomerulosclerosis *(caption opposite)*

Outcome of glomerular disorders

The renal disorders in which the major abnormality involves the glomerulus may subside spontaneously or with treatment. However, if they progress, glomerular blood flow is obstructed, glomerular filtration ceases and the tubules associated with affected glomeruli become involved; thus many nephrons may cease to function. When sufficient nephrons have been affected, the clinical features of the disease gradually progress to chronic renal failure.

By way of illustration, a patient with the nephrotic syndrome caused by diabetic glomerular disease may slowly develop the features of chronic renal failure as individual nephrons are destroyed. In contrast, a patient who initially presents with the acute nephritic syndrome caused by a rapidly progressive crescentic glomerulonephritis (Fig. 15.7) may quickly progress to acute renal failure as the glomeruli are rapidly destroyed by the disease process.

Disorders of the renal tubule and interstitium

The tubules and interstitium may be primarily damaged as a result of hypovolaemic shock, by inorganic and organic toxins, or as the result of infection. In hypovolaemic states and intoxication, tubular epithelial cells may exhibit marked cytoplasmic degenerative changes or frank necrosis leading to the pathological term *acute tubular necrosis* (Fig. 1.4) and producing the clinical syndrome of acute renal failure. Tubular epithelial cells have considerable powers of recovery and regeneration, and acute renal failure may be reversible under such circumstances if the patient can be sustained in the interim by dialysis and other supporting measures.

Another increasingly important cause of tubulointerstitial disease is drug toxicity giving rise to interstitial nephritis. In this condition, certain drugs have been implicated including certain antibiotics, non-steroidal anti-inflammatory drugs, thiazide diuretics and cimetidine. Onset may be acute or chronic. There is a mixed inflammatory infiltrate in the interstitium in which eosinophils may be prominent. Tubular damage occurs and the condition may proceed to chronic renal failure.

Infections of the kidney include acute and chronic pyelonephritis (see Fig. 15.10) and tuberculosis (see Ch. 4). Acute suppurative bacterial infections of the kidney (*pyelonephritis*) usually follow ascending infection from the lower urinary tract, particularly when there is obstruction to urinary outflow such as in benign prostatic hyperplasia or pressure from the fetus in pregnancy; in such cases, coliform organisms (such as *Escherichia coli* and *Proteus* species) are the most frequent infecting agents. Infection may also arise in the kidney by the haematogenous route during episodes of bacteraemia. Acute pyelonephritis may be complicated by the development of papillary necrosis (Fig. 15.11) or pus accumulation in a dilated, obstructed pelvicalyceal system (**pyonephrosis**). Acute pyelonephritis is illustrated in Figure 15.10. Tuberculous infection of the kidneys and lower urinary tract may also arise by similar routes of spread; renal tuberculosis is shown in Figure 4.7.

Patients with urinary reflux or obstruction are prone to develop recurrent pyelonephritis; repeated attacks lead to scarring and after many episodes the kidney becomes coarsely scarred, a phenomenon termed *chronic pyelonephritis*.

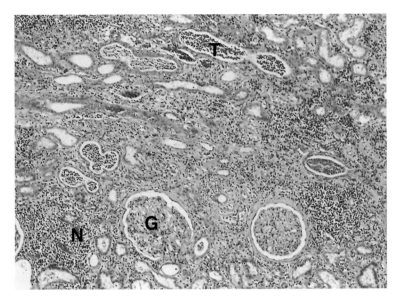

Fig. 15.10 Acute pyelonephritis (HP)

This micrograph illustrates established acute pyelonephritis. There is extensive infiltration of the kidney by small dark-staining neutrophil polymorphs **N**, which are also seen filling dilated tubules **T**. Abscess formation may ensue and, in untreated cases, multiple abscesses may merge to produce larger abscesses. These may discharge into the pelvicalyceal system to produce *pyonephrosis*, or through the capsule into perinephric fat to produce a *perinephric abscess*. Note that the glomeruli **G** are spared.

Vascular disorders

The kidney is especially vulnerable to the effects of arterial hypertension as seen in Figures 11.9 and 11.10, and irreversible damage to nephrons may result either acutely from accelerated hypertension or progressively over a period of years in benign essential hypertension. *Hypertensive nephrosclerosis* resulting from benign essential hypertension is illustrated in Figure 15.12a. Malignant or accelerated hypertension causes a different pattern of renal damage, which is very similar to the changes seen in acute *scleroderma*, and may result in acute renal failure.

Various forms of vasculitis including *polyarteritis nodosa* (Fig. 11.18), *microscopic polyarteritis* (Fig. 11.19 and Wegener's granulomatosis also affect the kidney. Analgesic abuse nephropathy owing to overuse of analgesic mixtures is characterised by a chronic interstitial nephritis and papillary necrosis.

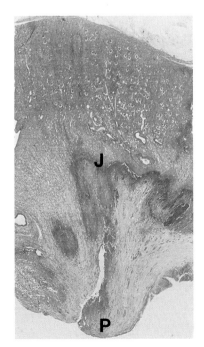

Fig. 15.11 Renal papillary necrosis (LP)

This low power micrograph shows the condition known as *papillary necrosis* or *necrotising papillitis*. The tip of the papilla **P** undergoes necrosis of a coagulative type, with preservation of ghost-like outlines of the papillary tubules and collecting ducts. In the early stages, there is a neutrophil inflammatory response at the junction **J** between normal and necrotic papillae but this largely disappears at a later stage when the necrotic papilla separates and is shed. This condition, which is probably ischaemic in nature, often occurs in association with acute infection of the urinary parenchyma and pelvicalyceal system, particularly when accompanied by an obstructive lesion in the lower urinary tract. It may also be seen with or without overt infection in diabetic nephropathy and in analgesic nephropathy. If there is sudden loss of many papillae, the patient may develop acute renal failure.

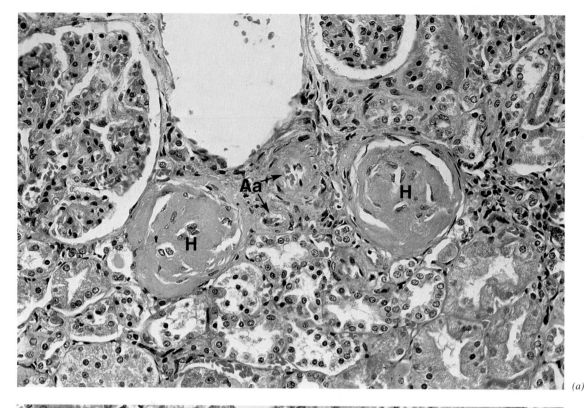

(a)

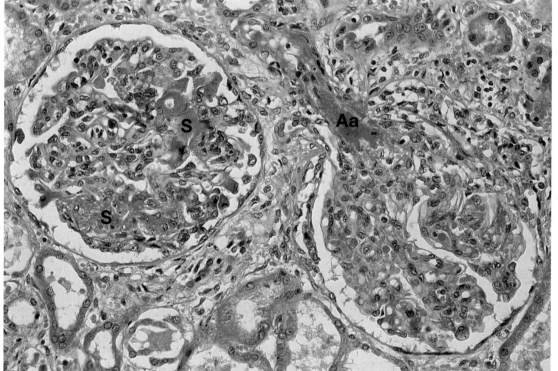

(b)

Fig. 15.12 Hypertensive nephrosclerosis *(caption opposite)*

Fig. 15.12 Hypertensive nephrosclerosis
(a) Benign hypertensive nephrosclerosis (HP)   (b) Malignant hypertensive nephrosclerosis (HP)

The vessel changes in systemic hypertension have been discussed and illustrated in some detail in Figures 11.9 and 11.10. The kidney is particularly vulnerable to the damaging effects of these vessel changes and renal failure is an important complication of untreated hypertension. The pathological changes in the kidney depend on the severity and rate of progress of the hypertension.

In *benign (essential) hypertension*, the hypertension is of gradual onset and progression with only moderately elevated diastolic pressure. Large and medium-sized renal arteries show marked thickening of their walls by a combination of medial hypertrophy, elastic lamina reduplication and fibrous intimal thickening; this is shown in Figure 11.9a; arterioles show hyaline thickening of their walls as seen in Figure 11.9b. These changes reduce the calibre of all renal afferent vessels and the resulting chronic ischaemia leads to progressive *sclerosis (hyalinisation)* of the glomerulus and subsequent disuse atrophy of the tubular component of the nephron.

Micrograph (a) shows a group of glomeruli, two of which have become converted into hyaline amorphous pink-staining masses **H** as a result of chronic ischaemia owing to hyalinisation of the walls of their afferent arterioles **Aa**; the other glomeruli are as yet unaffected. Slowly progressive loss of functioning nephrons may eventually lead to chronic renal failure and the morphological state known as end-stage kidney (Fig. 15.1).

In contrast, in *malignant (accelerated) hypertension*, where the rise in blood pressure is rapid and severe, the arterial and arteriolar changes are different. Large and medium-sized arteries may show only concentric thickening of the intima by loose, rather myxomatous, fibroblastic tissue as seen in Figure 11.10a, and there is no elastic lamina reduplication or significant medial hypertrophy. Small arteries may show marked concentric fibroblastic intimal thickening so that the lumen is often virtually obliterated. Arterioles frequently show patchy acute necrosis of their walls with the accumulation of amorphous, brightly eosinophilic proteinaceous material (*fibrinoid*) in the damaged walls; this is shown in Figure 11.10b. This change is known as *fibrinoid necrosis*. In the kidney as seen in micrograph (b), this often affects the afferent arterioles **Aa** at the glomerular hila and may extend into the glomerular tuft to affect some segments **S** of the glomerular capillary network. The onset of small vessel changes is acute and may produce an abrupt reduction in blood supply to the nephrons, often producing glomerular micro-infarction and tubular epithelial necrosis. The effect is to produce a catastrophic reduction in glomerular filtration, and the patient may develop acute oliguric or anuric renal failure. Not infrequently, the patient with longstanding benign hypertension may suddenly develop an accelerated phase, and the histological changes in the kidney may be those of mixed benign and malignant nephrosclerosis.

Pathology of renal transplantation

Renal transplantation has become a routine treatment for chronic renal failure in many countries. The transplant recipient is freed from a life of regular dialysis with a consequent improvement in quality of life. The function of the transplanted kidney may however be affected by a number of factors in the days, weeks and months following transplantation. The most important of these include:

- **Acute tubular necrosis** – this is identical to acute tubular necrosis from other causes (see Fig. 1.4). The major factor here is the 'cold ischaemic time', i.e. the length of time between harvesting of the kidney and re-establishment of vascular perfusion in the donor. Supportive measures may be needed in the immediate post-transplantation phase but usually this will resolve.
- **Rejection** – see Figure 15.13
- **Drug toxicity** – routinely used immunosuppressive agents, such as cyclosporin A and related compounds, may have a range of effects on the kidney. Histologically, there may be changes in the tubules and/or the blood vessels. Exquisite control of dosage and sometimes transfer to a different agent will usually control this problem.
- **Infection**
- **Recurrent glomerulonephritis.**

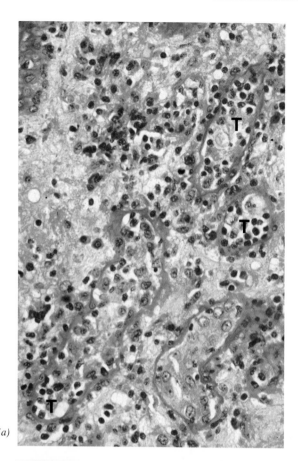

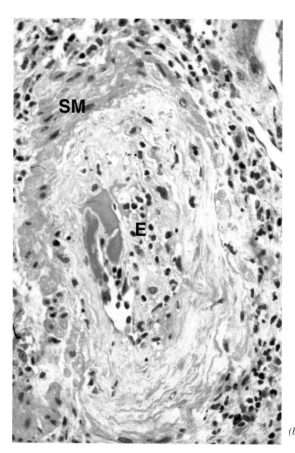

Fig. 15.13 Renal transplant rejection
(a) Acute cellular rejection (MP) (b) Acute vascular rejection (HP)

Rejection of a transplanted kidney or other organ, depends mainly on the degree of *human leucocyte antigen (HLA)* matching between donor and recipient. Obviously transplantation between identical twins has the best chance of success but this is rarely feasible. Tissue typing is routinely carried out on potential donors to identify recipients with the closest HLA match.

The Banff classification, designed by a panel of renal pathologists in Banff in Canada, is a semi-quantitative method for assessing rejection. Various features of rejection are graded numerically and the scores combined to classify according to the type and degree of severity of rejection. The classification is used for international trials of transplant immunosuppression and is regularly reviewed and updated.

Renal transplant rejection may be divided into four main categories:

- **Hyperacute rejection** (antibody-mediated) – occurs within minutes to an hour of transplantation and appears to be the result of preformed recipient antibodies binding to donor endothelial cells in the graft. Intravascular thrombosis quickly follows and the kidney becomes dusky (a feature which may be seen on the operating table) and infarcts. Treatment is generally ineffective.
- **Acute cellular rejection** (Banff type 1) – occurs within days to months after transplantation. As shown in micrograph (a), the interstitium is infiltrated by

lymphocytes that are also seen within the tubular epithelium (*tubulitis*) **T**. Tubulitis represents a cell-mediated immune response directed against donor tubular epithelial cells and results in destruction of tubules. The glomeruli are generally not affected. Pure acute cellular rejection can be reversed by increased immunosuppression.

- **Acute vascular rejection** (Banff types II and III) – represents an immune response against vascular endothelial cells. The typical features (micrograph (b)) include infiltration of the vascular endothelium by inflammatory cells, and swelling and proliferation of endothelial cells, a pattern known as *endotheliitis* **E**. The smooth muscle of the wall of the artery **SM** is relatively unaffected. When there is inflammation of the full thickness of the vessel wall or fibrinoid necrosis of the media, this is classified as Banff type III acute rejection. As seen here, this may result in intravascular thrombosis **Th** with consequent ischaemia of the kidney. As the condition becomes chronic, there is intimal thickening owing to fibrosis and proliferation of myointimal cells. Acute vascular rejection is generally difficult to treat successfully.
- **Chronic rejection** (chronic/sclerosing allograft nephropathy) – generally occurs after months to years and results in a fairly non-specific histological pattern resembling end-stage kidney (see Fig. 15.1) although specific features of acute rejection may be found.

Tumours of the kidney

The most common malignant tumour of the kidney in adults is the ***renal adenocarcinoma (renal cell carcinoma)*** derived from the tubular epithelial cells; this is illustrated in Figure 15.16. One of its important methods of spread is by venous invasion; this is shown in Figure 7.6. The kidney is also the site of an important malignant tumour of children, ***nephroblastoma*** or ***Wilms' tumour*** (Fig. 15.14); this is an example of a so-called '***small round blue cell tumour***' and is of embryological origin. Benign tumours of the kidney include ***oncocytoma*** and ***angiomyolipoma***.

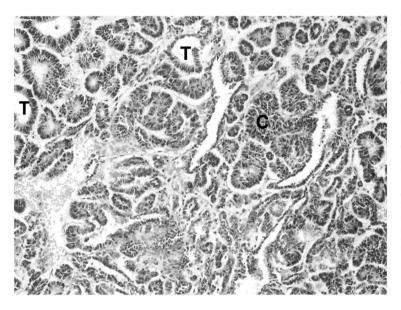

Fig. 15.14 Nephroblastoma (HP)

This is one of the most common malignant tumours of infants and children and is believed to originate from embryonic renal blastema. It is composed of a mixture of primitive and undifferentiated cells **C** and tubular structures **T** resembling primitive renal tubules; occasionally, structures resembling immature glomeruli are also found. There are many histological variants of this tumour, some of which contain primitive tissue cells such as skeletal muscle precursors (rhabdomyoblasts).

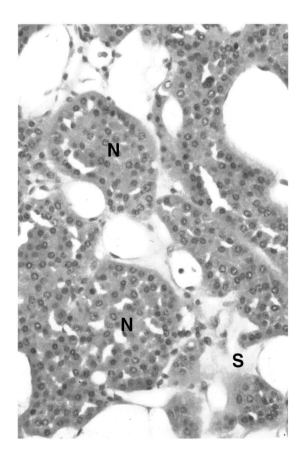

Fig. 15.15 Oncocytoma

Oncocytoma is a fairly common benign renal neoplasm, which can be difficult to differentiate clinically from renal cell carcinoma. Macroscopically, the tumour is a mahogany brown colour with a well-defined margin and arises in the renal cortex. There is often a central irregular fibrotic scar which may be identifiable radiologically. Necrosis and haemorrhage are very rare in contrast to renal cell carcinoma. Microscopically, the tumour is composed of small regular round cells arranged in nests **N** as shown in this micrograph. The cell nests are separated by an oedematous stroma **S**. There is little cellular pleomorphism and minimal if any mitotic activity. The cells have abundant granular eosinophilic cytoplasm, resulting from the very large numbers of mitochondria that pack the cytoplasm.

BASIC SYSTEMS PATHOLOGY

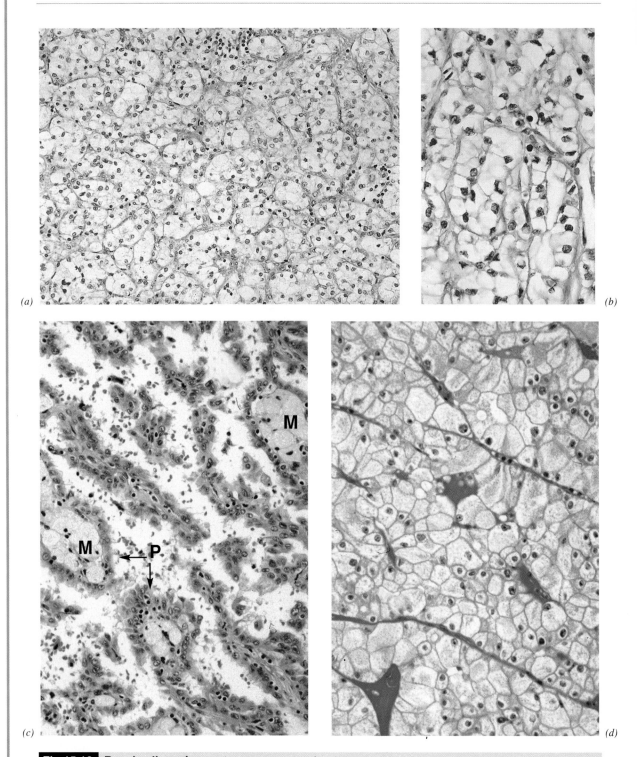

(a)

(b)

(c)

(d)

Fig.15.16 Renal cell carcinoma *(caption opposite above)*

Fig.15.16 **Renal cell carcinoma** (*illustrations opposite*)
(a) Clear cell carcinoma (MP) **(b) Clear cell carcinoma (HP)** **(c) Papillary carcinoma (MP)**
(d) Chromophobe carcinoma (MP)

The most common primary malignant tumour of the kidney is the ***renal cell carcinoma*** derived from renal tubular epithelium. Recently, renal cell carcinoma has been subclassified according to histological and cytogenetic criteria. All types of renal cell carcinoma present with one or more of the classical triad of signs: haematuria, flank pain and a palpable mass. A few renal cell carcinomas are hereditary and some are found in von Hippel–Lindau syndrome in association with cerebellar and retinal haemangioblastomas. However, the great majority of cases are sporadic. The major subtypes of renal cell carcinoma are:

- **Clear cell carcinoma** – this is by far the most common type and generally has the worst prognosis. As seen in micrographs (a) and (b), the tumour cells are large and polygonal in shape and the cytoplasm is clear because of the accumulation of cytoplasmic glycogen and lipid. In other areas of the tumour, the tumour cell cytoplasm is granular and pink-staining, more closely resembling the tubular epithelium from which these tumours are derived.
- **Papillary (chromophil) carcinoma** – the next most common variant, this tumour is composed of papillary

structures as shown in micrograph (c). The tumour is often surrounded by a thick fibrous capsule and there is typically extensive necrosis and haemorrhage. Microscopically, the tumour consists of papillary structures **P** surrounded by a layer of cuboidal to columnar malignant epithelial cells. The papillary cores are often packed with foamy macrophages **M**, as demonstrated here.

- **Chromophobe carcinoma** – this tumour consists of sheets of malignant epithelial cells with pale cytoplasm (as in micrograph (d)) and prominent cell boundaries. Note the difference between this tumour and clear cell carcinoma in micrograph (b).
- **Collecting duct carcinoma**.
- **Sarcomatoid carcinoma**.

Clear cell carcinoma tends to breach the walls of intrarenal venous tributaries and to grow as solid cords along the lumen of the renal vein towards and into the inferior vena cava. From here, venous emboli spread tumour deposits to the lung producing typical isolated '***cannon ball secondaries***'. Renal adenocarcinoma also has a particular propensity for metastasis to bone and brain.

Diseases of the lower urinary tract

The most important disorders of the lower urinary tract are infection and neoplasia.

Infections are common, but usually remain confined to the bladder (***cystitis***); ascending spread into the ureters and pelvicalyceal systems may result in renal parenchymal involvement (***acute pyelonephritis***) as shown in Figure 15.10. Persistent or repeated infection in the urinary tract predisposes to the development of urinary stones, particularly in the bladder and pelvicalyceal systems. Infections of the urethra (***urethritis***) are commonly sexually transmitted involving the organisms gonococcus and *Chlamydia*.

The pelvicalyceal system, ureters and bladder are lined by a specialised epithelium known as ***transitional epithelium (urothelium)***. Malignant tumours of the urothelium, known as transitional cell or urothelial carcinomas (Fig. 15.19), are common and of particular interest because of the possible role of chemical carcinogens such as aniline dyes in their pathogenesis. Urothelial carcinomas may be either invasive or non-invasive. Most of the deeply invasive tumours are high grade carcinomas. Malignant tumours are probably preceded by the development of urothelial dysplasia and carcinoma in situ (Fig. 15.18). Benign tumours include ***transitional cell papillomas*** and ***inverted papillomas***.

As in other areas of pathology, these tumours have recently been reclassified, with the hope that the new classification will more accurately reflect the clinical behaviour of the tumours and therefore provide a better indication of treatment requirements. At the time of writing, both old and new classifications are in use. The two classifications are outlined below.

Fig. 15.17 Classification of urothelial tumours	
WHO 1973 classification	**WHO/ISUP consensus classification 1998**
Papilloma	Papilloma
Transitional cell carcinoma Grade 1	Papillary urothelial neoplasm of low malignant potential (PUNLMP)
Transitional cell carcinoma Grade 2	Low grade urothelial carcinoma
Transitional cell carcinoma Grade 3	High grade urothelial carcinoma

BASIC SYSTEMS PATHOLOGY

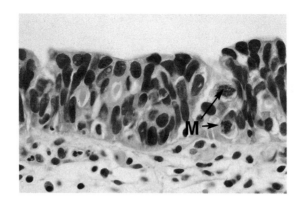

Fig. 15.18 Bladder carcinoma in situ (HP)

Carcinoma in situ of the urinary bladder is characterised by replacement of normal epithelium by cells indistinguishable from those seen in urothelial carcinoma. The epithelial cells are enlarged and crowded with enlarged hyperchromatic nuclei and prominent mitotic figures **M**, one of which is near the epithelial surface. The epithelium is not thickened and this area might, at cystoscopy, merely appear reddened. Urothelial carcinoma in situ may be found in isolation or in association with papillary urothelial carcinoma (Fig. 15.19). These lesions are likely to progress to invasive carcinoma.

(a)

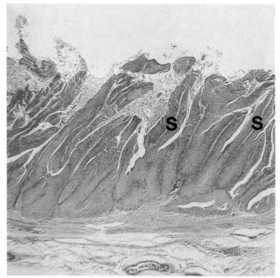

(b)

Fig. 15.19 Urothelial (transitional cell) carcinoma
(a) Low grade (LP) (b) High grade (MP)

Urothelial (transitional cell) carcinomas (TCC) are common. All are regarded as malignant despite the fact that many show no evidence of invasion when first detected.

As in the pelvicalyceal tumour shown in micrograph (a), low grade urothelial carcinomas (TCC grade 1) commonly form frond-like papillary outgrowths from the urothelial surface with a slender connective tissue stroma **S** supporting the layers of neoplastic cells which are enlarged and disorganised compared to normal urothelium.

In high grade urothelial carcinomas (TCC grade 3), there may be a surface papillary component but the lesion often forms a sessile ulcerated plaque and, as shown in micrograph (b), the tumour **T** invades deeply into the bladder wall, infiltrating between smooth muscle bundles **M**.

Urothelial carcinomas are frequently multifocal in origin, and there is a strong link between their development and exposure to certain industrial chemicals such as aniline dyes. Cigarette smoking has also been causally linked with the development of urothelial carcinomas.

The prognosis of urothelial carcinomas depends on their location, the grade of the tumour, and the extent of local invasion when the tumour is first detected. The cytology of urothelial carcinomas is shown in more detail in Figure 7.15. Occasionally, squamous carcinomas may develop in the bladder from metaplastic epithelium associated with chronic inflammation by a stone or parasitic infection (schistosomiasis). Rarely, adenocarcinoma arises from embryological urachal remnants.

16. Lymphoid and haemopoietic systems

Functions of the lymphoreticular system

The lymphoreticular system is composed of various organs and tissues which facilitate the interaction of lymphocytes with cells of monocyte-macrophage lineage in the generation of immune responses. The main tissues of the system are the thymus, spleen, lymph nodes, bone marrow and mucosal-associated lymphoid tissue (MALT) such as tonsils and Peyer's patches of the gut. Virtually every tissue in the body also has a resident population of specialised interstitial dendritic cells of macrophage type which have important roles in presenting new antigens to lymphocytes.

Lymphocytes are produced in the bone marrow, their number being selectively expanded, mainly in lymph nodes, in response to specific immunological requirements; many circulate through peripheral tissues via blood and lymphatic vessels in a constant search for antigens.

The monocyte-macrophage system includes the tissue macrophages (histiocytes) found in virtually every tissue; these become activated following tissue damage and, together with monocytes recruited from the blood, act as phagocytic cells in the process of organisation. This system also includes specialised dendritic antigen-presenting cells with a role in initiating new immune responses by presenting antigen to T lymphocytes.

Lymphoreticular disorders fall into four main groups: reactive changes caused by infection and inflammation, autoimmune diseases, immunosuppression (including HIV/AIDS) and neoplasia.

Reactive disorders of lymph nodes

The lymphoreticular system is remarkably labile and quickly responds to the presence of infective agents or foreign material in the activation of an immune response. There are two main patterns of immune response:

- The **cell-mediated response** – this involves the activity of *T lymphocytes* which are either directly or indirectly cytotoxic.
- The **humoral response** – this involves the activation of *B lymphocytes* which transform into antibody-secreting *plasma cells*; interaction of antibody with antigen leads to destruction of the antigen.

Following tissue damage, particularly infection, lymph nodes in the drainage area become particularly active and enlarged; this is termed *reactive hyperplasia* (Fig. 16.1). This may involve one or more of the principal cellular constituents of the node, depending on the nature of the foreign material encountered:

- In a predominantly humoral response, there is hyperplasia of the cortical follicles (mainly composed of B lymphocytes) with development of large B cell germinal centres (*follicular hyperplasia*).
- In a predominantly cell-mediated response, there is hyperplasia of the paracortical (parafollicular) region of the node which is mainly occupied by T lymphocytes (*parafollicular* or *paracortical hyperplasia*).
- Certain stimuli evoke intense phagocytic activity leading to dilatation of subcapsular and medullary sinuses with increased numbers and activity of macrophages and phagocytic sinus-lining cells (*sinus hyperplasia* or *sinus histiocytosis*).

Certain foreign agents stimulate characteristic patterns of reaction in lymph nodes which allow a diagnosis of disease to be made on lymph node biopsy, for example multiple minute granulomas in toxoplasmosis. In addition, lymph nodes are classically involved by specific chronic granulomatous inflammations such as tuberculosis, sarcoidosis and Crohn's disease syphilis (see Chs 3 and 4).

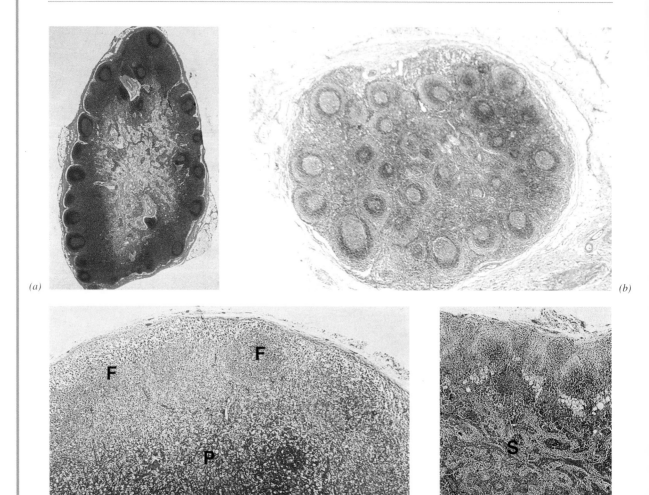

(a) *(b)* *(c)* *(d)*

Fig. 16.1 Reactive hyperplasia of lymph nodes

(a) **Normal lymph node (LP)**   (b) **Follicular hyperplasia (LP)**   (c) **Paracortical hyperplasia (MP)**
(d) **Sinus hyperplasia (MP)**

Damage or inflammation of any tissue may excite a reactive response in the draining lymph nodes. The three basic patterns of response, follicular hyperplasia, paracortical hyperplasia and sinus hyperplasia, may be seen separately or in combination according to the nature of the stimulus.

In *follicular hyperplasia*, illustrated in micrograph (b), there is an increase in number and size of cortical lymphoid follicles evident on comparison with the normal in micrograph (a). This reflects a B cell (humoral) response and results in the production and clonal expansion of antibody-secreting plasma cells.

In *paracortical (parafollicular) hyperplasia*, seen in micrograph (c), there is expansion of the T cell

parafollicular zone **P** with small B cell follicles **F** pushed to the periphery of the node beneath the capsule. This pattern is common in response to viral infection.

In *sinus hyperplasia* or sinus histiocytosis, shown in micrograph (d), there is no great increase in the lymphoid component of the node, but the medullary sinuses **S** are extremely prominent by virtue of dilatation, and by hyperplasia of histiocytic cells lining the sinuses. This reaction is seen in nodes draining tissues from which endogenous particulate matter such as lipid is released, for example a necrotic tumour.

Acquired immune deficiency syndrome (AIDS)

The *human immunodeficiency virus type 1 (HIV-1)* is a lymphotropic virus which gains access to cells by way of the CD4 surface protein normally found on T helper cells as well as most monocytes and other macrophages. Infection with HIV-1 is associated with several clinical and pathological syndromes. Some patients develop fever, weight loss, diarrhoea and generalised lymph node enlargement (**lymphadenopathy**) in which there is generalised follicular hyperplasia. In patients with the full-blown immunodeficient state of AIDS, lymph nodes commonly show loss of follicles, lymphocyte depletion, vascular proliferation and fibrosis.

The main consequences of the immune-deficient state seen in AIDS are:

Predisposition to opportunistic infections
Important opportunistic infections in AIDS patients are:-

- *Pneumocystis carinii* pneumonia (Fig. 4.23)
- *Cytomegalovirus* infection (Fig. 4.16)
- *Mycobacterial* infections, tuberculosis as well as atypical Mycobacteria (Fig. 4.10)
- *Mucocutaneous and other fungal infections* (Fig. 4.19), including *Cryptococcus* (Fig. 4.22)
- Toxoplasmosis

Predisposition to certain tumours
The most important are:-

- Kaposi's sarcoma (Fig. 11.16)
- Non-Hodgkin's lymphoma (see below).

Malignant disorders of the lymphoid system

Apart from reactive changes in which the lymphoreticular system is mounting an immune response to some foreign agent, the most common disorder encountered in the lymphoreticular system is the development of primary neoplastic proliferation of various lymphocytic cell lines. Such neoplastic proliferations are divided into two broad groups depending on histopathological identification of the type of neoplastic cell:

- **Hodgkin's disease (lymphoma)** is characterised by neoplastic proliferation of large activated lymphoid cells, which may be either T or B cells, eponymously termed *Reed-Sternberg cells*.
- **Non-Hodgkin's lymphomas** are derived from neoplastic proliferations of lymphocytes (either T or B) or rarely histiocytic cells.

These diseases usually present with involvement of a group of lymph nodes but then spread to involve multiple lymph node groups, spleen and bone marrow. Eventually, peripheral sites such as liver, skin or nervous system may also become involved. Non-Hodgkin's lymphomas may also arise in other organs, for example the gut, lung, brain, salivary gland, thyroid and testis. These conditions and their classification are discussed in detail later.

The lymphoreticular system is also the subject of a group of disorders termed *Langerhans cell histiocytoses (histiocytosis X)* which, although not certainly neoplastic, behave as disseminated infiltrative cellular proliferations. In these conditions, there is widespread infiltration of tissues by histiocytic cells with features of Langerhans cells, a type of dendritic antigen-presenting cell normally found in skin and its draining lymph nodes. There is a spectrum of severity from localised and benign to disseminated and fatal which may involve skin, viscera, bone marrow and lymph nodes.

Organs of the lymphoreticular system, in particular lymph nodes, are also commonly sites of metastatic deposits of tumour (Fig. 7.5).

BASIC SYSTEMS PATHOLOGY

Hodgkin's lymphoma

Hodgkin's lymphoma is a malignant neoplasm of the lymphoreticular system which usually first becomes manifest by lymph node enlargement but later by splenomegaly, hepatomegaly and bone marrow involvement. Hodgkin's lymphoma can be divided into several subtypes, each with a different histological pattern and clinical prognosis. The tumour cells in Hodgkin's lymphoma are morphologically distinctive and are named **Reed-Sternberg cells**. These cells are derived from activated lymphocytes and in some sub-types have been found to be activated B cells. Reed-Sternberg cells are divided into several main morphological types. The classical form is large and binucleate with two mirror image nuclei containing large pink-staining nucleoli (said to resemble an owl's eyes). Multinucleate and mononuclear variants of the Reed-Sternberg cell are also seen in different forms of Hodgkin's lymphoma.

Reed-Sternberg cells usually only form a small proportion of the cell population of lymph nodes in Hodgkin's lymphoma, and the neoplastic cells are hidden amongst a sea of reactive lymphoid cells, histiocytic cells and commonly eosinophils.

There are five histological subgroups of Hodgkin's lymphoma which correlate with prognosis and response to treatment: **nodular lymphocyte-predominant** and **lymphocytic-rich** (slowly progressive), **mixed cellularity** (intermediate progression), **lymphocyte-depleted** (aggressive disease) and **nodular sclerosing pattern** (slowly progressive).

The delineation of each type depends on the number of Reed-Sternberg cells and related cells relative to reactive cells in the node (Fig. 16.2). Nodular sclerosis is distinguished by a fibroblastic response in the node with the production of bands of collagen.

The prognosis and treatment of Hodgkin's lymphoma are not only related to the histological type but also to the extent of involvement of the lymphoreticular system as a whole. Investigation usually involves biopsy examination of lymph nodes, bone marrow and liver, with extent of nodal involvement being assessed by CT scan or lymphangiography.

Fig. 16.2 Hodgkin's lymphoma (*illustrations opposite*)
(a) Nodular lymphocyte-predominant pattern (HP) (b) Mixed cellularity pattern (HP)
(c) Lymphocyte-depleted pattern (HP) (d) Nodular sclerosing pattern (LP)

The subtype of Hodgkin's lymphoma with the best prognosis is the **nodular lymphocyte-predominant pattern** seen in micrograph (a). In this type, reactive lymphocytes make up the bulk of tissue in affected nodes and form extensive sheets within which are scattered relatively few mononuclear **Reed-Sternberg cells**; these cells are also termed 'popcorn' cells because of the lobulated contour of their nuclei. They have been shown to be a form of activated B cell. This subtype of Hodgkin's lymphoma may be difficult to differentiate from some types of non-Hodgkin's lymphoma. **Lymphocyte-rich Hodgkin's lymphoma** is not illustrated.

The next most favourable prognosis applies to the most common form, namely **mixed cellularity Hodgkin's lymphoma** shown in micrograph (b). Here classical Reed-Sternberg cells **RS** are mixed with a variable population of reactive cells including lymphocytes **L**, histiocytes **H**, eosinophils **E**, neutrophils **N** and fibroblasts **F**.

The type with the worst prognosis is **lymphocyte-depleted Hodgkin's lymphoma** illustrated in micrograph (c) in which there is little evidence of reactive cells. Affected nodes are replaced by sheets of large pleomorphic cells which are Reed-Sternberg cell variants with only a few classical Reed-Sternberg cells **RS**; lymphocytes **L** and other reactive cells are scanty.

Most commonly, Hodgkin's lymphoma destroys the normal architecture of the lymph node completely, producing a homogeneous appearance in which no trace of the original cortico-medullary demarcation and follicular pattern remains. However, one form of Hodgkin's disease, the **nodular sclerosing pattern** seen in micrograph (d), results in the deposition of broad irregular bands of pink-staining collagenous fibrous tissue which separates the cellular Hodgkin's tumour mass into islands, imparting a nodular appearance to the cut surface of the node. The nodular sclerosing pattern is associated with a good prognosis if diagnosed at an early stage.

With modern chemotherapy, it is now common to achieve complete cure of Hodgkin's lymphoma. Prognosis depends on histological type and clinical stage of disease. There is, however, a tendency for the lymphocyte-predominant type to present with localised disease (excellent prognosis) while the lymphocyte-depleted type presents with disseminated disease (poor prognosis). The prognosis for mixed-cellularity disease depends on stage; localised disease is associated with an excellent prognosis while disseminated disease, particularly involving extranodal tissues, is associated with a less favourable outcome.

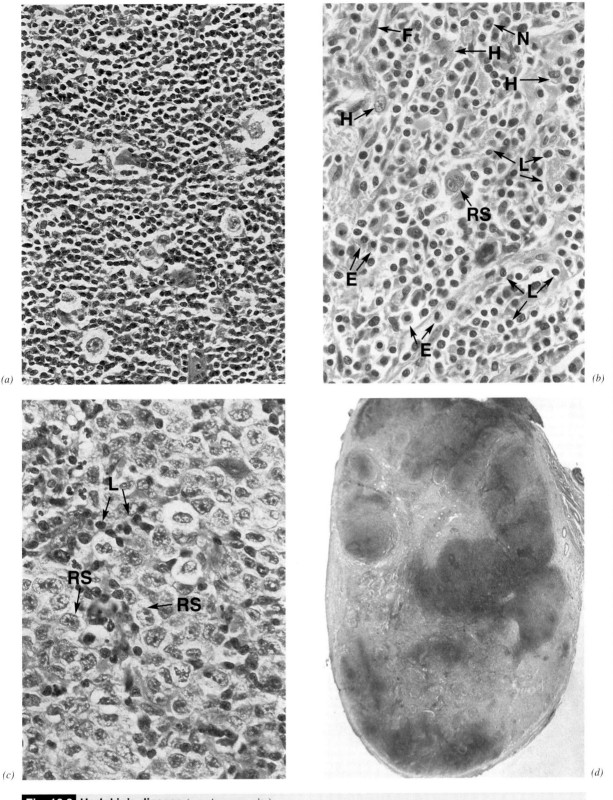

Fig. 16.2 Hodgkin's disease *(caption opposite)*

Non-Hodgkin's lymphomas

The non-Hodgkin's lymphomas are a group of neoplastic proliferations of lymphoid or, very rarely, histiocytic cells.

They are collectively known as *lymphomas* and, despite the suffix -*oma*, all are malignant in that they may become widely disseminated. The main features of non-Hodgkin's lymphomas are as follows:

- The usual clinical presentation is with enlargement of a group of lymph nodes; biopsy is usually performed to establish a diagnosis. As well as conventional histology, immunohistochemistry and molecular genetics are used to establish the precise type of cell forming the neoplastic proliferation.
- Early stage disease may be localised to one set of nodes or may affect lymph nodes in a generalised fashion.
- Tumours are derived from either T or B lymphocytes but hardly ever from true histiocytic cells. The majority of lymphomas arise in lymph nodes and are B cell in type.
- Non-Hodgkin's lymphoma may occur in the gut, lung, salivary gland or lacrimal gland in which case the neoplastic cells are derived from mucosal-associated lymphoid tissues (MALT). These specialised types tend to remain as relatively localised disease without systemic spread (see Fig. 13.12).
- T cell lymphomas most commonly occur in the skin as a disease termed *mycosis fungoides* (Fig. 21.17).

Classification of non-Hodgkin's lymphomas

There are many different subtypes of non-Hodgkin's lymphoma and as a result there have been a variety of different classifications based on either morphology, immunology or clinical behaviour. The WHO classification (Fig. 16.3) has now superseded the previous classifications such as Kiel, Lukes–Collins and the Working Formulation; however, it is also useful clinically to divide them into *low grade*, *intermediate grade* and *high grade* types corresponding to good, intermediate and poor prognosis. The following features are assessed in classification:

- **Cell morphology** – lymphoma cells may be classified according to cell size, i.e. *small* (about the size of a mature lymphocyte) or *large* (five to six times the size of a small lymphocyte). In general, a high proportion of small cells is associated with less aggressive disease while a high proportion of large cells is associated with aggressive disease.
- **Immunophenotype** – immunochemical reagents are now used routinely to classify lymphoid cells into functional subtypes. The main division is into B cell and T cell lymphomas; additional markers may then be employed to characterise the neoplastic cell population more precisely.
- **Growth pattern** – B cell lymphomas may be classified as being either *follicular* or *diffuse*. In the follicular pattern, the cells form aggregates which resemble lymphoid follicles but without germinal centres. In the diffuse pattern, there is diffuse distribution of cells with no evidence of follicular aggregation.
- **Lymphocyte maturation** – research on the normal cytology and function of follicular B lymphoid cells as they undergo transformation from small mature lymphocytes through to plasma cells has revealed characteristic cytological features which are recapitulated in the patterns of differentiation seen in non-Hodgkin's lymphomas. The *Kiel classification*, popular in Europe, identified lymphocytic, lymphoblastic, centrocytic, centroblastic, immunoblastic, lymphoplasmacytic and plasma cell variants of lymphoid cells. The *Lukes–Collins classification*, popular in the USA, applied the terms lymphocytic, lymphoblastic, small and large cleaved cell, small and large non-cleaved cell, and immunoblast to describe the same morphological features.
- **Molecular biology** – it is possible to obtain molecular confirmation of clonality of a lymphoid tumour by characterising the immunoglobulin or T cell receptor genes. In addition, specific cytogenetic abnormalities are seen in some tumours, reflecting activation of specific oncogenes.

In clinical practice, the histologist identifies cytological features of neoplastic lymphocytes, including size, shape, number and position of nucleoli, as well as amount and distribution of cytoplasm. The cell of origin (B or T cell) is then determined by immunochemical methods using antibodies which stain specific cell markers. On this basis, the type of lymphoma is determined. Based on this approach, several clinico-pathological classifications of lymphomas have been proposed, with different centres favouring each. The WHO classification of non-Hodgkin's lymphomas which has become accepted as an international standard is shown in Figure 16.3. It is not necessary to learn this classification, it is shown here to illustrate the range of entities presently recognisable.

There are several relatively common groups of non-Hodgkin's lymphomas which have distinct clinical and pathological features which are summarised as follows:

- **Small cell lymphocytic lymphomas** occur in elderly patients, often with widespread disease; they behave as indolent low grade neoplasms. Bone marrow involvement and an associated leukaemic component are common.
- **Follicular centre cell, follicular pattern lymphomas** with a predominance of small cells occur in older patients and present with generalised lymphadenopathy and frequent marrow involvement. They run a long indolent course; complete remission is difficult to achieve.
- **Diffuse large B cell lymphomas** occur particularly in adults and have a high cell proliferation rate. Aggressive chemotherapy is required to achieve remission.
- **Lymphoblastic lymphomas** (B and T cell types) present in childhood and have high cell proliferation rates associated with large masses of tumour. Aggressive chemotherapy is required to achieve remission.
- **Myeloma** (plasmacytoma) is a tumour of plasma cells (derived from B cells) usually presenting as osteolytic lesions in bones, or as a diffuse infiltration of bone marrow.
- **Cutaneous T cell lymphoma** (also known as *mycosis fungoides*) is a form of low grade T cell lymphoma involving skin (see Fig. 21.27). It has an insidious onset as persistent flat red patches which slowly progress to raised nodular lesions. At a late stage the lymphoma may become systemic.

Fig. 16.3 WHO classification of non-Hodgkin's lymphomas

B cell neoplasms	T cell neoplasms
Precursor B cell lymphoblastic leukaemia/lymphoma	**Precursor T cell lymphoblastic leukaemia/lymphoma**
Mature B cell neoplasms	**Mature T cell and NK cell neoplasms**
B cell chronic lymphocytic leukaemia/small lympho-cytic lymphoma	T cell prolymphocytic leukaemia
B cell prolymphocytic leukaemia	T cell large granular lymphocytic leukaemia
Lymphoplasmacytic lymphoma (lymphoplasmacytoid lymphoma)	NK cell leukaemia
Mantle cell lymphoma	Extranodal NK/T cell lymphoma, nasal-type (angio-centric lymphoma)
Follicular lymphoma (follicle centre cell lymphoma)	Mycosis fungoides
	Sezary syndrome
Marginal zone B cell lymphoma of mucosa-associated lymphoid tissue (MALT) type	Angioimmunoblastic T cell lymphoma
Nodal marginal zone lymphoma with or without monocytoid B cells	Peripheral T cell lymphoma (unspecified)
Splenic marginal zone B cell lymphoma	Adult T cell leukemia/lymphoma (HTLVI+)
Hairy cell leukaemia	Systemic anaplastic large cell lymphoma (T and null cell types)
Diffuse large B cell lymphoma	Primary cutaneous anaplastic large cell lymphoma
Sub-types mediastinal (thymic), intravascular, primary effusion lymphoma	Subcutaneous panniculitis-like T cell lymphoma
Burkitt lymphoma	Enteropathy-type intestinal T cell lymphoma
Plasmacytoma	Hepatosplenic γ/δ T cell lymphoma
Plasma cell myeloma (multiple myeloma)	

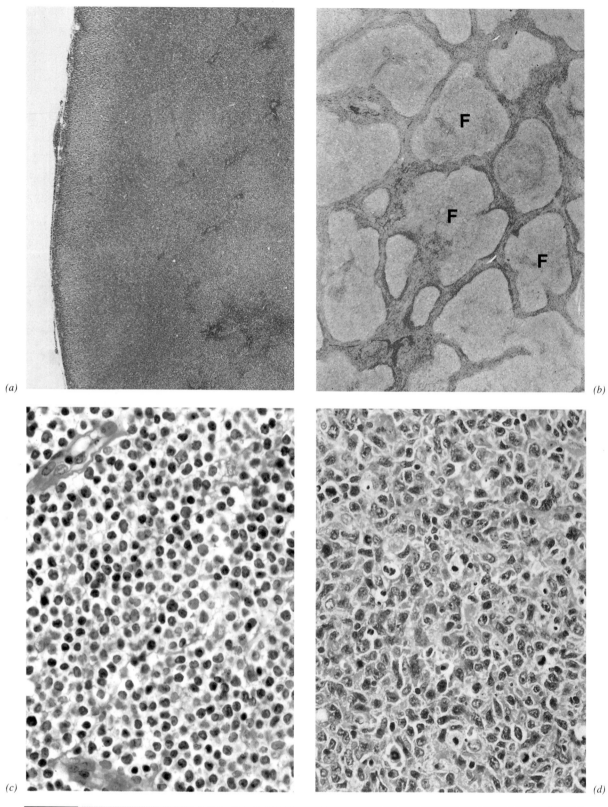

Fig. 16.4 Non-Hodgkin's lymphoma B cell type (*caption opposite*)

Fig. 16.4 Non-Hodgkin's lymphoma B cell type (*illustrations opposite*)
(a) Diffuse pattern (LP)   (b) Follicular pattern (LP)
(c) Follicular centre cell, predominantly small cells (HP)   (d) Large cell lymphoma (HP)

B cell lymphomas may be subdivided by pattern of growth into *follicular* and *diffuse types*, and also by size of cell into *small* and *large cell variants*. These micrographs show four variants of B cell lymphoma based upon these criteria.

In the diffuse pattern shown in micrograph (a), the normal architecture of the node has been completely effaced and replaced by uniform sheets of neoplastic lymphocytes. In contrast, in the follicular pattern illustrated in micrograph (b), the neoplastic cells are aggregated into irregular follicles **F**, larger and more variable in size and shape than normal follicles.

At a cellular level, the malignant lymphocytes come in a variety of shapes and sizes. Two common types are illustrated here. In the small follicle centre cell type as shown in micrograph (c), the tumour cells are like small lymphocytes with round darkly-staining nuclei often with a groove ('cleaved' cells) and only an insignificant rim of surrounding cytoplasm. The large cell variant shown in micrograph (d) exhibits less uniformity of nuclear shape, size and staining intensity, most nuclei being large with an open chromatin pattern and large nucleoli.

Bone marrow disease

The bone marrow spaces between the trabeculae of spongy bone are occupied by adipose tissue within which are collections of haemopoietic tissue responsible for the production of red blood cells, white blood cells and platelets. These cell lines are derived from a reservoir of haemopoietic stem cells which differentiate into the various specialised cell lines in response to specific growth factors. The bone marrow is able to respond rapidly to increased demands for the various blood cells by increased proliferative activity of the precursor and stem cells.

The main diseases involving the bone marrow are:

- primary and secondary abnormalities of haemopoiesis
- metastatic tumour deposition
- primary leukaemia/lymphoma, including myeloma
- myeloproliferative syndromes.

Haemopoietic disorders

Disorders of haemopoiesis are extremely common, but are largely outside the scope of this book, although cytological examination of smear preparations of aspirated bone marrow and histological examination of trephine biopsy specimens of bone marrow form an important method of investigating some diseases.

Most anaemias (lack of red cells) are the result of lack of iron or vitamin B_{12}/folate, or due to excessive red cell breakdown (haemolytic anaemia), but one type (leucoerythroblastic anaemia) is due to destruction of the haemopoietic tissue by tumour or fibrosis, and histological diagnosis of a bone marrow biopsy is a vital investigation to establish the cause.

Metastatic tumour in bone marrow

The bone marrow is a common site for blood-borne metastasis of certain malignant tumours. The tumours which most commonly spread to bone marrow are carcinomas; the following are the most frequent primary sites:

- adenocarcinoma of the breast
- carcinomas of bronchus and lung
- carcinoma of the kidney
- carcinoma of the thyroid (particularly follicular type)
- carcinoma of the prostate (see Fig. 16.5).

In most cases, the growth of metastatic carcinoma in the bone marrow leads to destruction of trabecular bone leading to osteolytic deposits which appear as lucent areas on X-ray. Carcinoma of the prostate often stimulates the active formation of new woven bone, producing osteosclerotic deposits which appear as increased areas of bone density on X-ray.

Another tumour which particularly metastasizes to bone marrow is neuroblastoma.

BASIC SYSTEMS PATHOLOGY

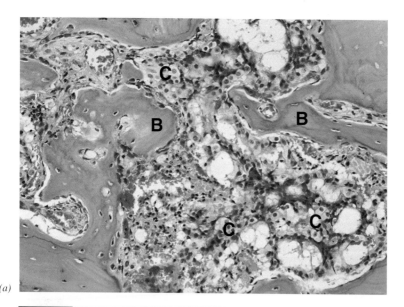

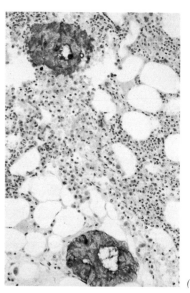

(a)   (b)

Fig. 16.5 Metastatic tumour in bone marrow: prostatic carcinoma
(a) H&E (MP)   (b) Immunoperoxidase method for prostate-specific antigen (PSA) (MP)

The bone marrow is a frequent site for deposits of metastatic carcinoma, the common primary tumours being from prostate, bronchus, breast, thyroid and kidney. Widespread replacement of bone marrow by metastatic tumour may induce extramedullary haemopoiesis in liver and spleen.

Most metastatic deposits cause bone destruction and, when widespread, can be associated with hypercalcaemia. Metastases from carcinoma of the prostate may, however, be associated with new bone

formation and result in osteosclerosis. This is shown in micrograph (a) where replacement of marrow by prostatic adenocarcinoma cells **C** is associated with reactive trabecular bone formation **B**. In micrograph (b), an immunoperoxidase method is employed to demonstrate *prostate-specific antigen (PSA)*, a specific marker for prostatic adenocarcinoma in metastatic tumour. The clumps of tumour cells are stained dark brown.

Leukaemias

The leukaemias are the most common neoplastic condition of white cells. The general characteristics of leukaemias are:

- neoplastic proliferation of marrow-derived cells, forming one or more neoplastic cell lines
- circulation of the neoplastic cells in the blood in almost all cases
- suppression of normal haemopoietic activity by the rapidly expanding leukaemic cell population.

Because the neoplastic leukaemic cells circulate in the blood, the cells are usually deposited in other tissues and organs, particularly lymph nodes, liver and spleen.

Leukaemias are classified according to the cell of origin, but a useful preliminary classification is into two main types, chronic leukaemias and acute leukaemias.

- **Chronic leukaemias** are characterised by neoplastic proliferation of nearly mature white cells. Typically, the clinical course is indolent, with a long natural history. Although the neoplastic cells predominate in the marrow, other haemopoietic cells can survive alongside, and adequate numbers of red cells and platelets are produced.
- **Acute leukaemias** are characterised by neoplastic proliferation of very immature cells of the white cell line (*blast cells*). The course of the disease is very rapid, with destruction of all other haemopoietic cell lines in the marrow. Without treatment these diseases are rapidly fatal.

Chronic leukaemias are mainly seen in adults over the age of 40; they may eventually transform into a more aggressive acute leukaemia.

Chronic lymphocytic leukaemia (CLL) is a neoplastic proliferation of small mature lymphocytes, similar to those seen in small cell (B cell) lymphocytic lymphoma. The two conditions overlap and are often considered together (see Fig. 16.3). *Chronic myeloid leukaemia (CML)* is a neoplastic proliferation of the more mature precursors of neutrophils (for example myelocytes and metamyelocytes), and occurs most commonly in adults. *Acute lymphoblastic leukaemia (ALL)* is a tumour of immature lymphocyte precursors (lymphoblasts), and occurs most commonly in children.

Some lymphomas which originate in lymph nodes may also eventually spread to involve the bone marrow, and there may be enough circulating lymphoma cells in the blood to be detected in a blood film. Thus there are some areas of overlap between some leukaemias and lymphomas.

Acute myeloid leukaemia (AML) is a tumour of immature precursor cells in the myeloid series (mainly myeloblasts), and is most common in adults. It is the most common of a group of acute leukaemias derived from various myeloid precursors, collectively called acute non-lymphoblastic leukaemias.

Myeloproliferative disorders

These diseases are the result of abnormal proliferation of the stem cells in the bone marrow; can differentiate into red cell (erythroid) precursors, white cell (myeloid or granulocytic) precursors, megakaryocytes or fibroblasts. There is frequent overlap between this group of diseases, which includes *polycythaemia rubra vera*, an excessive autonomous primary proliferation of red cells and their precursors; *primary thrombocythaemia*, an excessive proliferation of megakaryocytes and platelets and *myelofibrosis*, an excessive proliferation of marrow fibroblasts leading to obliteration of the marrow cavity by collagen and fibroblasts (see Fig. 16.9). *Chronic myeloid/granulocytic leukaemia* is also considered to be one of the myeloproliferative disorders.

The myeloproliferative disorders, as well as showing frequent overlap and transition from one form to another, have a tendency to terminate in an acute leukaemic phase.

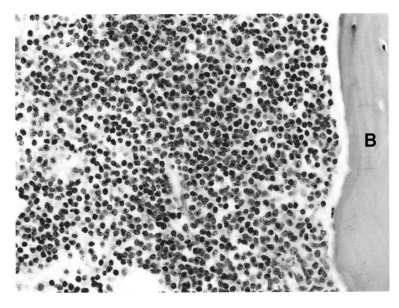

Fig. 16.6 Chronic lymphocytic leukaemia; bone marrow (HP)

In chronic lymphocytic leukaemia, the marrow between bone trabeculae **B** becomes infiltrated by small lymphocytes similar to those seen in small cell lymphocytic lymphoma and very large numbers of similar cells appear in the peripheral circulation.

Although occupation of the marrow is extensive, destruction of the normal haemopoietic marrow elements is not as rapid or severe as in acute lymphoblastic leukaemia and the condition runs an indolent course.

This is a disease seen mainly in later life. Lymphadenopathy, splenomegaly and anaemia are commonly encountered.

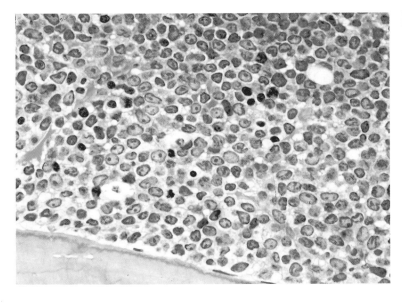

Fig. 16.7 Acute myeloid leukaemia; bone marrow (HP)

Acute myeloid leukaemia is characterised by proliferation of primitive myeloid cells in the bone marrow. There are several subgroups depending on degree of maturation of the neoplastic cells from primitive myeloblasts, through types with promyelocyte morphology, to types with both myeloid and monocytic morphology. As seen here, the marrow is replaced by large atypical myeloid blast cells with few maturing cells (compare with Fig. 16.8).

This type of leukaemia predominates in adults under the age of 60 and presents acutely with anaemia and bleeding secondary to thrombocytopaenia. Diagnosis is made on blood and marrow examination.

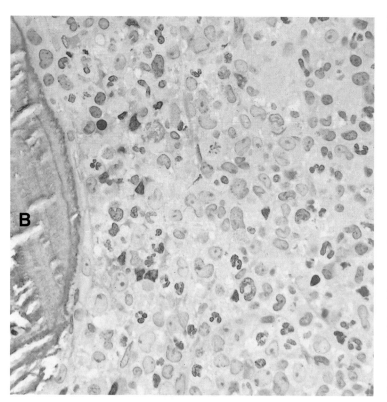

Fig. 16.8 Chronic myeloid (granulocytic) leukaemia; bone marrow (HP) (thin resin section)

In this disease, there is low grade neoplastic proliferation of neutrophil precursors. Increased numbers of myeloblasts produce greatly increased numbers of myelocytes, metamyelocytes and mature neutrophils, all of which appear in the peripheral blood in greatly increased numbers.

As seen in this micrograph, the marrow between bone trabeculae **B** is packed with neutrophils and late neutrophil precursors, particularly myelocytes and metamyelocytes; increased numbers of the most primitive precursor, the myeloblast, are also present, but they are a minority population compared to acute myeloid leukaemia (Fig. 16.7).

Despite the abnormal myeloid proliferation, normal haemopoietic activity continues, although at a reduced rate.

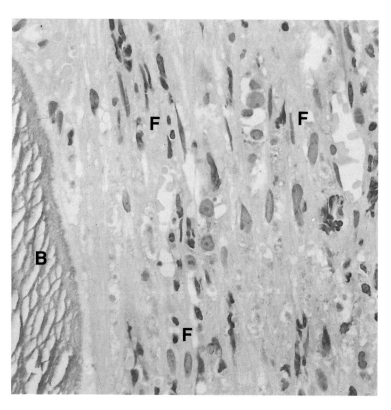

Fig. 16.9 Myelofibrosis (MP) (thin resin section)

In this disorder, replacement of haemopoietic bone marrow by progressive fibrosis leads to loss of capacity to produce erythrocytes, leucocytes and platelets. In this micrograph, the marrow space between bone trabeculae **B** is infiltrated by spindle-shaped fibroblastic cells **F**.

This is partly compensated for by extramedullary haemopoiesis, when other organs of the lymphoreticular system acquire again their fetal potential for haemopoiesis.

The spleen is the principal organ involved in this compensatory process and becomes greatly enlarged.

Histologically, the splenic red pulp is markedly expanded by the presence of immature erythropoietic and granulopoietic tissues.

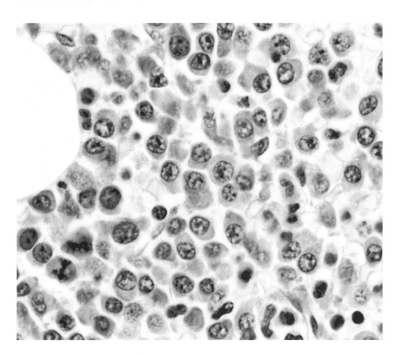

Fig. 16.10 Multiple myeloma (HP)

Myeloma is a tumour of plasma cells which may present with solitary, multifocal or diffuse bone marrow involvement. In this example from a patient with diffuse marrow involvement, the marrow space is replaced by abnormal plasma cells which, in normal marrow, are only a very minor constituent. Osteolytic lesions of myeloma lead to bone pain and sometimes fracture, whereas diffuse bone marrow infiltration may lead to destruction of normal haemopoietic cells, resulting in *leucoerythroblastic anaemia.* Solitary lesions in bone are termed plasmacytomas.

Each myeloma is derived from a single clone of plasma cells which produces a monoclonal antibody that can be detected in circulating blood by electrophoresis; light chains of the monoclonal antibody may appear in the urine (*Bence Jones protein*).

17. Female reproductive system

Introduction

The female reproductive tract comprises the vulva, vagina, uterus, Fallopian tubes and ovaries. As in other systems, a wide range of pathological conditions may occur in these organs. Malignant tumours and their precursor conditions are of major pathological importance. An interesting feature of the female genital tract is that there is a range of epithelial malignancies that can occur at almost any site in the tract. For instance, one might imagine that endometrioid adenocarcinoma would be found only in the endometrium, but primary endometrioid adenocarcinoma also occurs in the ovary, cervix, and very rarely, the vagina. Likewise, serous papillary adenocarcinoma is most commonly associated with the ovary, but also occurs in the endometrium, the cervix, the vagina and, occasionally, as a primary tumour of the peritoneum.

Disorders of the vulva

The vulva is subject to many of the conditions affecting skin elsewhere in the body, including various inflammatory conditions such as *dermatitis* (Figs 21.5 and 21.7) and *lichen planus*, but is also an important site for specific infective lesions which are transmitted sexually, including the *chancre of primary syphilis*. Many vulval inflammatory lesions lead to intense itching, so the histological features of these conditions are complicated by the effects of trauma from scratching (*lichen simplex chronicus*). In some post-menopausal women, the vulval mucosa tends to become thickened and white as a result of epithelial atrophy and sub-epithelial fibrosis, a condition known as *lichen sclerosus* (Fig. 17.1).

Many carcinomas of the vulva are preceded by human papillomavirus infection and epithelial dysplasia, known as *vulval intraepithelial neoplasia (VIN)*. Clinically, it can be difficult to differentiate these conditions from inflammatory lesions and biopsy is necessary for diagnosis.

Malignant vulval tumours are almost always slow-growing, well-differentiated squamous carcinomas similar to those of the skin and mucous membranes elsewhere (Fig. 7.14). Vulval tumours may originate in the labia majora, labia minora or clitoris, and may spread deeply into the underlying connective tissue and thence via lymphatics to superficial inguinal lymph nodes. Other tumours that may affect the vulva are benign naevi, malignant melanoma and, rarely, adenocarcinoma arising in Bartholin's glands.

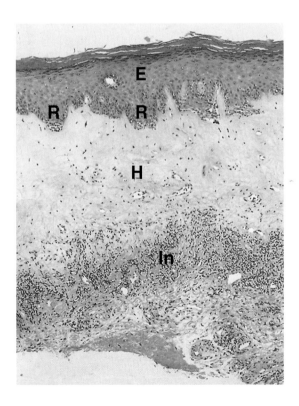

Fig. 17.1 Lichen sclerosus (HP)

This condition of unknown aetiology presents clinically as very itchy, smooth, whitish plaques around the vulva often with narrowing of the introitus. Histologically, there may be marked atrophy of the epidermis **E** with virtual disappearance of rete pegs **R** and skin appendages. Characteristically the dermis contains a band of inflammatory cells **In**, mainly lymphocytes and plasma cells, the inflammatory zone being separated from the epidermis by a layer of acellular hyalinised collagen **H** in the superficial dermis. Although this condition does not exhibit epithelial dysplasia, there is an association with invasive carcinoma.

Diseases of the vagina and uterine cervix

The vagina is rarely the site of important primary lesions of histopathological interest, although it is frequently the site of infections (*vaginitis*), especially by *Candida, Trichomonas* and *Gardnerella vaginalis*. Primary squamous carcinoma and adenocarcinoma of the vagina do occur but are rare.

The cervix frequently exhibits chronic inflammatory changes, described as *chronic cervicitis* (Fig. 17.2), which may also be associated with polypoid hyperplasia of the endocervical mucosa, sometimes with the formation of a large pedunculated *polyp* containing distended endocervical glands and stroma (Fig. 17.3). Clinically, the most important lesions of the cervix are *epithelial dysplasia* of varying degrees of severity and *squamous cell carcinoma*, all of which originate at the cervical squamocolumnar junction; these related conditions and their pathogenesis are considered in detail in Figures 17.4 to 17.7. *Adenocarcinoma in situ* and *invasive adenocarcinoma* of the cervix are less common than squamous cell carcinoma.

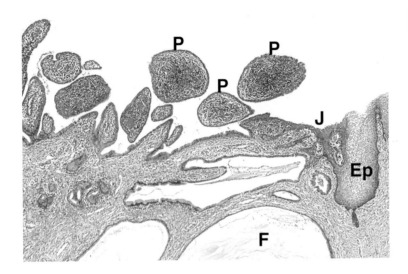

Fig. 17.2 Chronic cervicitis (MP)

In chronic cervicitis, the ectocervical squamous epithelium **Ep** is normal except for slight thickening. The major changes are seen in the endocervix immediately above the squamocolumnar junction **J** where there is *micropolyposis*, the core of each tiny polyp **P** showing a heavy chronic inflammatory cell infiltrate, composed mainly of lymphocytes and plasma cells. Cervical glands may develop cystic dilatation, often termed Nabothian follicles **F**. Long-standing inflammation may lead to *squamous metaplasia* of the endocervical surface epithelium (see Fig. 6.6a).

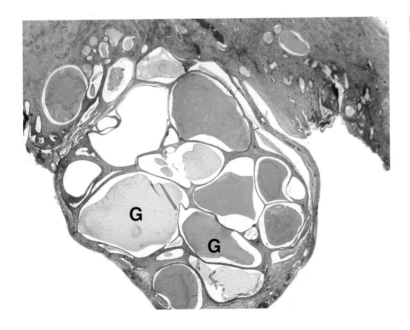

Fig. 17.3 Endocervical polyp (LP)

This micrograph shows a small benign endocervical polyp arising from the endocervical canal. The polyp is composed of cystically dilated glands **G** of varying sizes, each distended by mucin and lined by columnar endocervical mucin-secreting epithelium. As the polyp enlarges, it may develop a fibrous stroma between the cystic glands; extrusion through the external os may lead to surface ulceration.

Cervical polyps are thus an important cause of abnormal vaginal bleeding.

Aetiology and classification of dysplasia of the vulva, vagina and cervix

The vulva, vagina and ectocervix are lined by stratified squamous epithelium which is prone to sexually transmitted infection by **human papillomavirus (HPV)**. This virus has long been known to be associated with common skin warts, **verruca vulgaris** (Fig. 21.9) and venereal warts, **condyloma acuminatum**.

There are a large number of serotypes of HPV and recent evidence has shown a very close association between infection with certain serotypes and the presence of dysplasia and invasive carcinoma of squamous epithelia. The association was first discovered in the cervix where high risk HPV serotypes are associated with approximately 85% of invasive cancers but has also been shown to apply to the vagina, the vulva and to squamous lesions at other sites.

Infection with certain **low risk serotypes** of HPV, namely serotypes 6, 11, 42 and 44, results in condyloma acuminatum and low grade dysplasia. The **high risk serotypes**, serotypes 16, 18, 31, 33 and 35, are more likely to result in high grade dysplasia or invasive carcinoma. High risk serotypes are more likely to integrate their DNA into the host genome thereby introducing **viral oncogenes (v-oncogenes)** and allowing their transcription. The progression from latent infection to invasive carcinoma is also dependent on host factors such as the immune status of the host, nutritional factors and cigarette smoking, and only a small proportion of women infected with high risk serotypes progress to invasive carcinoma.

In the cervix, intraepithelial dysplasia is termed **cervical intraepithelial neoplasia** or **CIN** and graded as I, II or III (see Fig. 17.5). Similarly, **vulval intraepithelial neoplasia** is graded **VIN I, II or III** and **vaginal intraepithelial neoplasia** as **VAIN I, II or III**.

Cervical dysplasia and carcinoma

The vagina and the vaginal aspect of the cervix are covered by stratified squamous epithelium, which is well adapted to withstand the normal vaginal environment. The endocervical canal, on the other hand, is lined by a simple columnar, mucin-secreting epithelium; at a microscopic level, this is deeply folded so as to form gland-like invaginations into the cervical stroma, the endocervical glands, which are responsible for the elaboration of normal cervical mucus.

The junction between stratified squamous and columnar epithelium normally lies at the external os. The volume of the cervical stroma expands under the influence of hormones during each menstrual cycle, at menarche and during pregnancy, and this causes eversion of the vaginal end of the endocervical canal thus exposing some of the simple columnar epithelium to the vaginal environment. This exposed epithelium appears red in relation to the surrounding stratified squamous epithelium and hence became inaccurately known as a **cervical erosion**; more appropriate is the term **cervical ectropion**. Under the influence of the vaginal environment, the ectropic columnar epithelium may undergo squamous metaplasia (see Fig. 6.6a) to form stratified squamous epithelium indistinguishable from the lining epithelium native to the vagina. This metaplastic area, described as the **transformation zone**, appears to be unstable and susceptible to dysplastic changes induced by external factors. As described above, infection with certain HPV serotypes, as well as cigarette smoking and large numbers of sexual partners, is associated with a higher incidence of cervical dysplasia and carcinoma. The dysplastic changes may well regress if these predisposing factors are eliminated; however, it is believed that some undergo irreversible neoplastic change with the development of **CIN III**. Furthermore, a small proportion of untreated cases of CIN III progress to frank **invasive squamous cell carcinoma**.

The development of invasive squamous carcinoma may thus be prevented by intercepting the dysplastic process at an early stage and **cervical cytology** has been developed as a method of screening and monitoring this process in the population of women at risk. Once significant dysplasia has been demonstrated cytologically, histological examination of biopsy specimens taken at **colposcopy** is used to define accurately the degree of dysplasia and to plan appropriate treatment.

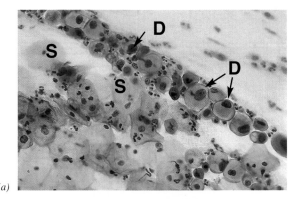

(a)

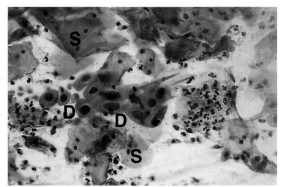

(b)

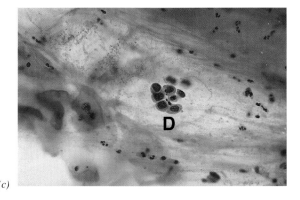

(c)

Fig. 17.4 Cervical smear cytology
(a) CIN I (b) CIN II (c) CIN III (Pap stain) (HP)

These micrographs are from preparations obtained by cervical smear stained by the *Papanicolaou method (Pap)*. Micrograph (a) of CIN I (*low grade squamous intraepithelial lesion (SIL)*) exhibits both normal cervical squamous cells **S** and clumps of mildly dysplastic cells **D** which have large dark-stained nuclei, a slightly irregular nuclear contour and a coarse pattern of nuclear chromatin.

Micrograph (b) shows CIN II (*high grade SIL*). In this smear, the abnormal epithelial cells **D** have larger nuclei and a higher nuclear to cytoplasmic ratio than in CIN I with coarser, more hyperchromatic nuclei. Normal epithelial cells are marked **S**. In CIN III (*high grade SIL*) as shown in micrograph (c), the nuclear to cytoplasmic ratio is even greater although the cells overall are smaller **D**. This corresponds to total lack of surface maturation so that cells resembling the basal layer cells are exfoliated at the surface. *Koilocytes* (virus-infected cells) may also be detected on cervical smears (see Fig. 17.6).

The abnormal surface cells of dysplastic epithelium are scraped off when a Pap smear is taken. Most dysplasia occurs at the transformation zone, which is an area of metaplastic squamous epithelium found at the squamocolumnar junction in most women of reproductive age; clinically, the transformation zone is correctly described as an ectropion or more colloquially as an 'erosion'. It is therefore important that endocervical cells are seen in the Pap smear to ensure that the correct area has been sampled.

Many pathologists use the Bethesda classification system when grading cervical cytology specimens. This system groups human papillomavirus-induced changes and CIN I into the category of *low grade squamous intraepithelial lesion (SIL)* and CIN II and III into *high grade SIL*. These slightly confusing grading systems are compared in Figure 17.5 below.

Figure 17.5 Comparison of grading systems for cervical dysplasia

Histological features	Traditional system	WHO system	Bethesda system
Koilocytes plus mild atypia	HPV infection	HPV infection	Low grade SIL
Dysplasia limited to lower third of epithelium	Mild dysplasia	CIN I	Low grade SIL
Dysplasia limited to lower two thirds of epithelium	Moderate dysplasia	CIN II	High grade SIL
Dysplasia extending into upper third of epithelium	Severe dysplasia	CIN III	High grade SIL
Dysplasia of full thickness of epithelium	Carcinoma in situ	CIN III	High grade SIL

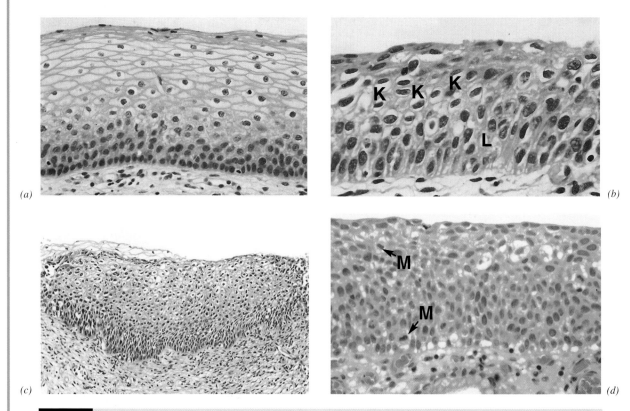

Fig. 17.6 Cervical intraepithelial neoplasia (CIN)
(a) Normal ectocervix (MP) (b) CIN I (MP) (c) CIN II (LP) (d) CIN III (MP)

Micrographs (a) to (d) illustrate the spectrum of cervical epithelial appearances from normal stratified squamous epithelium through to CIN III.

As seen in micrograph (a), normal ectocervical epithelium has a typical stratified squamous form with all cell division being confined to a single basal layer of small darkly staining cuboidal cells. As the cells undergo maturation, their eosinophilic cytoplasm expands greatly and the cells are pushed upwards into a stratum equivalent to the prickle cell layer of skin. Beyond this, the cells become flattened with further maturation, their nuclei becoming first pyknotic then undergoing karyorrhexis and karyolysis (Fig. 1.6); the cytoplasm becomes progressively flattened until the cells are finally shed from the surface.

In CIN I as seen in micrograph (b), the cells in the lower third of the epithelium **L** are enlarged, crowded and hyperchromatic and show increased mitotic activity. In this biopsy, there is also evidence of associated HPV

infection with plentiful *koilocytes* **K**; such virus-infected cells are characteristically found in the upper layer of the epithelium and have enlarged irregular nuclei with clear cytoplasm (see also Fig. 4.17).

When basal cell proliferation extends from one-third to two-thirds of the thickness of the epithelium as in micrograph (c), the lesion is termed CIN II. Numerous koilocytes are also seen in this example. These koilocytes represent productive infection by HPV.

In CIN III as seen in micrograph (d), the atypical cells extend into the upper third of the epithelium. As in this example, mitotic figures **M** are common and are seen well above the basal layer; abnormal mitotic figures may also be seen.

A critical feature of the dysplastic examples just discussed is that the basement membrane remains sharply defined and intact. With any evidence of *microinvasion* or more extensive spread into underlying tissues, the lesion is defined as *invasive carcinoma*.

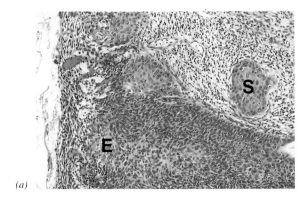

(a)

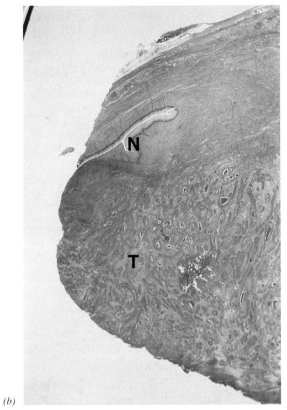

(b)

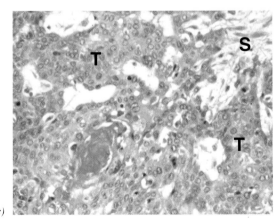

(c)

Fig. 17.7 Invasive squamous cell carcinoma of the cervix

(a) Microinvasive carcinoma (MP)
(b) Invasive carcinoma (LP)
(c) Moderately differentiated carcinoma (MP)

Most cases of invasive squamous cell carcinoma of the cervix are preceded by a long premalignant phase of dysplasia (CIN). The treatment for CIN is dependent on the grade of the lesion but high grade lesions (CIN II and III) are generally excised, most often by loop excision biopsy. On histological examination, a few of these specimens exhibit the earliest form of invasive carcinoma with only superficial invasion of the cervical stroma. When the lesion is limited in extent (invasion less than 5 mm deep), it is termed *microinvasive carcinoma* and relatively conservative surgery such as cone biopsy is adequate to achieve cure. As seen in micrograph (a), the dysplastic surface epithelium **E** is similar to that seen in CIN III (Fig. 17.6d). Similar dysplastic epithelium is seen in the lower half of the field extending more deeply into an endocervical gland. Small nests of squamous carcinoma **S** are seen lying separately within the supporting stroma, the tumour cells having breached the epithelial basement membrane.

More extensive and macroscopically obvious carcinoma of the cervix is treated by surgical removal of the uterus in toto (*hysterectomy*). Such an invasive squamous carcinoma of the cervix is illustrated at low magnification in micrograph (b). Note that purple-staining tumour **T** has replaced most of the cervical stroma and muscle, although a portion of normal vaginal mucosa **N** remains at the tumour margin. The surface of the tumour is ulcerated; this accounts for the frequent presenting feature of *postcoital bleeding*.

An area of a moderately differentiated cervical squamous cell carcinoma is shown in micrograph (c). The lesion consists of sheets of pleomorphic squamous cells **T** invading the cervical stroma **S**. The cells have plentiful eosinophilic cytoplasm, and are separated by a small space where intercellular bridges would be seen at higher magnification. Compare this example with well and poorly differentiated squamous cell carcinoma in Figure 7.14.

Squamous carcinomas account for about 90% of cervical malignancies, most of the remainder being adenocarcinomas arising in the endocervix. Invasive carcinomas of the cervix spread widely into local structures and become disseminated to lymph nodes in the pelvis.

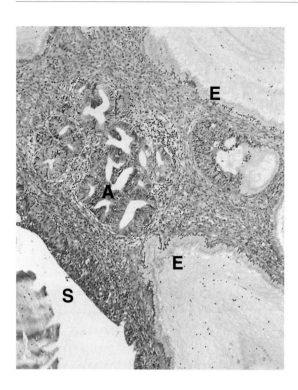

Fig. 17.8 Adenocarcinoma in situ of the endocervix (MP)

Adenocarcinoma of the cervix is less common than squamous carcinoma and arises from the endocervical glands. It is also often preceded by dysplastic changes in the glandular epithelium. This micrograph shows a small focus of *adenocarcinoma in situ* **A** (also known as *cervical glandular intraepithelial neoplasia, CGIN*). Compare the enlarged dysplastic columnar cells with those of the adjacent normal endocervical epithelium **E**. These glands show many of the features of adenocarcinoma but as yet have not developed the ability to invade the stroma. Adenocarcinoma in situ of the cervix commonly occurs in association with squamous dysplasia, as in this case where the surface epithelium **S** shows changes amounting to CIN III.

Disorders of the uterus

The uterine endometrium undergoes monthly cyclical changes under the influence of hormonal stimuli during the period between menarche and menopause, normally only being suspended in pregnancy. Before menarche, the endometrial glands and stroma are compact and inactive, a state they return to after the menopause. At menarche, around the menopause, and for the first few cycles after a pregnancy, the endometrium shows a mixture of inactive and normal functional patterns. Under the influence of oral contraceptive drugs and intrauterine contraceptive devices, the endometrium assumes various other histological patterns.

Endometrial infection is uncommon, but may follow genital tuberculosis or mechanical obstruction to the endocervical canal (e.g. by tumour), often leading to distension of the endometrial cavity by pus (*pyometra*). Fulminant infection of the uterus by coliform organisms was once a common fatal complication following childbirth (*puerperal fever*) but is now uncommon in developed countries.

Excessive or uncoordinated hormonal stimulation of the endometrium may produce *diffuse endometrial hyperplasia*. Two patterns are recognised, *simple (cystic) hyperplasia* and *complex hyperplasia*; these are illustrated in Figure 17.10. Localised areas of polypoid hyperplasia forming *endometrial polyps* are common and often contain cystically dilated endometrial glands (Fig. 17.9). The most common malignant tumour of the endometrium is *endometrioid carcinoma*, an adenocarcinoma derived from endometrial glands (Fig. 17.11). Other types of adenocarcinoma of the endometrium occur rarely, including tumours typical of the ovary such as serous papillary carcinoma and mucinous carcinoma.

The myometrium is the site of one of the most common benign connective tissue tumours, the *leiomyoma* (Fig. 17.12); in the myometrium, these smooth muscle tumours become progressively more collagenous as they enlarge, giving rise to the colloquial term *fibroid*. Leiomyoma must be differentiated from its much rarer malignant counterpart, *leiomyosarcoma* as well as tumours of borderline malignancy, known as *smooth muscle tumours of low malignant potential*.

The myometrium may also contain islands of ectopic endometrium known as *adenomyosis* (Fig. 17.13) which may give rise to pain and other menstrual disturbances. Such ectopic endometrial tissue may also be found in various other sites throughout the pelvis and sometimes the abdominal cavity when it is called *endometriosis* (Fig. 17.14). In this case, it may respond to the normal cyclical hormonal changes giving rise to bleeding into the tissues and consequent fibrosis.

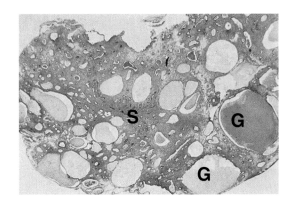

Fig. 17.9 Endometrial polyp (LP)

Endometrial polyps are an important but innocuous cause of abnormal uterine bleeding at or near the menopause; they are pedunculated and often multiple. Most are composed of cystically dilated glands **G** in a fibrotic endometrial stroma **S** and covered by a layer of flattened endometrial surface cells. The glands and stroma in some polyps are responsive to ovarian hormones, and may thus resemble proliferative, secretory or hyperplastic endometrium.

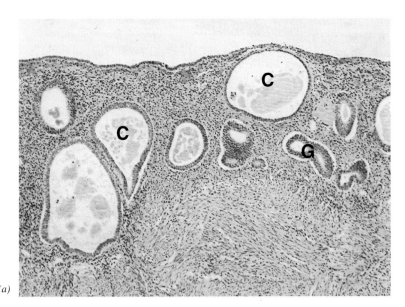

(a)

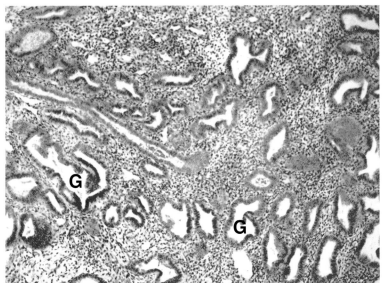

(b)

Fig. 17.10 Endometrial hyperplasia

(a) **Simple (cystic) hyperplasia (MP)**
(b) **Complex hyperplasia (MP)**

Endometrial hyperplasia appears to be a response to excessive or uncoordinated oestrogen production and may be either simple or complex in form.

In *simple (cystic) hyperplasia* as shown in micrograph (a), the endometrial lining becomes thickened by proliferation of the endometrial glandular tissue with the formation of numerous tiny cysts **C** scattered among normal-looking endometrial glands **G**; the cysts result from dilatation of endometrial glands. The intervening stroma frequently contains prominent thin-walled blood vessels (not shown here); heavy uterine bleeding is the most common presenting symptom.

In *complex hyperplasia*, shown in micrograph (b) there is also proliferation of the endometrial glands **G**, which show evidence of abnormal growth regulation. Many are irregular in shape and size, often with papillary infoldings. Adjacent glands may be so closely packed that there is little intervening stroma.

Marked cytological atypia may be superimposed upon simple, but more often complex, hyperplasia, with nuclear and cytoplasmic pleomorphism and increased mitotic activity. All types of hyperplasia are associated with an increased risk of invasive endometrial carcinoma. This is slight in the case of simple hyperplasia, greater with complex hyperplasia and greatest in *complex hyperplasia with atypia*.

BASIC SYSTEMS PATHOLOGY

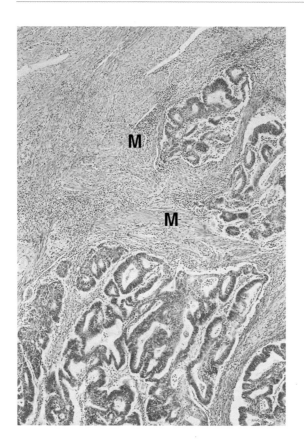

Fig. 17.11 Endometrioid adenocarcinoma (MP)

Endometrioid or *endometrial adenocarcinoma* is the most common malignancy of the endometrium, so-called because it resembles endometrial glands. It usually occurs in post-menopausal women and is the most important cause of post-menopausal bleeding.

Endometrioid adenocarcinoma often arises in endometrium with complex hyperplasia. It may be limited to the endometrium, forming a mass bulging into the endometrial cavity or it may invade the underlying myometrium **M**, as shown in this example. Distorted, irregular, glandular patterns are typical, and focal squamous metaplasia is seen frequently, known as *squamous morules*. The tumour spreads by local invasion through the myometrium and via lymphatics to iliac and para-aortic lymph nodes.

Endometrioid adenocarcinoma is graded on architectural and cytological criteria into grades 1, 2 and 3, with grade 1 having the best prognosis and grade 3 the worst. Other factors which determine the prognosis are depth of invasion into the myometrium, involvement of the cervix, lymph node metastases and distant metastases.

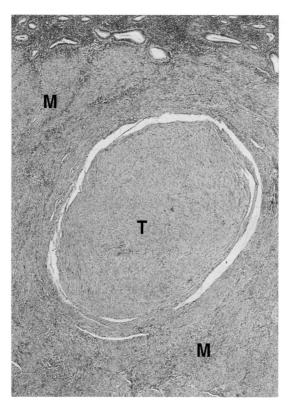

Fig. 17.12 Leiomyoma (fibroid) of myometrium (LP)

This benign tumour of myometrial smooth muscle is a very common cause of abnormal or excessive uterine bleeding and pelvic discomfort.

The tumour **T** is composed of fascicles of smooth muscle cells but larger tumours also show foci of collagen deposition particularly towards the centre of the tumour. Gradual expansion of the tumour compresses the surrounding myometrium **M** leading to atrophy of normal myometrial smooth muscle cells.

In this example, the tumour lies in the myometrium deep to the endometrium but some tumours arise near the endometrial cavity and may protrude into the cavity to produce a polypoid *submucous fibroid*. Secondary changes may also occur, including extensive collagenisation and calcification (especially with increasing age), and cystic degeneration. To an extent, the growth of these tumours is hormone-dependent, since they almost always shrink and partially regress after the menopause. These tumours are differentiated from *smooth muscle tumours of low malignant potential* and *leiomyosarcomas* of the myometrium on the basis of mitotic activity, cellular crowding and pleomorphism and invasive margins.

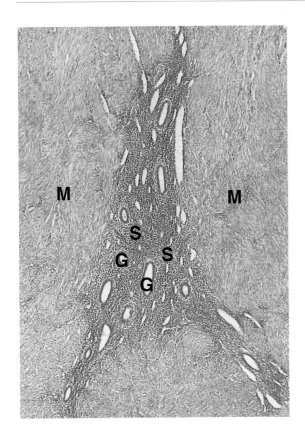

Fig. 17.13 Adenomyosis of the uterus (MP)

Adenomyosis is the term applied to a condition in which islands of ectopic endometrial glands **G** and stroma **S** are found embedded deep within the myometrium **M**, often at a considerable distance from the normal endometrium. Their presence is often associated with symmetrical increase in myometrial bulk thus enlarging the uterus; occasionally, they stimulate a more localised increase in smooth muscle to produce a leiomyoma-like mass containing endometrial islands, a lesion called an *adenomyoma*.

This ectopic endometrium represents an outgrowth of the basal endometrial layer and thus is not responsive in the normal manner to ovarian hormones. It is therefore not shed during menstruation, in contrast to endometriosis (Fig. 17.14), and thus no evidence of bleeding is seen in the tissue.

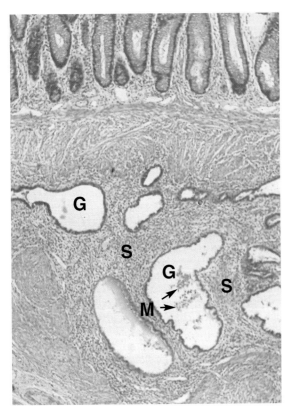

Fig. 17.14 Endometriosis (MP)

The Fallopian tubes, paratubal connective tissues and ovaries are the most frequent sites for the condition known as *endometriosis*, in which islands of ectopic endometrial glands and stroma are found outside the uterine body.

This micrograph shows endometrial glands **G** and stroma **S** embedded within the smooth muscle of the colon. Unlike adenomyosis, this endometrium is hormone-responsive and bleeds during menstruation causing pain. Evidence of bleeding may be seen as haemosiderin-laden macrophages **M** in the tissue and in the lumen of the glands as in this case. The presence of free blood within the tissue often causes a marked fibrotic reaction that may cause adhesions between loops of bowel. Fibrosis of the Fallopian tubes owing to endometriosis is a common cause of infertility and of tubal ectopic pregnancy. Endometriosis of the ovary may give rise to a cyst filled with altered blood, known as a *chocolate cyst*.

Placental disorders

Details of the various structural and functional abnormalities of the placenta, decidua, membranes and umbilical cord are generally outside the scope of this book; however, *hydatidiform mole* (Fig. 17.15) and *choriocarcinoma* (Fig. 17.16) are included as examples of disorders of placental growth. Ectopic pregnancy is discussed in Figure 17.18.

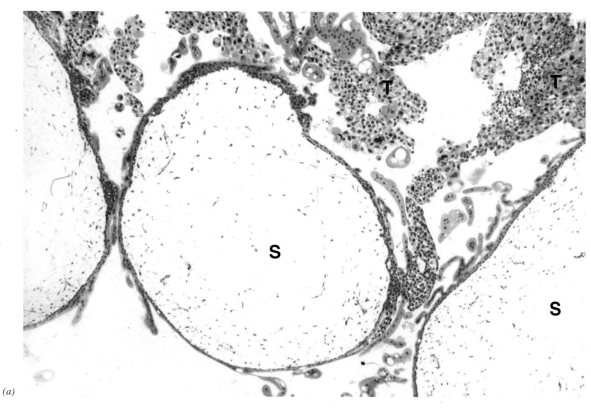

(a)

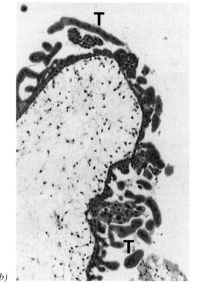

(b)

Fig. 17.15 Hydatidiform mole
(a) MP   (b) HP

The condition known as *hydatidiform mole* arises in a small proportion of pregnancies, after miscarriages or terminations of pregnancy or even years after a pregnancy. Moles may be *partial* or *complete*. In a complete mole, as seen in micrograph (a), the chorionic villi become oedematous with central cystic spaces (*cisternae*) **S**. The cisternae are invested by a layer of hyperplastic cytotrophoblast and syncytiotrophoblast. In addition to hyperplasia of the trophoblast there are disconnected masses of trophoblast cells **T** lying apparently free of the villi and showing mild cellular pleomorphism. Hydatidiform moles exhibit a wide spectrum of behaviour; some are eradicated by simple curettage, others persist despite repeated curettage, and a small number develop into undoubtedly malignant *choriocarcinoma* (Fig. 17.16).

Complete hydatidiform mole almost always has a 46,XX karyotype but all the chromosomes are derived from the spermatozoa with none from the ovum. Partial moles have similar but less prominent histological abnormalities, rarely develop into choriocarcinoma and have a triploid karyotype such as 69,XXY.

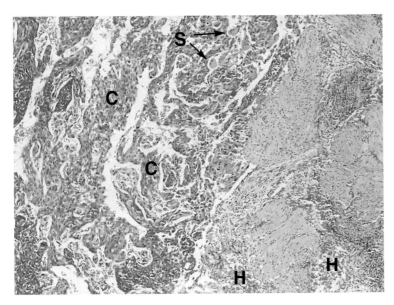

Fig. 17.16 Choriocarcinoma (HP)

Choriocarcinoma is a malignant tumour derived from trophoblast cells, usually from abnormal gestations. The tumour consists of malignant cells resembling either cytotrophoblast cells **C** or multinucleate syncytiotrophoblast cells **S**. The two cell types are arranged in alternating layers mimicking the structure of chorionic villi. No true chorionic villi are found. The tumour is typically haemorrhagic **H** because of the propensity of trophoblast cells to invade blood vessel walls. Choriocarcinoma is remarkably invasive, metastasising widely via lymphatics and the bloodstream, particularly to the lungs. Areas of necrosis in the tumour are common.

Choriocarcinoma may also occur rarely in the ovary and in the testis, in the latter case, usually as part of a mixed germ cell tumour.

Diseases of the Fallopian tubes

The Fallopian tubes may become infected by pyogenic bacteria, particularly the gonococcus and *Chlamydia*, and the acute inflammation, ***acute salpingitis*** (Fig. 17.17), may be complicated by obstruction of the tubal lumen, leading to chronic suppurative inflammation and abscess formation. Along with tuberculous infection of the Fallopian tube, these conditions constitute an important cause of female infertility owing to tubal lumen obliteration. Scarring of the tube and other disorders may prevent the free passage of a fertilised ovum into the endometrial cavity and implantation may occur in the oviduct leading to ***tubal ectopic pregnancy*** (Fig. 17.18); this usually culminates in massive haemorrhage caused by the placenta eroding through the tubal wall.

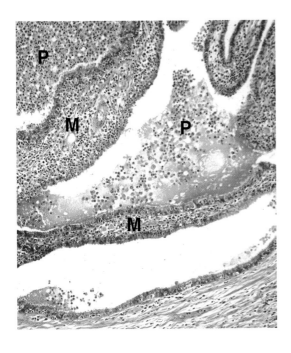

Fig. 17.17 Acute salpingitis (MP)

In ***acute salpingitis***, the tubal mucosa **M** becomes hyperaemic, oedematous, and infiltrated with neutrophils and the lumen becomes filled with purulent exudate **P**. Blockage of the tubal lumen often follows, preventing drainage and leading to distension of the tube by pus (***pyosalpinx***). Sometimes the inflammation produces ***adhesions*** between tube, fimbriae and ovary, and extension of suppuration to these areas may produce multiple locules of pus, the ***tubo-ovarian abscess***. Without the intervention of antibiotics, the combination of adhesions and suppuration rarely permits total resolution of the acute inflammation and a state of chronic inflammation generally ensues. This state, known as ***chronic salpingitis***, may persist for many years resulting in fibrosis and tubal obstruction and is an important cause of female infertility. Chronic salpingitis may be a component of more widespread chronic inflammation involving ovaries, clinically termed ***pelvic inflammatory disease***. Sometimes the inflammation dies down but the obstructed tube becomes massively distended by fluid, a condition termed ***hydrosalpinx***.

BASIC SYSTEMS PATHOLOGY

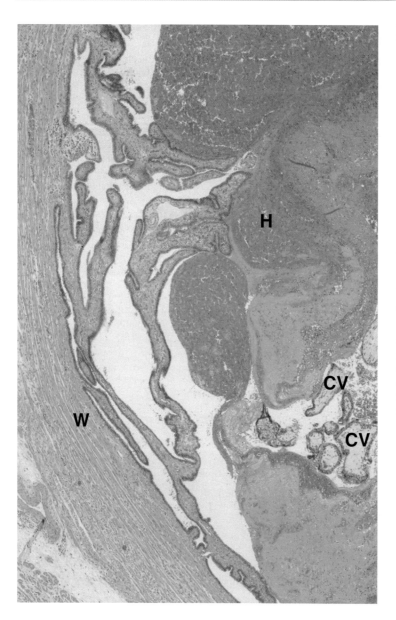

Fig. 17.18 Tubal ectopic pregnancy (LP)

The Fallopian tube is the most frequent location for ectopic implantation of the fertilised ovum resulting in *ectopic pregnancy*.

The tubal lumen becomes filled with the developing embryo (not seen in this micrograph) and associated membranes as well as the chorionic villi **CV** of the placenta. The distended tubal wall **W** is often deeply congested and thinned. There is extensive haemorrhage **H** into the lumen of the tube (*haematosalpinx*). The trophoblast burrows into the wall of the Fallopian tube leading to perforation.

Ectopic pregnancies usually become dramatically apparent by severe haemorrhage into the lumen often followed by tracking of blood into the peritoneal cavity. Thus tubal ectopics most often present as acute abdominal emergencies; only very rarely does the pregnancy continue to near normal term.

Disorders of the ovary

Non-neoplastic cysts

Under the influence of pituitary gonadotrophins, the ovary undergoes cyclical changes providing for the development and release of a mature ovum at the mid-point of each monthly menstrual cycle, and for the production of the ovarian hormones which control the menstrual cycle. During the proliferative phase of the menstrual cycle, a number of follicles enlarge culminating in maturation of one follicle that discharges its single ovum into the Fallopian tube (ovulation). The follicle, until this time also responsible for production of oestrogens, now develops into the corpus luteum responsible for producing progesterone until the beginning of the next menstrual cycle when the follicle atrophies to form the redundant collagenous corpus albicans. This regular sequence of changes is normally only interrupted by the advent of pregnancy, in which case the corpus luteum persists until the end of the first trimester. On occasion, however, the sequence is arrested at some stage and small *follicular* or *luteal cysts* may form. Some small cysts may also form by inclusion of islands of surface 'germinal' epithelium of the ovary; these are known as *germinal inclusion cysts*. These three types of cyst are shown in Figure 17.20.

Tumours of the ovary

Tumours may arise from each of the specialised elements that make up the ovary and may be classified into four broad groups. These groups of tumours and their major subtypes are listed in Figure 17.19 below.

- **Epithelial origin** – tumours of the surface ovarian epithelium are common and are usually cystic. These tumours may be either benign (often cystic) or malignant. A third group of epithelial tumours are of intermediate malignancy with a low but significant probability of metastasising. This group is called borderline or atypical proliferating tumours.
- **Stromal origin** – tumours may develop from *granulosa cells* and *theca cells* (Fig. 17.24) as well as from spindle cells of the ovarian stroma forming *fibromas*. These *sex cord-stromal tumours* may produce oestrogenic hormones and cause endocrine effects such as endometrial hyperplasia (Fig. 17.10).
- **Germ cell origin** – the classification and morphology of ovarian germ cell tumours are similar to those for testicular germ cell tumours (Fig. 19.3).
- **Metastatic** – the ovary is a common site for metastatic carcinoma. A well-known example is the so-called *Krukenberg tumour* in which there is infiltration of the ovary by mucin-secreting adenocarcinoma of signet ring pattern (Figs 7.16c and 13.11b); such tumours are usually derived from stomach or colon, and probably reach the ovary by either transcoelomic or lymphatic spread. Tumours from other parts of the genital tract, including uterus and cervix, commonly involve the ovaries. Breast cancer also frequently metastasises to this site. The ovaries may also be involved by lymphoma.

Fig. 17.19 Overview of ovarian tumours

Tumour type	Subtype
Epithelial	Serous – serous cystadenoma, borderline serous tumour, serous cystadenocarcinoma Mucinous – mucinous cystadenoma, borderline mucinous tumour, mucinous cystadenocarcinoma
	Endometrioid – almost all carcinomas
	Brenner tumour – benign, rarely malignant
	Clear cell – almost all malignant
Sex-cord-stromal tumours	Fibroma
	Thecoma
	Granulosa cell tumour
Germ cell	Mature teratoma (dermoid cyst)
	Dysgerminoma (testicular equivalent is seminoma)
	Yolk sac tumour
	Choriocarcinoma
Metastatic	Primary in stomach, colon, breast, uterus, cervix
	May also be involved by lymphoma

Other disorders of the ovary

The ovary may be involved in *endometriosis* (Fig. 17.14), as well as being involved by chronic inflammation in the form of tubo-ovarian abscesses caused by primary infection of the Fallopian tube (Fig. 17.17).

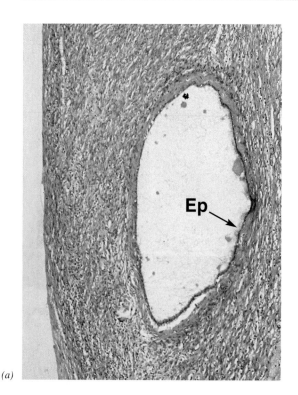

(a)

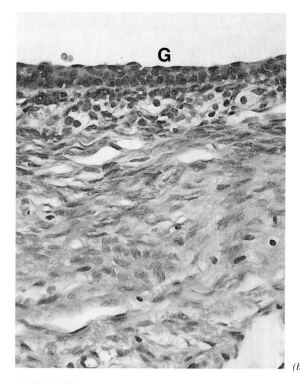

(b)

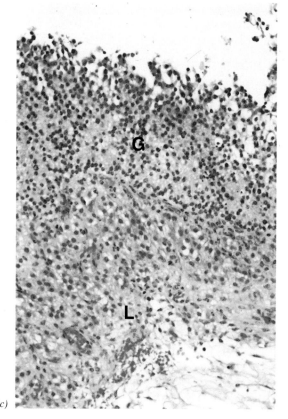

(c)

Fig. 17.20 Non-neoplastic ovarian cysts
 (a) Germinal inclusion cyst (MP)
 (b) Follicular cyst (MP) (c) Luteal cyst (MP)

The most common type of ovarian cyst is the so-called *germinal or epithelial inclusion cyst* illustrated in micrograph (a). These cysts are commonly multiple, small and lined by a simple cuboidal epithelium **Ep**. They are thought to be derived from entrapped portions of the ovarian surface epithelium, which is erroneously but traditionally referred to as germinal epithelium.

Follicular cysts, as seen in micrograph (b), are lined internally by granulosa cells **G** which usually form a thicker layer than do the flattened cells lining the germinal inclusion cyst. Continuing enlargement of the follicular cyst leads to atrophy of the lining cells so that distinction between a large follicular cyst and a germinal inclusion cyst may be difficult.

The *luteal cyst* is probably derived from a corpus luteum that has not undergone the normal transition to a corpus albicans. The cyst is usually ovoid with a slightly irregular outline. Microscopically, it contains clear or brownish fluid and is lined by a yellow-coloured layer of variable thickness. As shown in micrograph (c), the yellow layer is composed of plump luteal cells **L** with lipid-rich cytoplasm; the inner layer is composed of granulosa cells **G**, which are also luteinised.

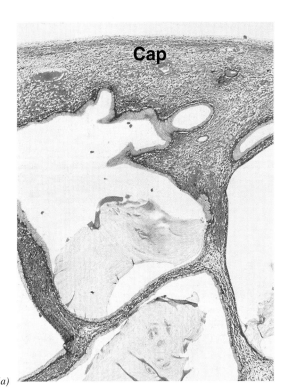

(a)

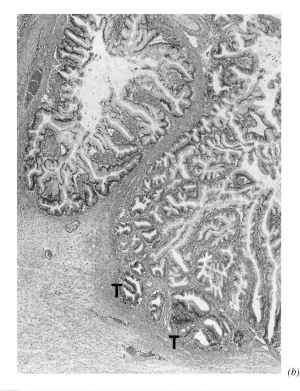

(b)

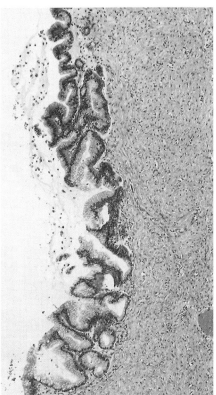

(c)

Fig. 17.21 Mucinous tumours of ovary
- **(a) Benign mucinous cystadenoma (MP)**
- **(b) Mucinous cystadenocarcinoma (MP)**
- **(c) Borderline mucinous tumour (MP)**

Mucinous tumours of the ovary may be benign or malignant. The *benign cystadenoma*, as shown in micrograph (a), has a characteristically smooth outer surface composed of the ovarian capsule **Cap**. The cystic locules are filled with mucin and lined by tall columnar epithelium with uniform basal nuclei and copious mucin-containing cytoplasm at the luminal aspect. These cells are thought to resemble endocervical epithelial cells.

The malignant variant, *mucinous cystadenocarcinoma*, illustrated in micrograph (b), is less common. The tumour is more solid, with smaller cystic spaces. The cells are usually recognisably columnar, but the nuclei are larger and more pleomorphic. The cells are crowded and show increased mitotic activity. Evidence of malignancy is usually demonstrated by invasion of tumour cells **T** into the supporting stroma.

Some mucinous tumours show many of the cytological features of mucinous adenocarcinoma without actual invasion of the stroma. These are called *borderline* or *atypically proliferating mucinous tumours* and their prognosis is better than for overtly malignant tumours; an example is shown in micrograph (c).

Fig. 17.22 Serous ovarian tumours

(a) Serous cystadenoma (HP)
(b) Serous papillary cystadenocarcinoma (MP)
(c) Borderline serous tumour (LP)

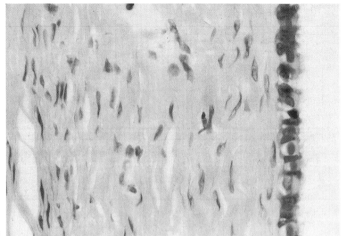

(a)

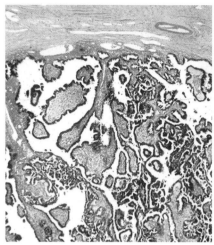

(c)

(b)

Benign serous cystadenomas, which may form very large cysts, are often unilocular and are filled with a clear watery (serous) fluid. The benign cysts are lined by columnar epithelium, which resembles that of the Fallopian tube. A variant on this theme is the serous *cystadenofibroma,* which has a similar epithelium but also includes a stromal component made up of bland spindle cells in a collagenous stroma. The appearances are reminiscent of *fibroadenoma* of the breast (see Fig. 18.6).

In malignant serous tumours (b), known as *serous cystadenocarcinomas*, the cystic cavity tends to be filled by complex branching papillary structures. These are covered by columnar cells that are crowded and dysplastic. The cells are stratified and form solid sheets. Essential for the diagnosis of malignancy is evidence of invasion of the stroma by tumour **T**; indeed the tumour may breach the capsule of the ovary, forming papillary outgrowths on the surface.

Tumours of borderline malignancy, known as *borderline* or *atypically proliferating serous tumours* (c), show many of the cytological and architectural features of serous cystadenocarcinoma but lack stromal invasion. Some papillary growths contain spherical, concentrically laminated, calcified bodies in their stroma; these *psammoma bodies* are typical of papillary tumours of the ovary, although they are also seen in papillary tumours of the thyroid and in meningiomas (Fig. 23.14).

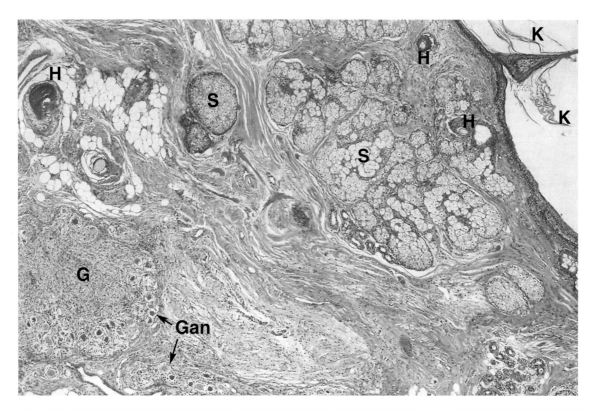

Fig. 17.23 Benign cystic teratoma (MP)

This tumour, formerly known as ***dermoid cyst of the ovary***, is an example of a mature teratoma in which ectodermal elements usually predominate. The lesion takes the form of a unilocular cyst filled with a thick, yellowish, pasty material composed of masses of degenerating keratin **K**, often containing hair. This is produced by the lining epithelium of the cyst, which is keratinising stratified squamous epithelium resembling skin. At one end of the cyst wall, there is often a raised area within which are other teratomatous components including hair follicles **H**, sebaceous glands **S** and occasionally teeth. Although ectodermal derivatives predominate, particularly skin and skin appendage components, mesodermal (e.g. cartilage and smooth muscle) and endodermal (e.g. respiratory and gut epithelium) elements occur in some tumours.

Neuroectodermal tissues may also be found; in this example, note the area of glial tissue **G** and a ganglion **Gan** alongside.

Cystic teratomas are most common in young women, and are almost always benign. Rarely, malignant change may occur in the squamous epithelial component; this is seen in elderly patients who have harboured a cystic teratoma for many years.

In addition to benign cystic teratomas discussed here, solid malignant ovarian teratomas occur in children and pubertal girls and are prone to widespread metastasis. Other germ cell tumours of the ovary such as dysgerminoma, choriocarcinoma and yolk sac tumour are rare and have the same histological appearances as their testicular equivalents (see Ch. 19).

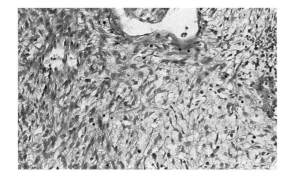

Fig. 17.24 Theca cell tumour (MP)

This is but one example of a number of ovarian sex-cord-stromal tumours. Other tumours in this group include granulosa cell tumours, ovarian fibromas and Sertoli–Leydig cell tumours, which may occur in the ovary (rarely) as well as in the testis. ***Theca cell tumours (thecomas)*** are lobulated solid tumours with a well-circumscribed margin and a bright yellow cut surface macroscopically. The tumour is composed of plump spindle cells containing fine lipid droplets, which make the cytoplasm appear foamy. This tumour usually secretes excessive amounts of oestrogens and may be associated with endometrial hyperplasia or even endometrial carcinoma. Thecomas are virtually always benign.

18. Breast

Introduction

The female breast is dependent for its normal activity on oestrogen and progestogens and thus exhibits considerable structural and functional variation throughout life. Apart from the overt changes occurring at puberty, pregnancy, lactation and menopause, more subtle changes also occur within the normal menstrual cycle. As a corollary, hormonal disturbances probably underlie various disorders of the breast, notably *benign breast disease*, but probably also play some part in the pathogenesis of more serious conditions such as *breast cancer*. Likewise, the male breast normally remains rudimentary unless breast enlargement, *gynaecomastia* (Fig. 18.5), is induced by exogenous or endogenous hormone imbalance; it may also result from the use of certain drugs, for example spironolactone.

Most clinically significant breast disorders present as a lump and the major imperative is to identify those which are malignant tumours so that the patient may be treated promptly. Several national screening programmes now use radiological techniques (*mammography and/or ultrasound*) to identify early suspicious breast lesions, including abnormal calcifications. A tissue diagnosis is then made by *fine needle aspiration biopsy (FNAB), core biopsy* or *excision biopsy* before definitive treatment is undertaken. It is expected that early removal of very small tumours will be curative.

Inflammatory disorders of the breast

Infections of the breast are uncommon and mainly occur during lactation; the organisms (usually *Staphylococcus aureus*) gain access through cracks and fissures in the nipple and areola. Without early antibiotic therapy, the resulting *bacterial mastitis* may be followed by the development of a *breast abscess* that may require surgical drainage. More commonly, localised areas of inflammation of the breast follow trauma, which may be of sufficient severity to produce a condition known as *fat necrosis* (Fig. 18.1).

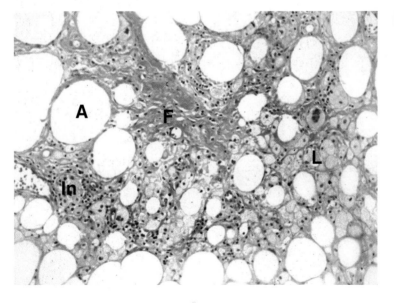

Fig. 18.1 Fat necrosis (MP)

Trauma to the breast, sometimes apparently quite trivial, may result in necrosis of mammary adipose tissue. The presence of necrotic adipose tissue **A** excites a chronic inflammatory cell infiltrate **In**, in which lipophages **L** (macrophages containing lipid giving their cytoplasm a foamy appearance) and plasma cells may be present in large numbers. Fibrosis **F** of the damaged area produces a hard, often irregular, breast lump, which may resemble a breast carcinoma on palpation. Similar, more localised, changes may be seen in the breast following FNAB, core biopsy or other surgical procedures.

Non-neoplastic breast disease

Non-neoplastic breast disease includes a number of disorders that may give rise to a palpable mass or a mammographic abnormality. These conditions may include alterations to the stroma, to the glandular architecture or to the glandular epithelium; usually more than one element is involved. Calcification is not uncommon in these benign lesions and must be differentiated from calcification seen in malignant breast disease. This is not always possible using imaging techniques and may require biopsy to determine the nature of the lesion.

Simple *fibrocystic change* involves cystic dilatation of ducts, apocrine metaplasia of the epithelium and fibrosis of stroma (Fig. 18.2). *Adenosis* refers to a benign proliferation of glands that may be combined with fibrosis (sclerosis) of the stroma to give rise to *sclerosing adenosis* (Fig. 18.3) which can be difficult to differentiate both clinically and pathologically from invasive carcinoma. Similar changes with proliferation and distortion of benign breast ducts and lobules along with fibrosis of the stroma may be seen in *radial scars* and *complex sclerosing lesions*. A third type of benign lesion is *ductal hyperplasia* involving the epithelium of the ducts without proliferation of the glands. In ductal hyperplasia there is an increase in the number of layers of cells lining the ducts, i.e. more than the normal two layers. This is generally graded as mild, moderate or florid ductal hyperplasia. *Atypical ductal hyperplasia (ADH)* (Fig. 18.4) is a condition intermediate between hyperplasia and *carcinoma in situ* and carries with it a small but significantly increased risk of developing carcinoma.

With the exception of atypical ductal hyperplasia and sclerosing adenosis, the above conditions carry little or no increased risk of malignancy. Benign breast disorders may be difficult to differentiate clinically from carcinoma; furthermore, these conditions are common and thus may occur concurrently with, but independently of, invasive carcinoma.

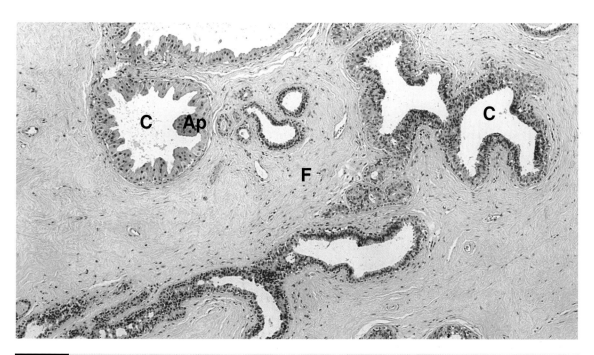

Fig. 18.2 Fibrocystic change (MP)

This breast lesion is so common that it is considered a normal physiological variant. It is nevertheless of great clinical importance since it may give rise to firm palpable masses and/or large cysts that require biopsy to exclude carcinoma. Calcification may also be seen in these lesions

Typically, as in this micrograph, there is dilatation of ducts to form cysts **C** accompanied by *apocrine metaplasia* **Ap** of ductal epithelial cells. In apocrine metaplasia, the epithelial cells have strongly eosinophilic cytoplasm often with apical buds and enlarged nuclei mimicking the apocrine secretory pattern of lactation. In addition, there is variable fibrosis **F** of the stroma which may give the mass an irregular outline.

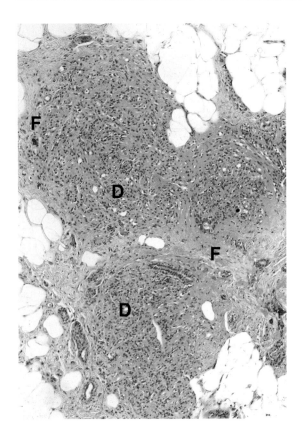

Fig. 18.3 Sclerosing adenosis (MP)

In this condition, there is fibrosis of the intralobular stroma in association with adenosis, i.e. proliferation of benign terminal duct-lobular units. This common lesion may give rise to a poorly defined palpable mass in the breast or to a mammographic abnormality including calcification. The lesion is centred on the lobules and the overall lobular pattern can still be discerned, in contrast to carcinoma in which it is usually lost. The condition is associated with a slight increase in risk of carcinoma.

As seen in this micrograph, there is a proliferation of small ducts **D** which are distorted by the surrounding fibrosis **F**.

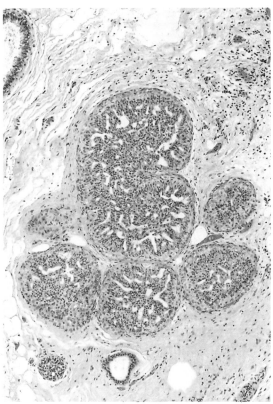

Fig. 18.4 Atypical ductal hyperplasia (MP)

Ductal hyperplasia is another common form of benign breast disease. In mild, moderate or florid hyperplasia (not illustrated), the thickness of the epithelial layer lining the ducts is increased from the normal two cells thick to three, four or more. In atypical ductal hyperplasia as illustrated in this micrograph, the ducts are distended by marked proliferation of epithelial cells forming a swirling pattern. The epithelial cells often exhibit a degree of cytological atypia manifest, as in this example, by cellular enlargement and mild nuclear pleomorphism.

Atypical ductal hyperplasia (ADH) is associated with a mildly increased risk of the development of invasive carcinoma but this is less than that associated with ***ductal carcinoma in situ*** (Fig. 18.9). ADH is also commonly seen in breast biopsies in association with both invasive and in situ carcinoma.

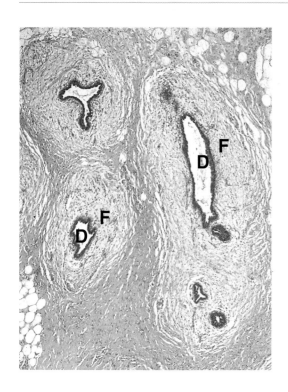

Fig. 18.5 Gynaecomastia of male breast (MP)

The male breast is normally rudimentary and inactive, consisting of fibroadipose tissue containing atrophic mammary ducts. Oestrogenic changes may result in breast hyperplasia (*gynaecomastia*). The simple mammary ducts **D** become enlarged, often with thickening of the epithelial layer and an increase in periductal fibrous tissue **F**.

Gynaecomastia may develop at puberty because of a rise in circulating oestrogens or by administration of exogenous oestrogens, for example sex change, drugs used in treatment of prostatic carcinoma. Various other drugs such as spironolactone, heroin and marijuana also cause gynaecomastia in some individuals. It may also result from alcohol abuse and, in particular, cirrhosis of the liver, which results in abnormal metabolism of androgens into oestrogens.

Neoplasms of the breast

The most common benign neoplasm of the breast is the *fibroadenoma* (Fig. 18.6), a localised proliferation of breast ducts and stroma. Such lesions occur most frequently in isolated form in women aged 25–35 ('breast mice'). The *phyllodes tumour* (Fig. 18.7) is related to the fibroadenoma except that it has a tendency to recur and some are frankly malignant. The only other benign tumour of much clinical significance is the *benign intraduct papilloma* (see Fig. 18.8), usually occurring as a solitary lesion in one of the larger mammary ducts. Histologically similar papillary lesions may also be multifocal, a condition known as *intraduct papillomatosis*. These lesions tend to occur in the smaller ducts and are associated with a small but definite increase in the risk of carcinoma.

Malignant tumours of the female breast are extremely common, with a peak incidence in the decade before the menopause. Most are adenocarcinomas arising from the epithelium of either the mammary lobules *(lobular carcinoma)* or the mammary ducts *(ductal carcinoma)*; the range of histological appearances is illustrated in Figs. 18.9 to 8.13. In many cases, the development of invasive breast cancer seems to be preceded by carcinoma in situ in which the malignant cells proliferate within the mammary ducts or lobules but do not breach the basement membrane (*ductal* or *lobular carcinoma in situ*).

In addition to the main groups of lobular and ductal carcinoma, there are several subtypes of ductal carcinoma that are associated with distinct clinical and pathological features, often with a good prognosis; examples are *tubular carcinoma* and *mucinous carcinoma* of the breast (Fig. 18.10). *Medullary carcinoma* is not illustrated but is a rare variant characterised by high grade histological features and a prominent inflammatory infiltrate.

In some cases of breast carcinoma, both in situ and invasive, malignant cells may spread along mammary and lactiferous ducts onto the surface of the nipple resulting in *Paget's disease of the nipple* (see Fig. 18.13).

Sarcomas also occur in the breast, the most common being *angiosarcoma*. Carcinoma of the breast does occur in males but is extremely uncommon.

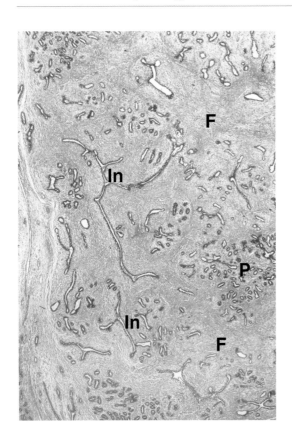

Fig. 18.6 Fibroadenoma (MP)

Fibroadenoma is a common benign solitary lesion found in the breasts of women of all ages but most often in women under 30. It is usually considered to be a tumour but may well represent a nodular form of benign mammary hyperplasia. The mass is well circumscribed with a pseudocapsule of connective tissue and is composed of both epithelial and stromal components. The epithelial components form glandular structures lined by mammary duct-type epithelium, whilst the stromal component is a loose, cellular form of fibrous tissue **F**. In some cases, the stroma may be myxomatous.

Two patterns of growth are seen, often in the same lesion. In the ***pericanalicular pattern*** **P**, the epithelial component takes the form of rounded ducts that remain small and undistorted, with the stroma arranged round them in a roughly symmetrical and regular manner. By contrast, in the ***intracanalicular pattern*** **In**, the ducts appear elongated but actually represent sections cut through flattened spaces compressed by nodular proliferation of the stromal component; in general, this latter pattern is more prominent in larger fibroadenomas. In both patterns of fibroadenoma, hormonal changes, such as occur in pregnancy and lactation, may induce hyperplasia of the epithelial component.

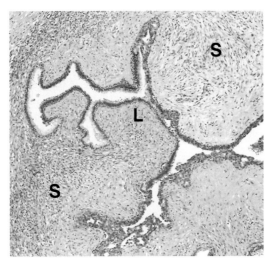

Fig. 18.7 Phyllodes tumour (MP)

The ***phyllodes tumour*** is related to the fibroadenoma, consisting of a mixture of epithelial and stromal elements. The stroma **S** is however more prominent in the phyllodes tumour, consisting of crowded atypical spindle cells. The stroma thus bulges into the lumen of the duct to give the characteristic leaf-like pattern **L** seen in this micrograph. Mitotic figures including abnormal mitotic figures may be present.

Most of these tumours are cured by complete excision, but some recur locally. A small proportion behave in a frankly malignant fashion with distant metastases. Hence, the old name, ***cystosarcoma phyllodes***, has been dropped in favour of the terms ***benign*** and ***malignant phyllodes tumour***. It is not always possible to predict which of these lesions are likely to be malignant from the histological appearances alone.

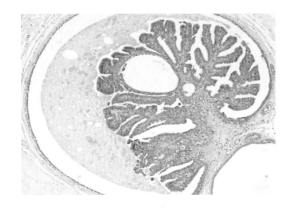

Fig. 18.8 Intraduct papilloma (LP)

Papillomas of mammary duct epithelium may arise as solitary or multiple lesions. Solitary lesions, as shown here, are usually located in the larger lactiferous ducts near the nipple and present with a blood-stained discharge from the nipple. The lesions are usually small, consisting of a delicate pink-staining supporting stroma covered by a single or double layer of cuboidal or low columnar epithelial cells resembling those lining the mammary duct from which the papilloma has arisen; with larger lesions, the duct is often dilated. Multiple duct papillomata (***florid duct papillomatosis***) may also occur. Malignant change is rare but carcinomas with a papillary architecture are sometimes seen. Carcinoma in situ may also arise in a breast papilloma.

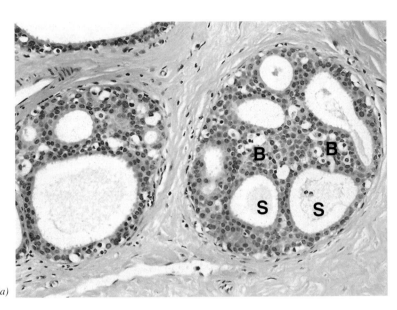

(a)

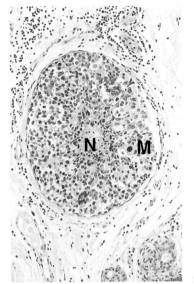

(b)

Fig. 18.9 Ductal carcinomas of the breast

(a) Low grade ductal carcinoma in situ (MP)
(b) High grade ductal carcinoma in situ (MP)
(c) Invasive ductal carcinoma (MP)

Ductal carcinoma is divided into invasive and in situ types depending on whether the malignant cells have breached the basement membrane of the duct and invaded the stroma. Both invasive and in situ carcinomas may be associated with abnormal calcifications that may provide the only mammographic clue to the presence of small tumours.

Ductal carcinoma in situ (DCIS) is graded according to the cytological and architectural features of the lesion, with low grade lesions conferring a moderate increase in the likelihood of invasive carcinoma while high grade lesions are associated with a marked increase in the likelihood of invasive carcinoma. Micrograph (a) shows an example of low grade DCIS. The epithelial cells fill and expand the ducts forming sharply defined glandular spaces **S** separated by 'rigid' bridges **B** of cells; this is also known as the ***cribriform pattern***. The cells are very uniform in size and very regularly placed in relation to each other. Another low grade variant is the ***micropapillary pattern*** (not illustrated here) which commonly occurs in association with the cribriform pattern.

In contrast, in high grade ductal carcinoma in situ, the duct is expanded by a proliferation of large highly pleomorphic cells. As seen in micrograph (b), mitotic figures **M** are common as is central necrosis **N** (often called ***comedo necrosis***), which may be calcified (not in this example). DCIS is usually detected by mammographic screening programmes and only gives rise to a palpable mass when extensive.

Invasive ductal carcinoma (often called ***ductal carcinoma, NOS***, i.e. *N*ot *O*therwise *S*pecified) is the most common form of invasive carcinoma and has the worst prognosis. As seen in micrograph (c), the invading malignant epithelial cells form small ductal structures **D**, solid nests **N** and even solid sheets of cells. The stroma **S**, as in this example, is frequently very fibrotic which gives the characteristic firm texture on palpation. Another example of invasive ductal carcinoma is shown in Figure 7.3.

Several grading schemes have been developed over the years to help predict the clinical behaviour of invasive breast carcinomas. The most commonly used scheme

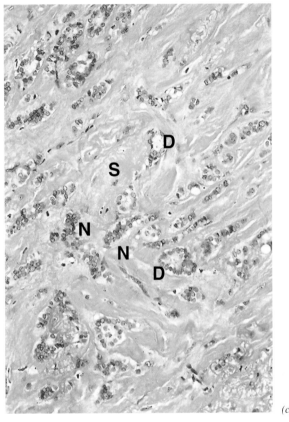

(c)

assigns a numerical grade to each of three features of the tumour; namely, the degree of gland formation, the nuclear features of the tumour cells and the frequency of mitotic figures. The sum of these grades is then converted to a numerical grade 1,2 or 3, with grade 1 being a low grade lesion with a better prognosis and grade 3 being a high grade lesion.

BASIC SYSTEMS PATHOLOGY

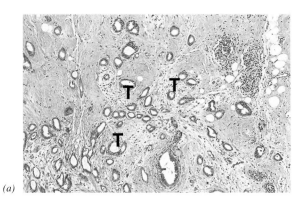

(a)

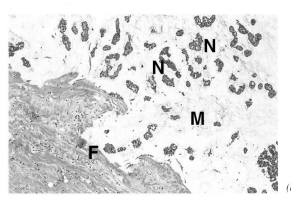

(b)

Fig. 18.10 Variants of invasive ductal carcinoma
(a) Tubular carcinoma (MP)   (b) Mucinous (colloid) carcinoma (MP)

Certain variants of invasive ductal carcinoma have a much better prognosis than invasive ductal carcinoma, NOS. These are much less common than invasive ductal carcinoma, NOS but two of the commoner types are invasive *tubular carcinoma* and *mucinous* or *colloid carcinoma*. Tubular carcinoma, as shown in micrograph (a), consists of malignant epithelial cells which form well-defined tubular or ductal structures **T** with no solid nests of cells or single cell invasion. The tubules are lined by a single layer of mildly pleomorphic cells and invade into the surrounding fat with no evidence of an overall

lobular architecture; this is in contrast to sclerosing adenosis (Fig. 18.3) which may be confused with tubular carcinoma.

Mucinous carcinoma, as seen in micrograph (b), is characterised by pools of mucin **M** in which nests of malignant cells **N** are suspended. Mucinous carcinoma is characteristically soft to palpation and has a well-defined margin of fibrous tissue **F**.

Other ductal carcinoma variants with a good prognosis that are not illustrated here include invasive *cribriform carcinoma* and *medullary carcinoma*.

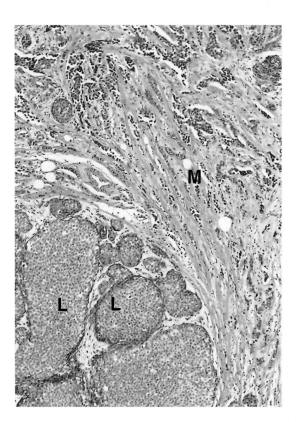

Fig. 18.11 Lobular carcinoma of the breast (MP)

Like their ductal counterparts, cancers arising from breast lobules are divided into in situ and invasive forms; both are often present in the same lesion. This micrograph shows *lobular carcinoma in situ (LCIS)* at the lower left adjacent to an area of invasive carcinoma.

In the in situ area, the lobules **L** are expanded and filled by small, evenly spaced epithelial cells that do not form ducts. In the upper right part of the micrograph, *invasive lobular carcinoma* consists of similar malignant cells **M** infiltrating the stroma in rows of cells (often described as *Indian files*) and as single cells which do not form ducts.

Lobular carcinoma in situ is often found incidentally in biopsies taken for another purpose as it usually does not give rise to a mammographic or palpable lesion. LCIS is often multifocal and is considered as a marker lesion for invasive carcinoma rather than a premalignant lesion. Invasive lobular carcinoma carries a better prognosis than invasive ductal carcinoma NOS, but is more likely to be bilateral.

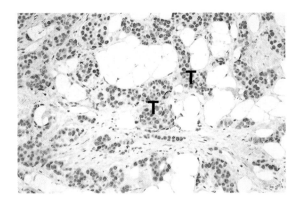

Fig. 18.12 Oestrogen receptors in breast carcinoma (MP)

Many factors influence the prognosis of patients with breast carcinoma. Most important among these are the histological type of the tumour, the histological grade of the tumour, tumour size, lymphatic or vascular invasion and the presence and number of lymph node metastases. Tumours that express receptors for oestrogen and/or progestogens also have a better prognosis and furthermore are more likely to respond to hormonal treatment.

This micrograph shows a section of invasive ductal carcinoma which has been stained by the immunoperoxidase method using a monoclonal antibody specific for oestrogen receptors. Most of the tumour cells **T** show strong brown staining of the nuclei indicating oestrogen receptor positivity and thus a relatively improved prognosis.

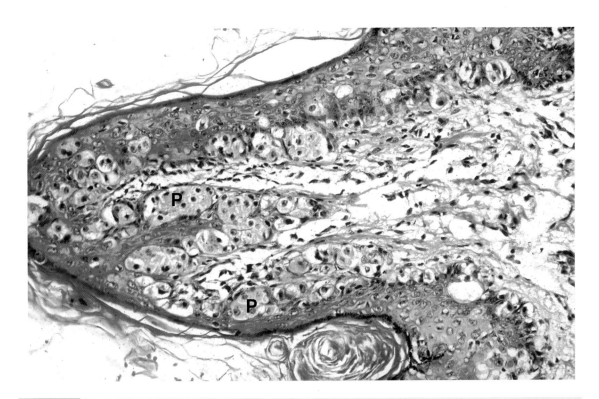

Fig. 18.13 Paget's disease of the nipple (HP)

Some patients with carcinoma of the breast (usually of ductal origin) develop reddening and thickening of the skin of the nipple and areola, occasionally followed by ulceration. The epidermis of the nipple and areola becomes infiltrated by malignant epithelial cells with hyperchromatic nuclei and pale cytoplasm. These cells, known as *Paget's cells* **P**, are breast carcinoma cells that have spread along the epithelium of the mammary and nipple ducts to the epidermis from an underlying in situ or invasive ductal carcinoma.

19. Male reproductive system

Introduction

The male reproductive system includes the testes with their related duct systems, the prostate and the penis. These organs are responsible for the production, storage and periodic emission of the male gametes, spermatozoa, as well as the production of male sex hormones, principally testosterone. The organs of this system are prone to the full range of pathological conditions seen in other organ systems. However, clinically the most important pathological conditions are inflammation (mainly caused by infection) and tumours.

Disorders of the testis and epididymis

Inflammation of the testis *(orchitis)* may result from virus infections, for example mumps; the testis may also be the site of a gumma in the tertiary stage of syphilis (Fig. 4.13). Other bacterial infections usually arise as a complication of infection of the lower urinary tract or following surgical instrumentation. A non-infective cause of testicular inflammation is *granulomatous orchitis,* which may follow an episode of trauma to the testis (Fig. 19.1). Focal granulomatous inflammation, known as *sperm granulomas* may also occur because of sperm retention, for example after vasectomy. Venous infarction of the testis owing to *torsion* is an important cause of testicular pain in childhood and young adulthood and is illustrated in Figure 19.2.

The most important pathological lesions of the testes are tumours, most of which are derived from germ cells; a system of classification is shown in Figure 19.3 and examples are illustrated in Figures 19.4 to 19.8.

Like the testis, the epididymis may become infected by pyogenic bacteria associated with lower urinary tract infection and/or surgical instrumentation. When infection occurs, usually both the testis and epididymis are involved, a condition known as *acute epididymo-orchitis*. The epididymis is occasionally the site of metastatic tuberculous infection, *tuberculous epididymitis*, usually secondary to active pulmonary or renal tuberculosis.

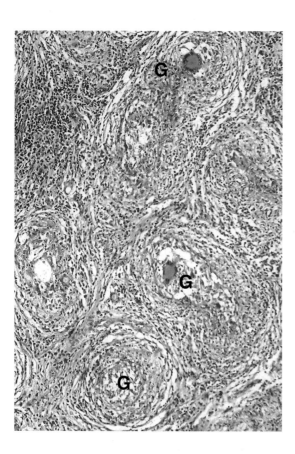

Fig. 19.1 Granulomatous orchitis (MP)

This form of inflammatory disease of the testis most commonly follows trauma to the testis or surgery to the spermatic cord. The testis becomes uniformly firm and enlarged and the cut surface has a homogenous pallid appearance.

Histologically there is a diffuse chronic inflammatory cell infiltrate, consisting mainly of lymphocytes and plasma cells, with numerous granulomata **G** containing giant cells. These inflammatory changes are associated with destruction and atrophy of the seminiferous tubules, which in this specimen have been almost entirely destroyed. The cause of this inflammation is not known but it may represent an abnormal response to extruded spermatozoa.

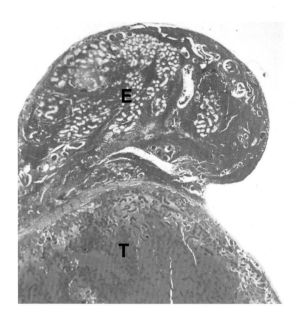

Fig. 19.2 Torsion of the testis (LP)

The arterial supply and venous drainage of the testis pass in the long course of the spermatic cord from and to the major vessels in the abdomen and pelvis. The spermatic cord is liable to twist, leading to compression of the thin-walled veins and obstruction of venous drainage from the testis. If this state persists for several hours or more without correction, the testis **T** and epididymis **E** may become deeply congested and subsequently undergo venous infarction in which necrosis is associated with severe congestion and extravasation of blood. Two small embryological remnants, the appendix testis and the appendix epididymis, are also liable to torsion. The histological changes are similar to those seen in venous infarction of the bowel following volvulus or strangulation (Fig. 10.5).

Testicular tumours

Testicular tumours may arise in any of the normal components of the testis but the most common are the **germ cell tumours** thought to be derived from multipotential germ cells of the seminiferous tubules. Most testicular germ cell tumours are thought to arise from in situ malignancy of the cells lining the seminiferous tubules which is known by the term **intratubular germ cell neoplasia (ITGCN)**. Foci of ITGCN are commonly found in the testis adjacent to tumours. The WHO classification is now widely used (Fig. 19.3). Approximately two-thirds of testicular tumours contain elements of two or more different tumour types, for example **seminoma** plus **embryonal carcinoma**. Many similarities exist between testicular and ovarian germ cell tumours; this is also demonstrated in Figure 19.3.

Testicular tumours are often divided into two major types:

- **Seminomas** – these consist of cells resembling the normal cells lining the seminiferous tubules. This group includes **classical seminomas** (Fig. 19.4) and the less common **spermatocytic seminoma**.
- **Non-seminomatous germ cell tumours** – this group includes a variety of tumours that exhibit differentiation towards embryonal or extraembryonal structures.

A small proportion of testicular tumours arise from the other cells in the testes, for example Leydig cells and Sertoli cells; the majority are benign and may secrete inappropriate sex hormones. In older men, the most common tumour of the testis is **lymphoma**, usually in association with lymphoma at other sites in the body. Rarely, a testicular mass may be the first indication of lymphoma. Testicular lymphomas are almost always non-Hodgkin's diffuse large cell lymphomas (see Ch. 16).

Fig. 19.3 Classification of germ cell tumours of the testis

Tumour type	WHO classification	Ovarian equivalent
Seminoma	Classical seminoma Spermatocytic seminoma	Dysgerminoma None
Non-seminomatous germ cell tumours	Teratoma — mature — immature — with malignant transformation Embryonal carcinoma Choriocarcinoma Yolk sac tumour	Teratoma/dermoid cyst Embryonal carcinoma Choriocarcinoma Yolk sac tumour
Mixed tumours	Embryonal carcinoma with teratoma (teratocarcinoma) Others named according to the components present	

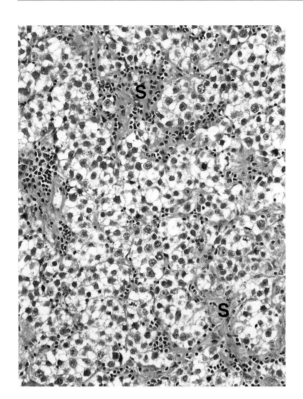

Fig. 19.4 Classical seminoma (HP)

Seminoma is the most common tumour of the testis, with a peak incidence between 30 and 45 years. Macroscopically, the tumour is well circumscribed, pale, creamy-white and homogeneous with a faint lobular pattern; necrosis and haemorrhage are rare unless the tumour is very large. Seminoma is a malignant tumour and tends to spread via lymphatics, initially to iliac and para-aortic lymph nodes.

Histologically, most seminomas show the classical appearance illustrated in this micrograph. The tumour consists of sheets of uniform polygonal cells with clear cytoplasm and a round central nucleus. The cells are divided into clusters by fine fibrous septa **S** which are usually infiltrated by small lymphocytes. In the past, attempts have been made to predict the behaviour of seminomas by grading the lesions according to a variety of criteria. The highest grade lesions under this system were called anaplastic seminomas. This grading system has little prognostic value and is no longer used. Another type of seminoma, the *spermatocytic seminoma*, occurs in older men than classical seminoma; these tumours usually have a benign clinical course.

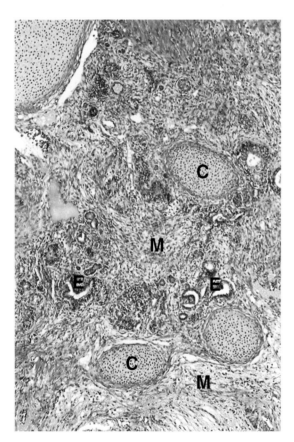

Fig. 19.5 Immature teratoma (MP)

In adults, most testicular teratomas are immature, consisting of fetal type tissues such as cartilage **C**, poorly differentiated epithelial structures **E** and primitive mesenchyme **M** as shown in this micrograph. These tumours tend to behave in a malignant fashion in contrast to ovarian teratomas which are almost always benign (Fig. 17.23). Some teratomas in adults show frank malignant transformation with areas of carcinoma or sarcoma. Teratoma is a common component of mixed germ cell tumours.

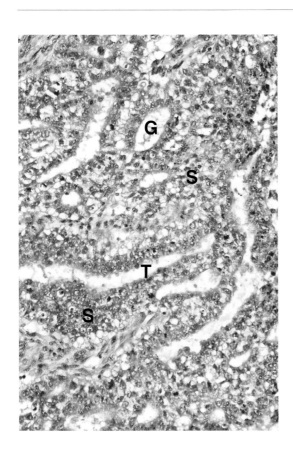

Fig. 19.6 Embryonal carcinoma (MP)

These tumours most often occur in men aged 20–30, and tend to be more aggressive than seminomas. Grossly, the tumour is often poorly circumscribed with areas of haemorrhage and necrosis.

The large anaplastic tumour cells may form sheets **S**, gland-like structures **G** or tubular structures **T** as seen in this micrograph. Mitotic figures are frequent. This tumour may invade through the tunica albuginea into the epididymis.

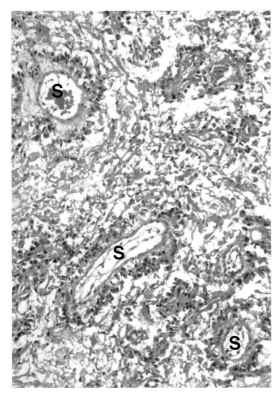

Fig. 19.7 Yolk sac tumour (MP)

Pure *yolk sac tumour* (or *endodermal sinus tumour*) is rare in adult men but is the most common malignant germ cell tumour in male infants and young boys. Yolk sac tumour resembles the yolk sac of the developing embryo. In practice, there is a wide range of histological patterns, the most common being a lace-like (*reticular*) pattern of large poorly differentiated cells as seen in this micrograph. The characteristic, but not common, feature is the *Schiller–Duvall body* **S.** Yolk sac tumour is fairly common as an element of mixed germ cell tumours in adults.

Yolk sac tumour secretes *alpha-fetoprotein (AFP)* which is easily measured in blood to monitor tumour progression.

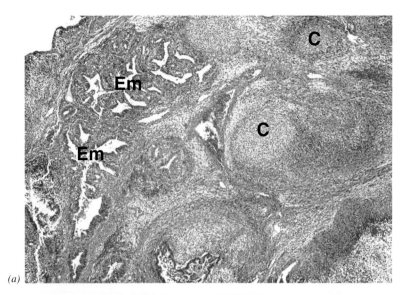

(a)

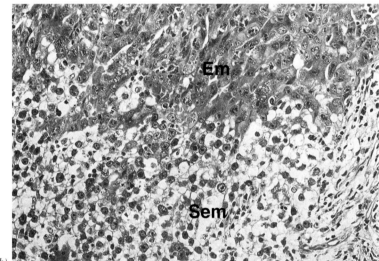

(b)

Micrograph (a) shows a germ cell tumour consisting of immature teratoma and embryonal carcinoma **Em**. Other areas show some tendency to differentiation into organoid structures though rarely as well differentiated as in a mature teratoma; in this example, there is some immature cartilage **C**.

Certain germ cell tumours are composed of a mixture of elements as in micrograph (b) in which pale-staining cells of the seminoma component **Sem** contrast with darker-staining cells of an embryonal carcinoma **Em**. This tumour is classified as *embryonal carcinoma with seminoma.*

Mixed germ cell tumours may also contain foci of *choriocarcinoma* or *yolk sac tumour. Beta-HCG* is produced by trophoblastic elements and can be used as a biochemical marker for the presence of choriocarcinoma, as well as to detect tumour recurrence.

Disorders of the prostate

The prostate gland undergoes *benign nodular hyperplasia (hypertrophy)* in almost all men from middle age onwards, probably because of an alteration in hormone balance. This important lesion, shown in Figure 19.9, produces obstruction to bladder outflow as a result of pressure on the prostatic urethra; in turn, the obstruction may produce pressure effects on the proximal conducting system of the urinary tract, leading to *hydroureter* and *hydronephrosis* with pressure atrophy of the renal parenchyma. Prostatic hyperplasia also predisposes to infection and stone formation.

Invasive carcinoma of the prostate is a common and important malignant tumour in men, and is illustrated in Figure 19.11. Carcinoma of the prostate may be associated with dysplasia of the glandular epithelium. This has been named *prostatic intraepithelial neoplasia (PIN)* and is shown in Figure 19.10. The prognosis of carcinoma of the prostate can be predicted quite accurately by careful grading and staging. Staging takes into consideration the size (volume) of the tumour, the degree of spread within the prostate, extension beyond the prostate, and lymph node and distant metastases. Perineural and vascular invasion also contributes to assessment of prognosis. Some of these features may only be assessable on radical prostatectomy specimens while others can be assessed on core biopsies. Imaging is also important for the detection of distant metastases, for example to bone. Small foci of low grade tumour that are not palpable may be found in prostates removed for benign hyperplasia. Most of these tumours progress too slowly for them to cause clinically significant disease in elderly patients and, for this reason, are often called *latent carcinomas.*

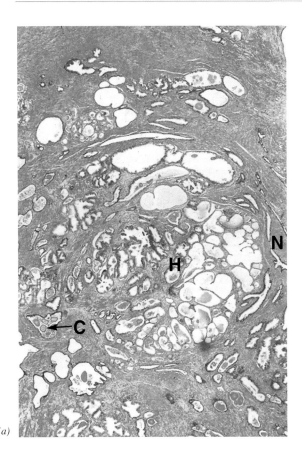

(a)

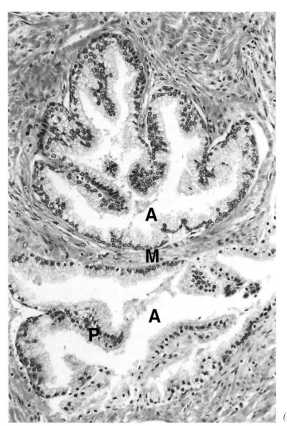

(b)

Fig. 19.9 Benign prostatic hyperplasia
(a) **LP** (b) **HP**

Benign prostatic hyperplasia is a common condition
affecting middle-aged to elderly men in which the
transitional and para-urethral components of the prostate
gland undergo glandular hyperplasia accompanied by
hypertrophy of the intervening fibromuscular stroma of
the gland. The peripheral zone of the prostate is not
involved in the hyperplastic process and becomes
compressed and atrophic at the outer margin.

At low magnification in micrograph (a), note the
rounded nodules of hyperplastic prostatic tissue **H** in the
transitional/para-urethral part of the gland, and the
compressed peripheral zone **N** at the periphery. Since the
para-urethral component of the prostate gland is
involved, compression of the urethral lumen is a frequent
occurrence, and is responsible for typical clinical features

such as hesitancy, poor urinary stream and urinary
retention. Macroscopically, the typical hyperplastic
prostate has a nodular microcystic appearance, the tiny
cysts representing enormously dilated hyperplastic
prostatic glandular acini, which often contain small
laminated concretions known as ***corpora amylaceae* C**.

At high magnification as in micrograph (b), the acini
A are lined by tall columnar prostatic epithelial cells with
small basal nuclei. The cells have a regular arrangement
but are sometimes thrown up into papillary folds **P**.
Adjacent acini are separated by a variable amount of
fibromuscular connective tissue **M** in which the muscular
component may be hypertrophied; muscular hypertrophy
is often particularly prominent in the region of the
bladder neck.

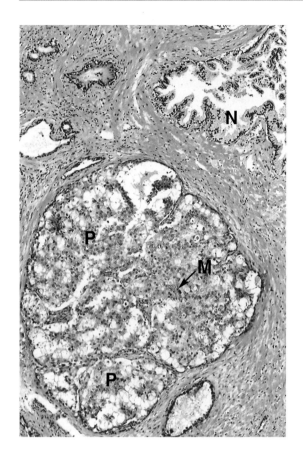

Fig. 19.10 Prostatic intraepithelial neoplasia (MP)

Prostatic intraepithelial neoplasia (PIN) represents dysplasia of the tall columnar epithelium. PIN may be subclassified as high or low grade. In clinical practice, as the significance of low grade PIN is uncertain, it can usually be ignored. High grade PIN, however, tends to occur in prostates with invasive carcinoma and therefore the finding of high grade PIN should prompt an intensified search for invasive carcinoma.

The large gland occupying the lower two-thirds of this micrograph is expanded and filled by papillary structures **P** consisting of highly atypical epithelial cells. These cells, in contrast to the normal prostatic epithelium **N** above, have a high nuclear to cytoplasmic ratio and prominent nucleoli. Mitotic figures **M** are easily seen. Although these cells show many of the features of malignant cells, there is no evidence of stromal invasion and a layer of basal cells can be detected around the periphery of the gland. However, a careful search of this prostatectomy specimen, which was removed for urethral obstruction because of benign hyperplasia, revealed a small focus of invasive carcinoma (not illustrated).

Fig. 19.11 Carcinoma of the prostate *(illustrations opposite above)*
(a) Well differentiated (HP) (b) Poorly differentiated (MP)

This common tumour usually arises in the peripheral zone of the prostate gland, as opposed to benign prostatic hyperplasia, which characteristically develops in the peri-urethral and transitional zones of the gland (Fig. 19.9). This tumour, which is derived from glandular cells of the prostatic acini, takes the form of an adenocarcinoma.

Prostatic carcinomas are graded according to their architectural features. This is known as the *Gleason grading system*. Gleason grade 1 lesions consist of nodules of small, well-defined glands with limited infiltration of the surrounding tissue. In contrast, grade 5 lesions consist of sheets of malignant cells with no discernible glandular differentiation and which infiltrate widely. Grades 2, 3 and 4 are intermediate. Most prostatic tumours include components of two or more of these patterns and therefore current practice gives the grade of the two most prominent components and their sum. This is known as the *combined Gleason grade or score*, for example combined Gleason score 3 + 5 = 8,

with the first number representing the most common component. As mentioned above, accurate grading along with staging is important to estimate the prognosis of prostatic adenocarcinoma and therefore gives a guide for treatment.

Micrograph (a) shows an area of Gleason grade 3 carcinoma. Small round malignant glands **M** lined by enlarged atypical epithelial cells are seen infiltrating between benign glands **B**. The contrast between the benign and malignant cells is particularly well demonstrated, the malignant cells being larger with prominent nucleoli and less cytoplasm. A very important feature is that the malignant glands lack the basal cell layer **E,** which is prominent in the benign glands.

Micrograph (b) shows an area of Gleason grade 5 prostatic adenocarcinoma where the malignant cells form sheets **S** of pleomorphic cells invading the stroma. No glandular structures are seen and there is extensive tumour necrosis **N**.

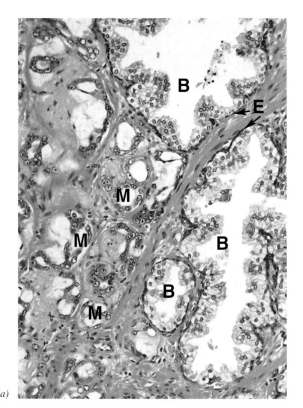

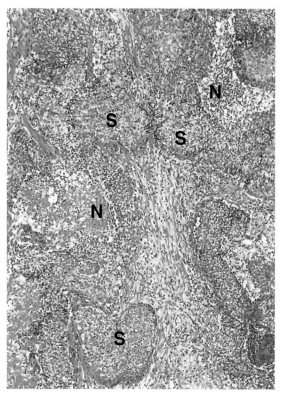

(a)

(b)

Fig. 19.11 Carcinoma of the prostate *(caption opposite below)*

Disorders of the penis

The most important pathological lesion of the penis is ***squamous cell carcinoma*** (Fig. 19.12) which is usually located on the glans or prepuce. The glans penis is also the site of a form of carcinoma in situ known as ***erythroplasia of Queyrat***, histologically similar to ***intraepidermal carcinoma*** of skin elsewhere (Fig. 21.15); it may precede invasive carcinoma. Genital warts or ***condyloma acuminatum*** are also found on the penis and are caused by infection from certain types of human papillomavirus as in the lower genital tract in the female. Phimosis is a common clinical condition. In some cases this is caused by an inflammatory and fibrosing condition of the foreskin termed ***balanitis xerotica obliterans***. This is histologically identical to the vulval disorder lichen sclerosus (Fig. 17.1).

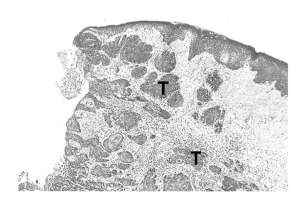

Fig. 19.12 Squamous carcinoma of penis (LP)

This micrograph illustrates, at low magnification, a well-differentiated keratinising squamous carcinoma of the glans penis with islands of tumour **T** extending deeply into the stroma of the glans. Metastatic spread is by lymphatics to superficial inguinal nodes.

Carcinoma of the penis is rare in circumcised men and chronic irritation and poor hygiene may be predisposing factors. However, evidence is accumulating that squamous carcinoma of the penis is associated with infection by human papillomavirus (serotypes 16 and 18), the same serotypes associated with invasive carcinoma of the female cervix.

BASIC SYSTEMS PATHOLOGY

20. Endocrine system

Pituitary gland disorders

Structural defects of the pituitary gland are few, although functional abnormalities are potentially numerous, leading to under-or overproduction of one or more of the many hormones produced by the pituitary and its target endocrine glands.

The most important histopathological lesions of the pituitary gland are benign *adenomas* derived from the anterior pituitary (adenohypophysis). These commonly secrete anterior pituitary hormones and result in the development of endocrine syndromes. Adenomas may be derived from any of the normal anterior pituitary cell types:

- **Prolactinomas** – lead to infertility, and occasionally inappropriate breast milk production
- **Corticotroph adenomas** – secrete ACTH and result in *Cushing's syndrome* (Fig. 20.1)
- **Somatotroph adenomas** – secrete excess growth hormone and lead to *gigantism* or *acromegaly*
- **Thyrotroph and gonadotroph adenomas** – both types are rare
- **Non-secretory adenomas** – a large number of pituitary adenomas have no demonstrable hormone secretion; such tumours thus only become manifest by impinging on vital local structures such as the optic chiasma causing visual disturbance, or by expanding to a size large enough to destroy the surrounding normal functioning tissue, resulting in clinical *hypopituitarism*.

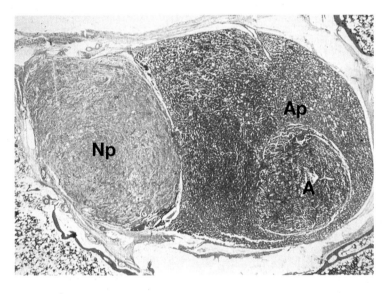

Fig. 20.1 Pituitary adenoma (LP)

The micrograph shows a pituitary gland in situ in the pituitary fossa and cut in sagittal section, showing the anterior pituitary (adenohypophysis **Ap**) and the posterior pituitary (neurohypophysis **Np**). Within the substance of the anterior pituitary lies a small benign *pituitary adenoma* **A** composed of cells of a uniform type. The tumour is benign as evidenced by its well-circumscribed, non-invasive, spherical appearance, and small enough to have caused no distortion of the pituitary outline or undue compression of adjacent normal pituitary cells. In this particular case, the tumour cells secreted ACTH in gross excess and the patient died as a result of the metabolic and cardiac complications of Cushing's disease; in all, the illness lasted no more than 7 or 8 weeks despite its 'benign' pathogenesis.

Disorders of the thyroid and parathyroid glands

The thyroid gland is subject to a variety of pathological processes which may lead to either diminished or excessive output of thyroxine. *Hypothyroidism (myxoedema)* may result from a number of causes, some of which have an autoimmune basis, for example *Hashimoto's thyroiditis* (Fig. 20.2). In cases of longstanding hypothyroidism, by the time the thyroid is examined histologically, it often shows only shrinkage, fibrosis and destruction of most of the thyroid acini, with a sparse residual infiltrate of chronic inflammatory cells. This change, known as *primary atrophic thyroiditis*, is analogous to the 'end-stage' of longstanding kidney damage (Fig. 15.1) and provides little evidence of the nature of the original thyroid abnormality.

Hyperthyroidism is usually the result of diffuse hyperplasia of the thyroid acinar cells, most commonly in the condition known as *Graves' disease* (Fig. 20.3). Sometimes the hyperplasia is confined to a single *benign thyroid adenoma*, or to one or two nodules in an otherwise inactive *multinodular goitre*; 'goitre' is the term now applied indiscriminately to almost any thyroid swelling. Nevertheless, the vast majority of thyroid adenomas and multinodular goitres are non-functional and do not lead to disturbances of thyroid hormone output. Examples are shown in Figures 20.4 and 20.5.

Four main forms of *thyroid carcinoma* occur, namely *follicular*, *papillary*, *anaplastic* and *medullary*. The first three types arise from cuboidal follicular lining cells and are illustrated in Figure 20.6. Medullary carcinoma of the thyroid is an uncommon malignant tumour of calcitonin-producing (parafollicular) cells and is particularly notable for its production of amyloid (Fig. 5.7). *Lymphoma* may also arise in the thyroid gland, usually following Hashimoto's thyroiditis.

The parathyroid glands show only two important pathological abnormalities, namely *hyperplasia* and *benign adenoma* (Fig. 20.7); in both cases, there are associated primary or secondary abnormalities of parathormone and calcium metabolism, leading to bone disease and hypercalcaemia. Carcinoma of the parathyroids is very rare.

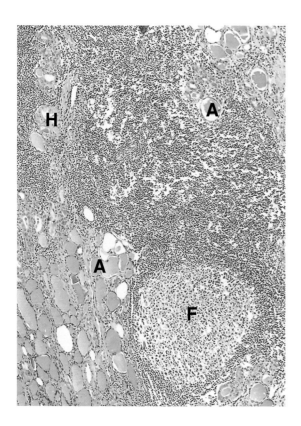

Fig. 20.2 Hashimoto's thyroiditis (MP)

This disease is an autoimmune thyroiditis in which thyroid acini **A** are progressively destroyed by immunological processes and the gland becomes diffusely infiltrated by lymphocytes and plasma cells. In some areas, the small darkly staining lymphocytes aggregate to form typical lymphoid follicles **F** often with germinal centres. In the early stages of the disease, the extensive lymphoid infiltrate produces a diffusely enlarged firm thyroid gland with a pale cut surface appearance. Thyroid epithelial cells in this condition commonly show *oncocytic* or *Hurthle cell transformation*, the Hurthle cells **H** having strongly eosinophilic granular cytoplasm and slightly enlarged nuclei.

As thyroid follicles are progressively destroyed over the years, the patient, who at the outset is euthyroid or even mildly hyperthyroid, becomes increasingly hypothyroid (myxoedematous). When almost all thyroid acini are destroyed, the lymphoid infiltrate becomes less obvious and fibrosis supervenes, with progressive reduction in size of the gland.

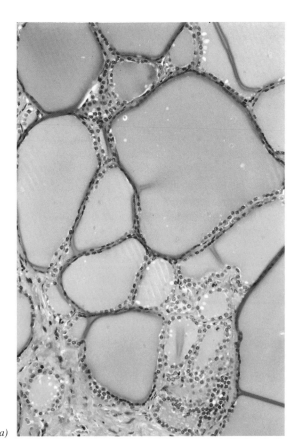

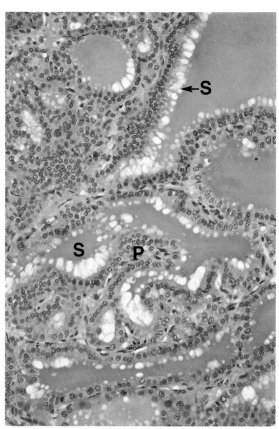

(a)   *(b)*

Fig. 20.3 Thyrotoxic hyperplasia
(a) Normal thyroid (HP)   (b) Hyperplastic thyroid (HP)

Thyroid function is normally under the control of the hypothalamic-pituitary system via the release of thyroid stimulating hormone (TSH) which stimulates thyroid acinar cells to liberate thyroxine. The resulting level of circulating thyroxine then regulates TSH production by a negative feedback mechanism.

Certain circumstances disrupt this balance, resulting in prolonged excess production of TSH or a functionally similar substance which then promotes hyperplasia and hypertrophy of thyroid acinar cells; this gives rise to the histological appearance known as ***thyroid hyperplasia***. Depending on the underlying cause, the patient may be clinically euthyroid or thyrotoxic.

Graves' disease is by far the most common cause of pathological thyroid hyperplasia. In this autoimmune disease, a circulating immunoglobulin called ***thyroid stimulating immunoglobulin–TSI***, formerly called ***long-acting thyroid stimulator (LATS)*** is produced which binds to TSH receptors on thyroid acinar cells,

mimicking the effects of TSH and resulting in excess secretion of thyroxine. The resulting glandular appearance is described as ***thyrotoxic hyperplasia*** and is illustrated in micrograph (b).

Compared to the normal thyroid shown in micrograph (a), the hyperplastic acinar cells are tall and have large nuclei reflecting a greater degree of metabolic activity. The acini themselves are smaller than normal because of the reduced amount of colloid resulting from increased thyroxine secretion. The hyperplastic acinar cells may crowd up on one side of the acini so as to project into the lumen as papillary structures **P**. The colloid in hyperplastic follicles shows peripheral scalloping **S** reflecting the increased utilisation of stored thyroid colloid to produce thyroxine by the hyperactive thyroid acinar cells. In Graves' disease, the thyroid may sometimes contain prominent lymphocytic aggregates (not shown in this specimen).

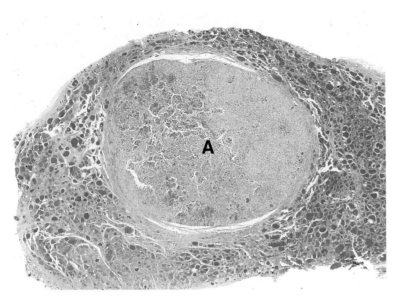

Fig. 20.4 Thyroid adenoma (LP)

Thyroid adenomas are benign tumours of follicular epithelium. They form encapsulated nodules which are usually round. The architectural pattern may be classified as ***colloid*** (macrofollicular), ***microfollicular***, ***fetal*** or ***embryonic***; however, mixed patterns are common and all behave in a benign fashion and are completely cured by local excision. This example of a thyroid adenoma **A** is of the microfollicular pattern. Follicular adenomas may be difficult to differentiate from encapsulated well-differentiated ***follicular carcinoma*** (Fig. 20.6b).

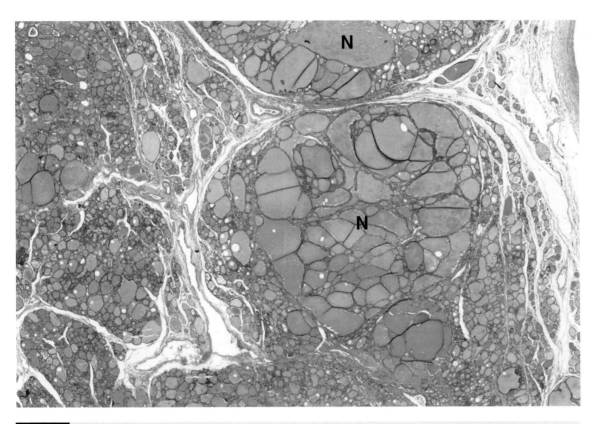

Fig. 20.5 Multinodular goitre (MP)

Multinodular goitre is thought to be caused by hyperplasia of the thyroid gland resulting from subclinical iodine deficiency. Thus, to maintain the euthyroid state, the gland becomes enlarged, initially because of the formation of larger than normal follicles; this is known as ***colloid goitre*** (not illustrated). This may progress to ***multinodular goitre***, as illustrated in this micrograph, in which the gland consists of multiple nodules **N** composed of follicles of varying size.

Fibrosis, haemorrhage and calcification (not illustrated) are common. Some cases of multinodular goitre have a ***dominant nodule***, a single very large nodule which may be difficult to distinguish clinically from an adenoma. However, histologically, the nodular appearance of the rest of the gland will usually identify the lesion as part of multinodular goitre.

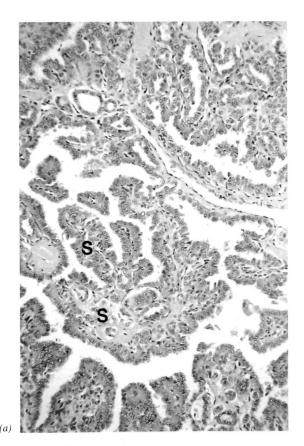

(a)

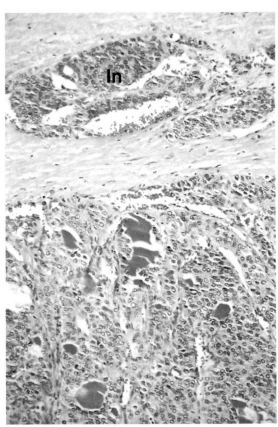

(b)

(c)

Fig. 20.6 Thyroid carcinoma
(a) Papillary (MP)   (b) Follicular (MP) (c)   Anaplastic (HP)

Carcinoma of the thyroid takes three common histological forms.

Papillary adenocarcinoma, shown in micrograph (a), is the most common type, found particularly in young women under 40. The tumour forms complex papillary structures, each composed of a narrow stromal core **S** covered with a layer of glandular epithelium. The stromal cores sometimes contain small calcified laminated bodies known as *psammoma bodies* (not shown here). This slow growing tumour tends to spread via lymphatics to regional nodes, and has the best prognosis of all thyroid cancers.

Follicular carcinoma, illustrated in micrograph (b), has a well-structured follicular pattern and may be difficult to distinguish from a benign follicular adenoma (Fig. 20.4); evidence of vessel invasion **In** at the tumour edge provides clear evidence of malignancy. Bloodstream spread is the major mode of metastasis, with lung and bone as common sites of secondary tumour deposits.

Anaplastic carcinoma, as shown in micrograph (c), usually occurs in the very elderly and is composed of sheets of small, very poorly differentiated cells with little cytoplasm; such tumours may be confused with large cell malignant lymphomas as seen in Figure 16.4d. These tumours grow very rapidly and extensively invade local tissues, often presenting as a bulky mass in the neck associated with symptoms of tracheal compression.

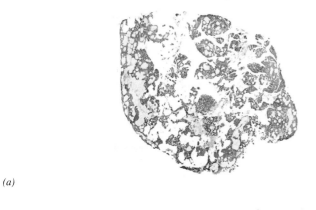

(a)

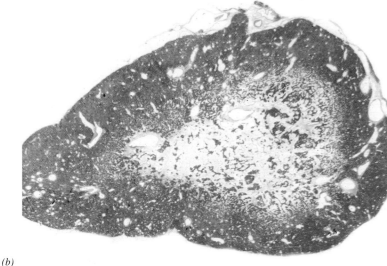

(b)

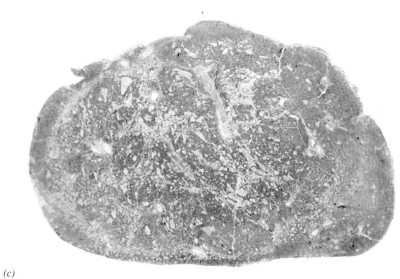

(c)

Fig. 20.7 Parathyroid hyperplasia and adenoma

(a) **Normal gland (LP)**
(b) **Hyperplastic gland (LP)**
(c) **Parathyroid adenoma (LP)**

The normal adult parathyroid gland contains small endocrine cells arranged in clumps or cords intermixed with adipose tissue; with increasing age, more of the gland becomes replaced by adipose tissue. Should the need arise for a greater output of parathormone, for example in cases of excessive urinary calcium loss in chronic renal failure, the endocrine cells undergo hyperplasia with loss of the adipose tissue.

Compare the hyperplastic gland in micrograph (b) with the normal parathyroid in micrograph (a); the hyperplastic gland is not only larger than the normal gland, but the hormonally active endocrine component has also increased markedly by replacing the adipose tissue component. If demand for excess parathormone persists, the gland may become markedly enlarged; these hyperplastic changes usually affect all four parathyroid glands uniformly.

In contrast, autonomous benign tumours of the parathyroid gland, *parathyroid adenomas*, usually affect only one of the four parathyroid glands, although occasionally they may be multiple. In micrograph (c), a parathyroid adenoma replaces the whole gland; often a fragment of normal parathyroid tissue remains at the periphery (not seen in this example). The cellular arrangement in parathyroid adenoma is variable, with the cells arranged in sheets or in a microacinar pattern. The finding of a peripheral rim of compressed normal gland is a useful clue in distinguishing an adenoma from hyperplasia.

In cases of parathyroid adenoma, the non-involved glands may show the suppressed parathyroid pattern, in which the endocrine component atrophies and is replaced by adipose tissue; the non-involved glands become much smaller, more adipose, and difficult to find at exploratory surgery.

Disorders of the adrenal glands

The adrenal gland has two distinct morphological and functional components:

- The **cortex** – this secretes three groups of steroid hormones, namely glucocorticoids (e.g. cortisol), mineralocorticoids (e.g. aldosterone), and small quantities of sex hormones. With the naked eye, the adrenal cortex appears yellow because of its high content of lipid (mainly cholesterol) which is the substrate for synthesis of steroid hormones.
- The **medulla** – this forms part of the neuroendocrine system and is responsible for the production of the catecholamines, adrenaline and noradrenaline.

Disorders affecting the adrenal cortex

In response to stress, the normally lipid-rich cells of the adrenal cortex metabolise lipid in the production of steroid hormones and become *lipid-depleted*. This is commonly seen in adrenal glands at post-mortem, particularly when a patient has died with features of shock. It is manifest by loss of the normal lipid vacuolation in the zona fasiculata cells seen with microscopy.

Atrophy of the adrenal cortex (Fig. 20.8b) may result from primary autoimmune disease, but is now more commonly iatrogenic, the result of steroid therapy. Hyposecretion of adenocortical steroids, known clinically as *Addison's disease*, may also rarely result from bilateral destruction of the glands by tuberculosis.

Hyperplasia of the adrenal cortex (Figs 20.8c and d) is usually caused by prolonged stimulation of the adrenal cortex by pituitary ACTH or a tumour-derived ACTH-like substance; this results in *Cushing's syndrome* (excess cortisol production).

The adrenal cortex may be the site of benign *adrenal cortical adenomas* (Fig. 20.9) or rarely malignant *adrenal cortical carcinomas*. These tumours of the adrenal cortex may be functional and result in the following endocrine syndromes:

- **Cushing's syndrome** – caused by tumours which secrete cortisol
- **Conn's syndrome** – results from tumours that secrete aldosterone
- **adrenogenital syndrome** – owing to excess production of androgens.

Often, cortical hyperplasia is nodular rather than diffuse, and it may be difficult to distinguish between a benign cortical adenoma and a large nodule forming part of nodular cortical hyperplasia.

Disorders affecting the adrenal medulla

The most important lesions of the adrenal medulla are tumours. *Phaeochromocytoma* (Fig. 20.10) produces excessive adrenaline and noradrenaline and is usually benign. *Neuroblastomas* (Fig. 20.11) are highly malignant embryonal tumours of neuroblasts seen in childhood. Both types of adrenal medullary tumour may also arise elsewhere in the abdomen in sites corresponding to components of the paraganglionic system such as the organ of Zuckercandl.

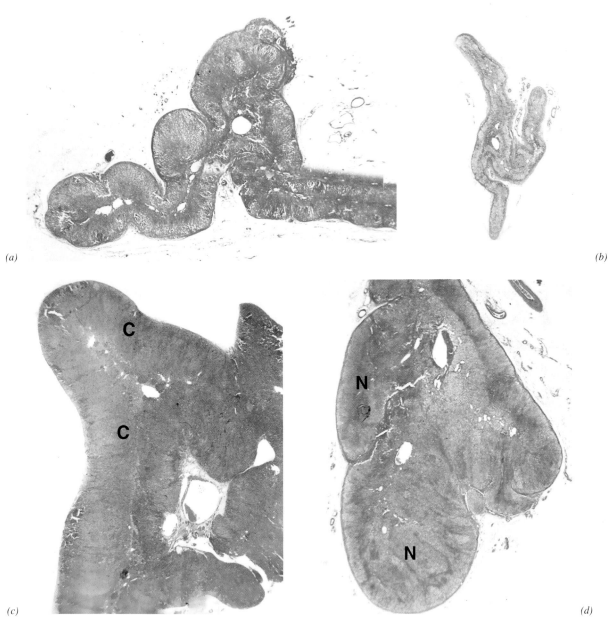

(a)

(b)

(c)

(d)

Fig. 20.8 Adrenal cortical atrophy and hyperplasia
(a) Normal gland (LP) **(b) Atrophic gland (LP)** **(c) Diffuse hyperplasia (LP) (d) Nodular hyperplasia (LP)**

These micrographs, taken at the same magnification, compare adrenal atrophy and hyperplasia with the normal.

In *adrenal atrophy* as shown in micrograph (b), marked reduction in gland size is due to atrophy of the cortex. In this example, the atrophy was caused by long-term administration of corticosteroids resulting in suppression of pituitary ACTH.

Adrenal cortical hyperplasia occurs in either *diffuse* or *nodular* forms as illustrated in micrographs (c) and (d) respectively. In the diffuse form, the cortex **C** is uniformly and regularly thickened, often by cells of one type. In the much more common nodular form, the cortex contains adenoma-like nodules **N** of hyperplastic cortical cells, usually of zona fasciculata type. Diffuse adrenal cortical hyperplasia is usually caused by excess stimulation by ACTH from the pituitary (*Cushing's syndrome*) or by an ACTH-like substance, for example from a small cell carcinoma of lung; rarely, it results from a congenital enzyme deficiency. Nodular hyperplasia is commonly idiopathic and non-functional.

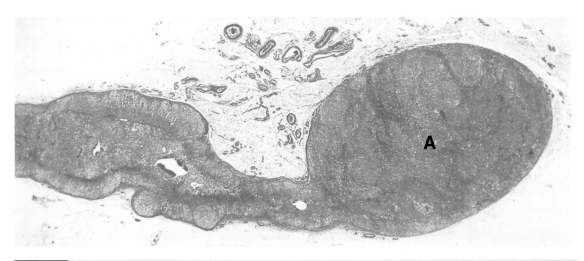

Fig. 20.9 Adrenal cortical adenoma (LP)

Hyperadrenal syndromes may result from excessive secretion of hormones by a solitary benign ***adrenal cortical adenoma***, the activity of which is independent of regulation by pituitary ACTH. These tumours form a circumscribed, spherical mass **A** within the cortex and may be composed of a single cell type (e.g. zona glomerulosa cells in ***Conn's syndrome***) but more often contain a mixture of cortical cell types. Note how similar the adenoma is to the nodules in nodular cortical hyperplasia seen in Figure 20.8d.

Cortical adenomas are a fairly frequent incidental finding at necropsy, a fact which leads to the belief that most are non-functioning and asymptomatic. Almost all cortical adenomas have a yellow cut surface, thereby distinguishing them from phaeochromocytomas which appear brown.

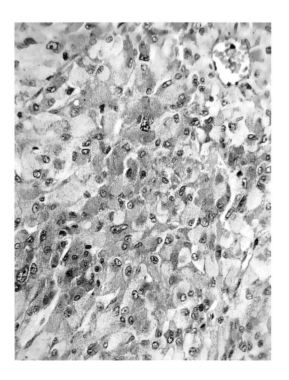

Fig. 20.10 Phaeochromocytoma (HP)

Phaeochromocytoma is a tumour arising from the adrenal medulla which secretes adrenalin and noradrenaline. Most tumours are benign in their growth characteristics but excess catecholamine secretion may cause potentially lethal hypertension. Macroscopically, the cut surface of the tumour is pale brown in colour. Histologically, the tumour is composed of nests of plump irregular cells, often with pink granular cytoplasm reflecting a high content of endocrine granules. True malignant variants do occur, but diagnosis must be based on evidence of invasion and spread since purely cytological criteria are unreliable.

These tumours commonly secrete catecholamines; a diagnostic marker is ***vanillyl mandelic acid (VMA)***, a metabolite which can be measured in the urine.

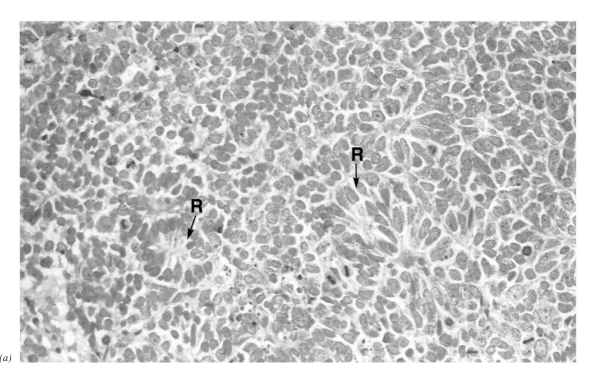

(a)

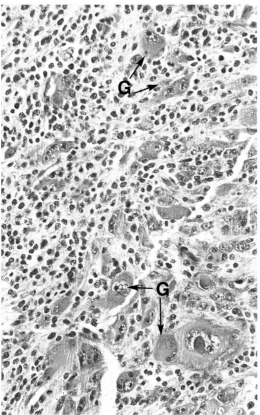

(b)

Fig. 20.11 **Adrenal embryonal tumours**
(a) Neuroblastoma (HP)
(b) Ganglioneuroblastoma (MP)

Neuroblastoma is an example of a small round blue cell tumour (Fig. 7.19) and is believed to be derived from primitive neuroblasts in the adrenal medulla. It occurs in children and is highly malignant, spreading mainly via the bloodstream to internal organs, especially the liver, and to the bones, particularly those of the face and skull.

The typical appearance of neuroblastoma is shown in micrograph (a). There is usually extensive haemorrhage and necrosis, but the viable areas (as shown here) are composed of small undifferentiated tumour cells in a pink-staining fibrillary stroma; the cells have a densely stained nucleus with scanty cytoplasm. A characteristic feature is occasional clumps of cells arranged in the form of a Homer Wright rosette **R** surrounding a central zone of neurofibrils.

A somewhat less aggressive form of this tumour is the *ganglioneuroblastoma*, illustrated in micrograph (b). These tumours exhibit some degree of differentiation with ganglion cells **G** of varying degrees of maturity found mixed with the small dark-staining undifferentiated neuroblasts. Such tumours have a rather better prognosis than those composed entirely of the undifferentiated neuroblasts.

BASIC SYSTEMS PATHOLOGY

21. Skin

Introduction

Many systemic diseases have manifestations in the skin. For example, skin rashes are a feature of many generalised viral infections such as measles, chicken pox and herpes virus infection (Fig. 4.14). Systemic autoimmune diseases such as scleroderma, systemic lupus erythematosus and dermatomyositis, and some vasculitic disorders such as Henoch–Schönlein purpura, have major manifestations in the skin. In addition, the skin is the subject of many specific primary disorders, mainly inflammatory or neoplastic in nature.

While there are many different causes of damage, the skin has only a limited repertoire of reactions; the most important of these are illustrated in Figures 21.1 to 21.4. Various skin disorders show these basic changes in different combinations and with varying degrees of severity. Few skin conditions have any absolutely pathognomonic histological features, and in most cases a precise diagnosis can only be made when the clinical history, macroscopic features, distribution and duration of the lesions are considered in conjunction with the histological appearances.

Dermatitis is a commonly used clinical term used to describe a variety of inflammatory conditions with many causes. Histologically, non-specific features of acute or chronic inflammation are seen (Figs 21.5 and 21.6); in some cases, there are additional histological changes which give a clue to the precise diagnosis or most likely cause. Two specific and relatively common types of dermatitis with characteristic histological features are *lichen planus* (Fig. 21.7) and *psoriasis* (Fig. 21.8).

Viruses are responsible for many common skin lesions; some, like *viral warts* (Fig. 21.9), *kerato-acanthoma* (Fig. 21.10) and *molluscum contagiosum* (Fig. 21.11), are probably primary skin lesions. Others, such as the vesicular lesions of herpes simplex, chickenpox and herpes zoster, are merely the cutaneous manifestations of a generalised viral illness, the last two being different manifestations of infection by the same virus. *Pyogenic granuloma* (Fig. 21.12) is a common, localised, nodular inflammatory lesion which frequently follows trauma.

Epithelial tumours derived from the epidermis and its appendages are common, the most frequent being *basal cell carcinoma* (Fig. 21.13), an invasive tumour of low grade malignancy derived from the basal cells. This has characteristic histological features which enable it to be easily distinguished from *squamous cell carcinoma* (Fig. 21.14), a rather more aggressive malignant tumour with appearances similar to the prickle cell layer of the epidermis.

Invasive squamous carcinoma may be preceded by *carcinoma in situ* (*intraepidermal carcinoma*, Fig. 21.15) in which the full thickness of the epidermis shows dysplasia of keratinocytes, thus being the skin equivalent of CIN III (see Fig. 17.6). There is a lesser degree of epidermal dysplasia, called *solar* or *actinic keratosis* in which the dysplasia is not full-thickness but is confined to the lower one-third or one-half of the epidermis, i.e the skin equivalent of CIN I or CIN II. Basal cell carcinoma, squamous cell carcinoma, intraepidermal carcinoma and solar keratosis all occur most frequently on sun-exposed skin, and excessive exposure to UV light is an important carcinogenic factor.

The skin is also the site of an unusual pattern of lymphoma due to malignant proliferation of T lymphocytes, *cutaneous T cell lymphoma* or 'mycosis fungoides' (Fig. 21.27).

Two common skin lesions which are difficult to classify are *epidermal cysts*, *pilar cysts* and the so-called *seborrhoeic keratosis* of the elderly; these are illustrated in Figures 21.16 to 21.18.

Numerically, the commonest skin lesions of all are the ubiquitous pigmented lesions known colloquially as 'moles'. This term encompasses a range of lesions called *naevi* characterised by the presence of aggregates of pigmented (melanin-producing) cells in various sites in the skin. Three important histological types, *junctional, intradermal* and *compound naevi*, are compared in Figures 21.19 to 21.21. Clinically, the most important pigmented lesion is *malignant melanoma* (Figs 21.24 to 21.26), potentially a highly malignant tumour of epidermal melanocytes. Melanocytic lesions of borderline malignancy include *dysplastic naevi* (Fig. 21.22) and *lentigo maligna* (Fig. 21.23).

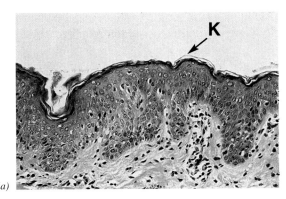

(a)

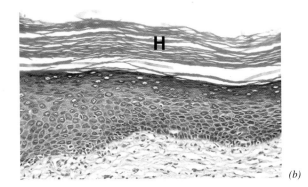

(b)

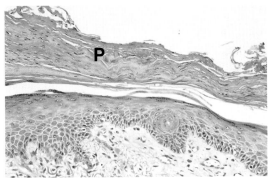

(c)

Fig. 21.1 Abnormalities of surface keratin (MP)

(a) **Normal keratin**
(b) **Hyperkeratosis**
(c) **Parakeratosis**

These photomicrographs compare the appearance of normal keratin **K** of thin skin (a) with two common abnormalities of keratin. In *hyperkeratosis* **H**, the keratin layer is thickened but otherwise histologically normal (*orthokeratosis*); it is usually associated with thickening of the granular layer underneath it. In *parakeratosis* **P**, the keratin is histologically abnormal in that it contains spindly nuclear remnants; parakeratosis is usually associated with loss or severe thinning of the underlying granular layer.

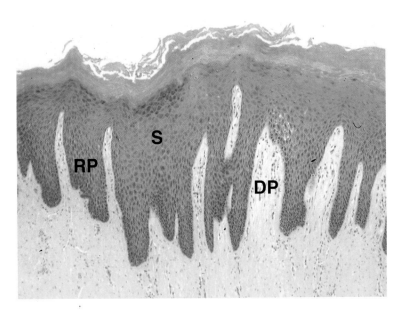

Fig. 21.2 Abnormal epidermal thickening – acanthosis (MP)

Acanthosis is the term given to thickening of the epidermis, usually to an increase in the thickness of the stratum spinosum **S** (prickle cell layer). It is a common feature of many skin conditions, particularly chronic inflammatory conditions (Figs 21.6 and 21.7). The thickening of the epidermal layer is particularly marked in the rete pegs **RP** which are expanded and elongated with prominent interdigitating dermal papillae **DP**. Note that there is associated thickening of the granular layer and overlying orthokeratotic hyperkeratosis.

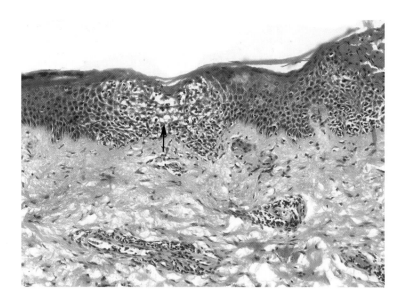

Fig. 21.3 Intraepidermal oedema – spongiosis (MP)

Oedema of the epidermis causes separation of epithelial cells, particularly in the prickle cell layer, a condition known as *spongiosis*. Accumulation of fluid between epidermal cells causes gaps to appear (arrow), which may coalesce to form fluid-filled intraepidermal vesicles. Spongiosis with vesicle formation is a feature of acute dermatitis (Fig. 21.5).

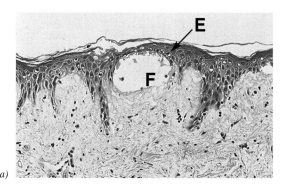

(a)

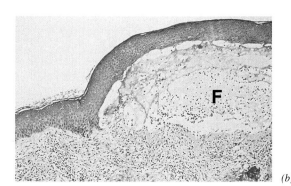

(b)

Fig. 21.4 Other epidermal inflammatory reactions
(a) Vesicle (MP)   (b) Bulla (MP)   (c) Pustule (MP)

Accumulations of fluid beneath or within the epidermis may cause small raised blebs on the skin; most are due to inflammation in the epidermis. When small, such lesions are termed *vesicles*; in micrograph (a), note the area of fluid accumulation **F** elevating and thinning the epidermis **E**. Larger collections of fluid are termed *bullae*. A bulla is shown in micrograph; (b) the collection of serous fluid **F** is larger and may include small numbers of inflammatory cells.

The term *pustule* is used to describe a collection consisting mostly of neutrophils, with some serous fluid, within or beneath the epidermis. Micrograph (c) shows a pustule **P** beneath the corneal layer of the epidermis.

Bullae and pustules are further categorised by their location, which may be *subepidermal*, *intraepidermal* or *subcorneal*.

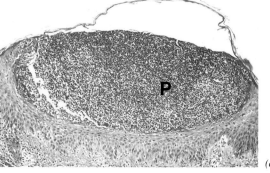

(c)

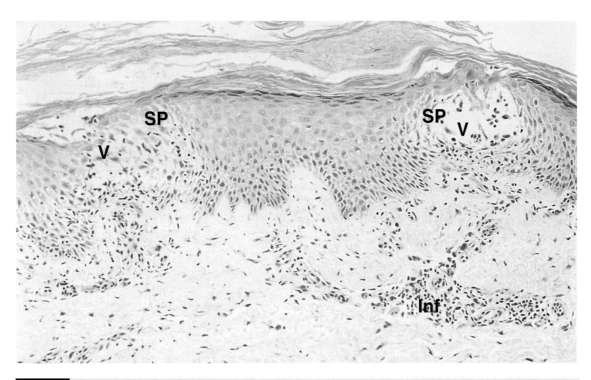

Fig. 21.5 Acute dermatitis (MP)

In early ***acute dermatitis***, the major changes involve the epidermis with fluid accumulating between the prickle cells causing spongiosis **SP**. As the lesion progresses, the spongiotic areas may become converted into fluid-filled vesicles **V** containing a few inflammatory cells, mainly lymphocytes and neutrophils, and there is variable infiltration of the epidermis by these cells. If the vesicles rupture onto the surface, crusts or scabs composed of

fibrin and polymorph nuclei form. In the earlier stages, the upper dermis shows only oedema, but later there may be a mixed acute and chronic inflammatory cell infiltrate **Inf**, particularly around upper dermal blood vessels.

This pattern is seen in the acute phase of the common inflammatory skin disease ***eczema***, which is thought to have an allergic aetiology.

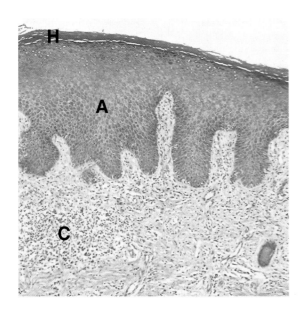

Fig. 21.6 Chronic dermatitis (MP)

The histological features of ***chronic dermatitis*** are seen in many skin rashes with a variety of causes. The characteristic feature is epidermal thickening, i.e. acanthosis **A** and a variable degree of hyperkeratosis **H**. There is no infiltration of the epidermis by inflammatory cells, but the upper and mid dermis show a moderate to heavy infiltrate of chronic inflammatory cells **C**, mainly lymphocytes and plasma cells, particularly around blood vessels. The acanthosis and hyperkeratosis may produce the clinical appearance of ***lichenification***. This feature is recognised in the term ***lichen simplex chronicus*** applied to one of the variants of this chronic non-specific dermatitis that occurs mainly in response to scratching of skin affected by acute dermatitis. When the dermatitis is still active, the thickened epidermis will contain the same sort of spongiotic vesicles seen in Fig 21.5, for example in long-standing eczema.

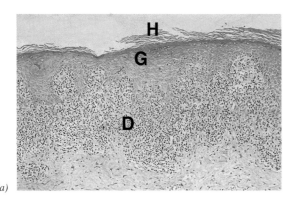

(a)

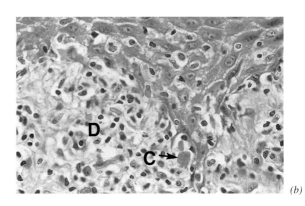

(b)

Fig. 21.7 Lichen planus
(a) **MP**   (b) **HP**

Lichen planus is a clinically and histologically distinct type of dermatitis. In the epidermis, as seen in micrograph (a), there is hyperkeratosis H, and thickening of the granular layer **G**. A characteristic feature is the disruption of the normally regular basal layer by hydropic degeneration and destruction of basal cells. As seen in micrograph (b), this leaves a ragged and irregular dermoepidermal junction in which *colloid* or *Civatte bodies* C (dead basal cells) may be seen. The dermis **D** shows a dense chronic inflammatory cell infiltrate mainly confined to the upper third. Lichen planus may affect the mucosal surfaces of the mouth and vulva where basal cell layer damage may lead to blistering and erosion.

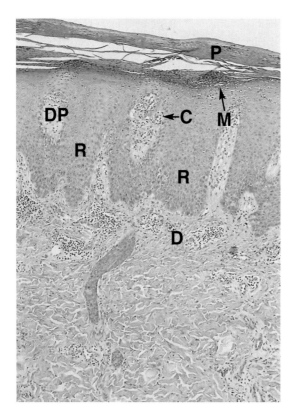

Fig. 21.8 Psoriasis (MP)

Psoriasis is a chronic skin disease characterised by well-demarcated, erythematous scaly lesions. Histologically, the major feature is acanthosis with greatly elongated, narrow rete pegs **R**. Between the rete pegs, the epidermis is thinned over oedematous and expanded dermal papillae **DP** in which dilated capillaries **C** are prominent. The alternately thick and thin epidermis is covered by a parakeratotic layer **P** of keratin which contains small aggregations of the nuclear debris of inflammatory cells, forming 'microabscesses' **M**.

There is a variable chronic inflammatory infiltrate in the upper dermis **D**.

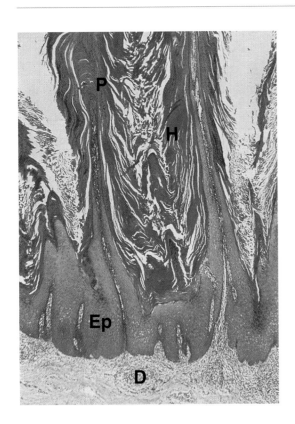

Fig. 21.9 Viral wart (MP)

Viral warts on non-traumatised skin have an exophytic papillary form. Histologically, the epidermis **Ep** is irregularly thickened and covered by a thick layer of hyperkeratosis **H** in which there are 'parakeratotic spires' **P** over the tips of the more prominent papillary epidermal outgrowths. The epidermal cells in an active viral wart usually show focal prominence of the granular layer, with occasional areas of large, pale vacuolated cells in the upper stratum spinosum (not seen at this magnification). The dermis **D** shows a chronic inflammatory cell infiltrate. In skin areas prone to trauma, warts have a much less papillary form and may be dome-shaped (e.g. in juvenile warts of the hands) or inverted (e.g. plantar warts of the sole of the foot).

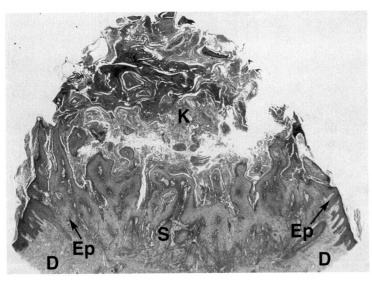

Fig. 21.10 Keratoacanthoma (LP)

The aetiology of *keratoacanthoma* is unknown but it has clinical features suggesting a viral lesion, in that it erupts suddenly and regresses spontaneously within weeks. A localised proliferation of squamous cells **S** produces a nodule in the skin with a central crater containing large masses of keratin **K**.

At its periphery, the nodule has a collar of thin but normal epidermis **Ep** and the junction between normal and proliferating epidermis is abrupt. The proliferating squamous cells may exhibit marked atypia, with large swollen cells showing abnormal nuclei and increased mitotic activity; this feature often leads to confusion with squamous carcinoma in biopsy specimens. The surrounding dermis **D** shows a heavy chronic inflammatory infiltrate with some inflammatory cells extending into the base of the lesion.

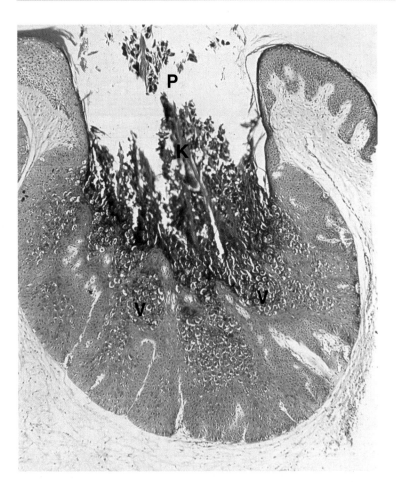

Fig. 21.11 Molluscum contagiosum (LP)

Molluscum contagiosum, like keratoacanthoma, is a localised nodular thickening of epidermis. In this condition, however, the viral aetiology is unquestioned since viral inclusion bodies **V** are easily visible, both in the proliferating epidermis, where they stain a reddish colour, and in the overlying keratin plug **K**, where they stain blue-black. The keratinous plug extrudes through a central pit **P** at the apex of the dome-shaped nodule which is surrounded by normal epidermis.

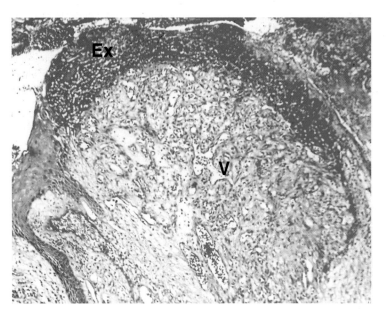

Fig. 21.12 Pyogenic granuloma (LP)

Pyogenic granuloma is a common inflammatory lesion which may follow a minor penetrating injury, for example by a rose thorn. It consists of a raised nodule of highly vascular tissue **V** somewhat resembling a capillary angioma and may represent an abnormal overgrowth of the vascular element of normal granulation tissue. The surface of the lesion is frequently ulcerated; in this example, the surface is covered by an inflammatory exudate **Ex**. A characteristic histological feature is a collar of proliferating epidermis at the margin of the lesion.

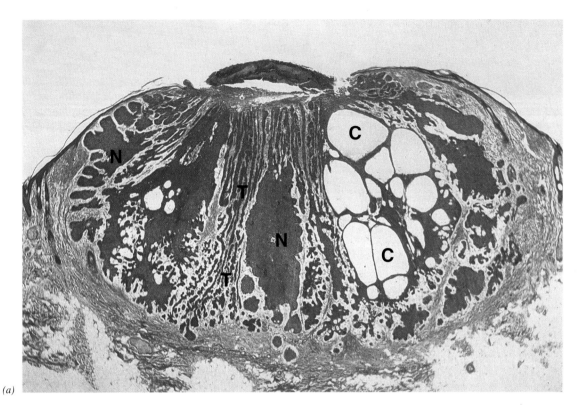

(a)

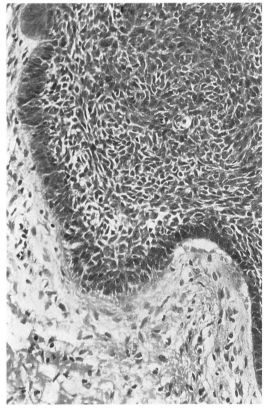

(b)

Fig. 21.13 Basal cell carcinoma
(a) LP (b) HP

Basal cell carcinoma is a common tumour composed of cells with deep blue-staining nuclei centrally located in sparse, poorly defined cytoplasm. Micrograph (a) shows the typical appearances of the common nodular form, with a mixture of solid nodular **N**, microcystic **C** and trabecular **T** growth patterns. Not all basal cell carcinomas are of this nodular pattern; some (***morphoeic pattern***) present as flat hard areas of skin, sometimes depressed, and others as a flat reddish scaly lesion (***superficial pattern***). As seen in micrograph (b), the cells at the periphery of the tumour clumps are characteristically arranged in a palisade pattern, whereas the central cells are more haphazardly arranged.

Basal cell carcinoma arises from the basal cells of the epidermis or epidermal appendages; it behaves as a malignant tumour in that it invades dermis and any deeper underlying structures, but almost never metastasises.

Basal cell carcinomas occur most frequently on the light-exposed areas of skin, particularly the face, and usually present as nodular lesions which may undergo ragged ulceration giving rise to the colloquial term ***rodent ulcer***.

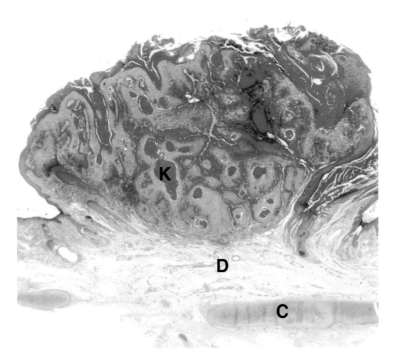

Fig. 21.14 Squamous cell carcinoma (LP)

Squamous cell carcinomas of the skin histologically resemble squamous cell carcinomas in many other sites (see Fig. 7.14). The skin tumours are usually well differentiated and highly keratinising, containing numerous keratin pearls **K**. The tumour may invade the dermis **D** and underlying structures, and may spread via the lymphatics to regional lymph nodes. Invasive squamous cell carcinomas of the skin may develop from intraepidermal carcinoma, the skin equivalent of carcinoma in situ (Fig. 21.15). In this micrograph, the tumour has arisen on the pinna of the ear, but has not yet invaded the underlying cartilage **C**.

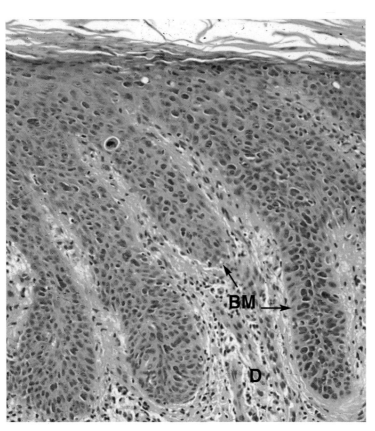

Fig. 21.15 Intraepidermal carcinoma (HP)

Invasive squamous carcinoma may be preceded by epidermal dysplasia. When the dysplasia is severe and involves the full thickness of the epidermis, it is termed *intraepidermal carcinoma*, *carcinoma in situ* or *Bowen's disease*. In this micrograph, note the severe dysplasia extending through the full thickness of the epidermis with the loss of normal organisation and stratification. The basement membrane **BM** is intact with no invasion of the dermis **D**.

When the epidermal dysplasia is restricted to lower levels of the epidermis, the condition is known as *actinic (solar) keratosis*.

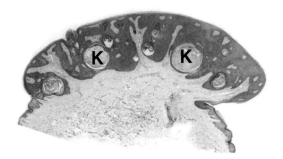

Fig. 21.16 Seborrhoeic keratosis (LP)

Seborrhoeic keratosis is a common lesion of the elderly, composed of a localised proliferation of basal cells forming a raised warty lesion. Such outgrowths are vulnerable to chronic trauma leading to overlying hyperkeratosis and formation of keratin nests **K** in the lesion. The aetiology of seborrhoeic keratosis is unknown, although in the past it has been regarded as a benign skin tumour (basal cell papilloma).

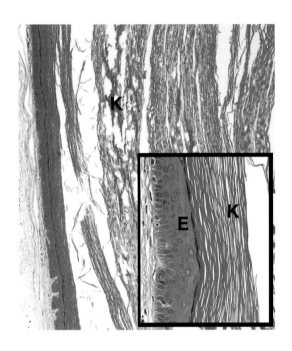

Fig. 21.17 Epidermal cyst (LP)

Epidermal cysts occupy the dermis and sometimes the subcutis, and may open to the exterior through a punctum. The cyst contains masses of degenerating keratin **K**, and is lined by a thin, flattened, stratified squamous epithelium **E** which, like the epidermis, has a granular layer (inset).

Trauma to the cyst may lead to rupture of the thin wall with escape of keratin into the surrounding dermis where its presence excites a foreign body giant cell granulomatous reaction (see Fig. 3.10) with swelling, tenderness and redness around the cyst.

Clinically these lesions are often (inaccurately) called 'sebaceous cysts', and traumatised ruptured cysts are said to be 'infected sebaceous cysts', again inaccurately. The clinical features of inflammation around ruptured cysts are due to the florid foreign body giant cell reaction to leaked keratin.

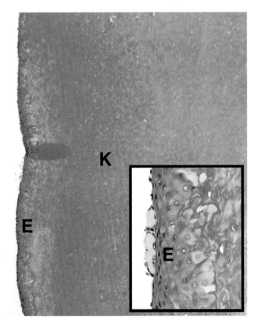

Fig. 21.18 Pilar cyst (LP)

Pilar cyst is another common skin cyst, clinically similar to an epidermal cyst, but occuring almost entirely in the scalp. It differs from epidermal cyst in the nature of the keratin **K**, which is compact, cohesive and non-degenerate, and in the lining squamous epithelium **E** which resembles that found in hair follicles, but lacking a granular layer (inset). These lesions are also mistakenly called 'sebaceous cysts'.

Melanocytic lesions

In normal skin, melanocytes are scattered in the basal layers of the epidermis, their fine cytoplasmic processes ramifying between the keratinocytes towards the skin surface. Melanocytes are responsible for the synthesis of the brown pigment, melanin, which is then transferred to adjacent keratinocytes. There are significant racial and genetic differences in the melanin synthetic activity of melanocytes, resulting in the varying degrees of normal pigmentation seen in the skin. Exposure to sunlight enhances melanin synthesis and transfer into keratinocytes.

Clinically, the most important and common disorders of melanocytes are the benign melanocytic proliferations known as *naevi* , and the malignant tumour of melanocytes known as *malignant melanoma*.

Benign melanocytic naevi

These are of three main types according to the location of the melanocytic nests:

- *Junctional melanocytic naevus* – nests of melanocytes are confined to the lower epidermis.
- *Compound melanocytic naevus* – melanocyte nests are located in both the lower epidermis and upper dermis.
- *Intradermal melanocytic naevus* – nests of melanocytes are present in the dermis only.

Benign naevi have a predictable natural history. Most begin as flat pigmented *junctional naevi* (see Fig 21.19), with nests of pigmented melanocytes confined to the lower levels of the epidermis, sitting on the dermo-epidermal membrane; purely junctional naevi are therefore most commonly found in children. As the child grows older, some of these junctional melanocytes migrate across the basement membrane into the upper dermis where they lose most of their pigment and the cells become smaller and tightly packed together. There are some remaining pigmented junctional nests in the epidermis and smaller non-pigmented naevus cells in the dermis; at this stage the naevus is called a *compound naevus* (see Fig. 21.20) and the intradermal nests produce a lesion which is raised above the level of skin to form a brown raised nodule. In early adulthood most of the junctional nests of melanocytes migrate into the dermis until no more are present in the epidermis; at this stage the naevus is a completely *intradermal naevus* (see Fig. 21.21). All of these lesions are completely benign, but rarely a previously benign naevus will convert into a malignant melanoma. This usually occurs by a well-recognised route. Sometimes the junctional nests do not completely migrate into the dermis, but proliferate abnormally and show features of cytological and architectural atypia, producing a *dysplastic naevus* (see Fig. 21.22). If untreated, a proportion of these eventually become superficial spreading malignant melanoma (see Figs 21.24 and 21.25).

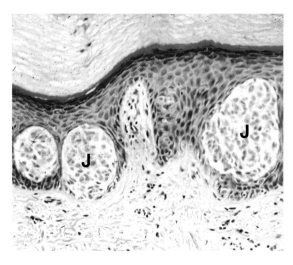

Fig. 21.19 Junctional naevus (MP)

In a junctional naevus, the melanocytes aggregate in nests **J** in the lower layers of the epidermis but do not encroach into underlying dermis. The nests are round to oval and well-circumscribed, and the melanocytes are pigmented.

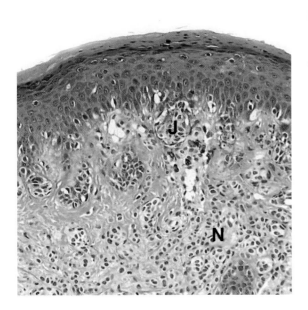

Fig. 21.20 Compound naevus (MP)

A compound naevus contains both intra-epidermal junctional nests **J** and collections of naevus cells in the upper dermis **N**; the cells in the dermis become small and densely packed, and are said to be 'maturing'. As time passes, more and more naevus cells occupy the dermis, and there are fewer junctional nests in the epidermis.

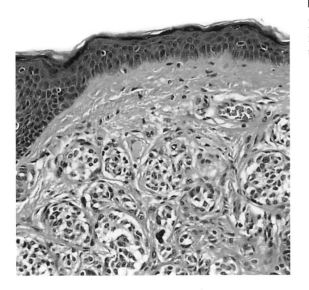

Fig. 21.21 Intradermal naevus (MP)

Eventually all the naevus cells which formed the intra-epidermal junctional nests have migrated into the upper dermis to form an entirely intradermal naevus.

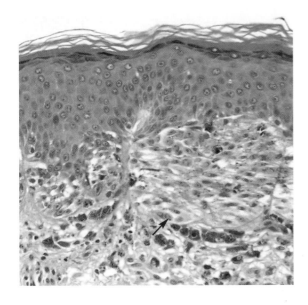

Fig. 21.22 Dysplastic naevus (MP)

Sometimes the junctional nest melanocytes do not migrate completely into the dermis, but develop features of both cytological and architectural atypia, with cytoplasmic and nuclear pleomorphism. The architectural atypia often takes the form of enlongated nests composed of spindle-shaped melanocytes running transversely, bridging adjacent epidermal rete ridges (arrow).

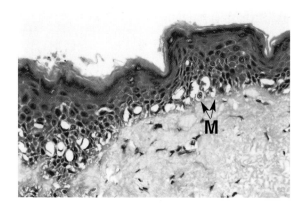

Fig. 21.23 Lentigo maligna (MP)

Another melanocytic lesion in which melanocytes in the basal layer of the epidermis show dysplastic change is *lentigo maligna*, which usually occurs as an enlarging flat pigmented patch on the faces of elderly people. Histologically, there is an almost continuous line of dysplastic melanocytes **M** in the basal layer, the cells showing cytological atypia with pleomorphism and enlarged hyperchromatic nuclei. Sometimes these abnormal melanocytes extend part way down the basal layer of skin appendages such as hair follicles, and eventually invasion of the dermis by the dysplastic melanocytes may occur (*lentigo maligna melanoma*). This is usually manifest clinically by the development of a raised nodule in the previously flat pigmented lesion.

Malignant melanocytic lesions (malignant melanoma)

Malignant melanoma is a malignant tumour of melanocytes, the incidence of which is increasing dramatically in white-skinned people around the world; excessive sun exposure, particularly sunburning, is believed to be the principal cause. Neglected malignant melanomas have frequently metastasized at the time of presentation but public awareness is leading to patients presenting earlier such that many malignant melanomas may now be completely cured by primary excision of the lesion. Malignant melanoma spreads initially via lymphatics to regional lymph nodes and subsequently via the bloodstream, by which time control of the disease is extremely difficult.

Predisposition to metastasis, and therefore prognosis, depends mainly on the following factors:

- **Pattern of growth**
  - whether or not there is invasion of the dermis. This classifies lesions as *invasive* or *in situ* respectively; in situ lesions have no metastatic potential.
  - whether the growth pattern is *radial* (i.e. horizontal or lateral) or *vertical*. Lesions are thus classified as *superficial spreading* or *nodular* variants respectively; both patterns may be seen in the same lesion. Lesions with a radial growth pattern have a good prognosis provided excision is complete; when a vertical growth pattern develops the prognosis is less good.
- **Tumour thickness**: the deeper the lesion, the worse the prognosis.
  - the *Breslow thickness* measures the greatest depth of tumour below the granular layer; lesions less than 0.76 mm are unlikely to have metastasized.
  - *Clarke's level* describes the depth of invasion in terms of histological layers, for example Clarke's level 2 indicates invasion of the papillary dermis only and indicates a good prognosis.
- **Vascular or perineural invasion**: histological evidence of tumour cells within blood or lymphatic vessels, or in perineural spaces, are bad prognostic indicators because of the high risk of metastasis to lymph nodes and blood stream spread.

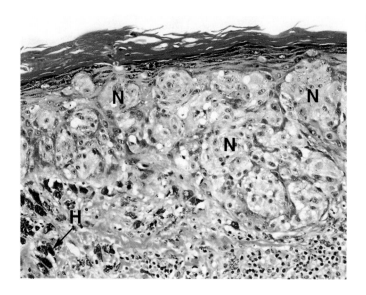

Fig. 21.24 Superficial spreading malignant melanoma in situ (HP)

The epidermis contains nests of melanocytes **N** which occupy all levels of the epidermis, unlike in junctional naevus (see Fig. 21.19) where they are confined to the basal layers. The nests are numerous, irregular in size and shape, and the melanocytes they contain are atypical and pleomorphic. The dermis contains histiocytes **H** which are packed with melanin ('melanophages') but there is no invasion of the dermis by the malignant melanocytes.

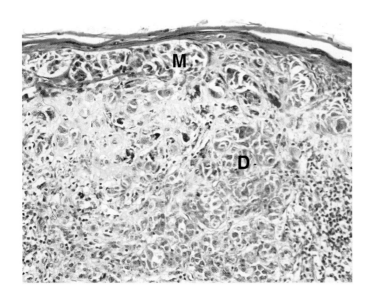

Fig. 21.25 Superficial spreading malignant melanoma – dermal invasive (MP)

As in superficial spreading malignant melanoma in situ shown in Fig. 21.24, there are nests of atypical melanocytes in all layers of the epidermis **M**, but in one area they have broken through the epidermal basement membrane to invade the dermis **D** in a radial/horizontal growth pattern.

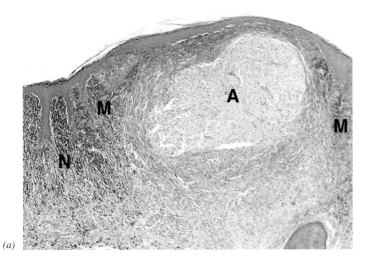

Fig. 21.26 Malignant melanoma – nodular
(a) LP (b) MP

The low power photomicrograph (a) shows the architectural pattern of a malignant melanoma with a nodular (vertical) growth phase component **A** which is largely amelanotic, surrounded by highly pigmented melanoma **M** and collections of macrophages which have phagocytosed melanin ('melanophages') **N**. Clinically this was a rapidly growing paler nodule arising in a previously flat, irregularly pigmented lesion.

At higher magnification (b) from the edge of the melanoma, the non-pigmented malignant melanocytes **A** can be seen extending deep into the dermis. The Breslow thickness is much greater than 1.5 mm, and the prognosis is poor, with a high chance of metastatic spread.

(a)

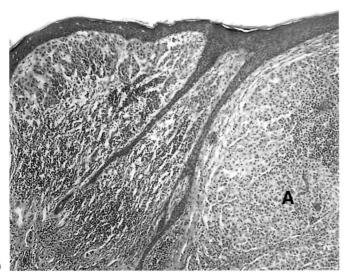

(b)

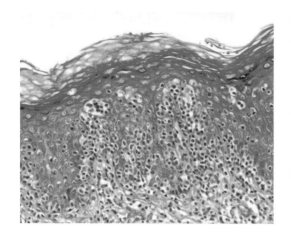

Fig. 21.27 Cutaneous T cell lymphoma (MP)

The most common type of lymphoma in the skin is T cell lymphoma; it begins as unexplained persistent red patches in the skin which slowly, often over years, enlarge and become slightly raised into red plaques. At a late stage the lesions become multiple raised red nodules (*mycosis fungoides*). This photomicrograph shows the disease in the early plaque stage; large numbers of atypical T lymphocytes are invading the epidermis from the dermis.

B cell lymphoma in the skin is much less common, and presents as (usually) solitary raised purple-red nodules.

TUMOURS OF THE DERMIS AND SUBCUTIS

Neurofibromas (see Fig. 23.16), schwannomas (see Fig. 23.15), leiomyomas, angiomas, and metastatic carcinomas can all occur in the dermis and subcutaneous tissue. However the commonest tumour to occur in the dermis is the benign fibrohistiocytic tumour, *dermatofibroma*; its malignant counterpart, *dermatofibrosarcoma protruberans* sarcoma protruberans, is much rarer. The commonest tumour of the subcutaneous tissue is the benign *lipoma*.

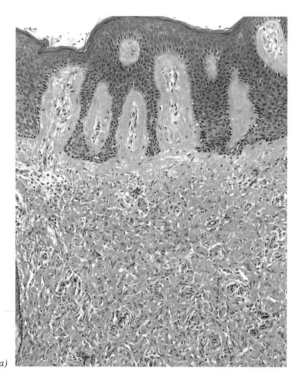

Fig. 21.28 Dermatofibroma
(a) MP (b) LP

This is a common tumour in the skin, usually on the limbs of young and middle-aged people in the form of a single raised firm nodule, ranging in colour from white to brown. Histologically the tumour lies in the dermis and has ill-defined margins, being composed of irregularly arranged spindle cells resembling fibroblasts, with scattered foamy histiocytes in some lesions. The overlying epidermis is often irregularly thickened (as seen in (a)).

(a)

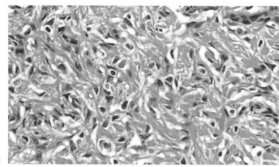

(b)

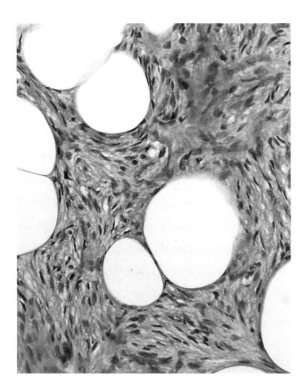

Fig. 21.29 Dermatofibrosarcoma protruberans (HP)

This low grade malignant tumour is also thought to be derived from fibrohistiocytic cells. It occurs most commonly on the trunk as a hard slowly enlarging plaque. The tumour is composed of fasciculated spindle cells showing variable pleomorphism. Although originating in dermis it enlarges by infiltrating laterally into adjacent dermis and deeply into subcutaneous adipose tissue, as in this photomicrograph. It often infiltrates much more extensively than is apparent clinically, and complete excision at first attempt can be difficult. Incomplete excision is always followed by recurrence and continued local spread.

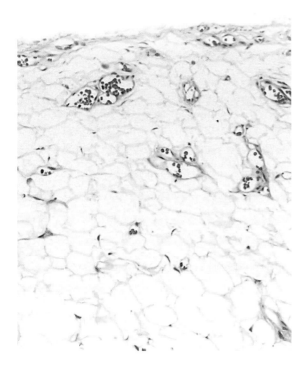

Fig. 21.30 Lipoma (LP)

The commonest tumour of the subcutaneous tissue is the benign *lipoma*, which presents as soft, often unsightly, tumours on the trunk and limbs. They may be single or multiple, painless or tender, ill-defined or well-circumscribed. The tumours are composed of adipose tissue, but the multiple tender tumours often contain large numbers of prominent blood vessels, as in this photomicrograph. This type is often called *angiolipoma*.

22. Skeletal system

Bone

Bone is a highly specialised tissue composed of a special type of collagen embedded in a ground substance matrix; this comprises *osteoid*. Osteoid becomes mineralised by the deposition of calcium salts in the form of hydroxyapatite. The osteoid is synthesised by specialised cells called *osteoblasts* which in their resting state are inactive spindle-shaped cells lying unobtrusively on bone surfaces; when there is a need to synthesise more osteoid, osteoblasts become cuboidal and actively synthesise protein. Bone is constantly being remodelled by removal of old bone by resorptive cells called *osteoclasts* and deposition of new osteoid by osteoblasts. Thus, the bulk and architectural arrangement of bone can be modified in response to changing functional demands and stresses. The calcified bone provides a large calcium pool from which calcium can be withdrawn (by resorptive activity of osteoclasts) to maintain serum calcium homeostasis.

Bone fracture

Bone fracture is a common and important result of trauma. Where there is some underlying bone abnormality, for example osteoporosis, osteomalacia, Paget's disease or metastatic tumour, the trauma or extra stress required to produce bone fracture may be minimal; this is termed *pathological fracture*. The healing of a bone fracture is briefly outlined in Figure 2.12 as an example of a specialised form of tissue repair.

Bone infections

Infections of the bone are now comparatively uncommon, although bacterial osteomyelitis, both pyogenic and tuberculous, were formerly important crippling diseases. *Acute osteomyelitis* caused by pyogenic bacteria, usually *Staphylococcus aureus* (Fig. 22.1), usually occurs in infants and young children, the bacteria gaining access to the marrow cavity via the bloodstream; it may also follow penetrating trauma in people of any age, for example after compound fracture. Pathologically, acute osteomyelitis represents abscess formation in the medullary space of the bone, but the course of the disease in bone is complicated by two factors. First, increased pressure in the confined space causes infarction of further large areas of bone; second, masses of dead bone (*sequestra*) behave as foreign bodies inhibiting normal repair processes and providing a haven for bacteria inaccessible to body defence mechanisms. *Chronic osteomyelitis* may follow if treatment is delayed or inadequate. *Tuberculous osteomyelitis* is illustrated in Figure 4.8.

Metabolic bone diseases

Osteoporosis (osteopenia) is a condition in which total bone mass is decreased by reduction of bone trabeculae in number or size (usually both) and thinning of cortical bone; nevertheless, the bone otherwise appears structurally normal. *Osteomalacia* is a disease in which osteoid fails to undergo normal mineralisation, usually because of deficiency of vitamin D, although other causes of total body calcium depletion may also be responsible; *rickets* is the childhood equivalent of osteomalacia. The appearance of normal bone, osteoporosis and osteomalacia are compared in Figure 22.2.

Paget's disease of bone (Fig. 22.3) is a condition of unknown aetiology occurring in the elderly; it is characterised by haphazard inappropriate osteoclastic erosion of formed bone and concurrent haphazard osteoblastic deposition of new bone. *Hyperparathyroidism*, due to excessive secretion of parathormone by a parathyroid adenoma or parathyroid hyperplasia, may cause somewhat similar haphazard osteoclastic erosion of bone.

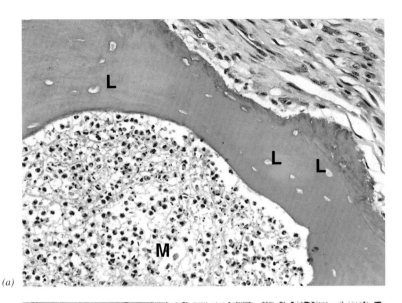

(a)

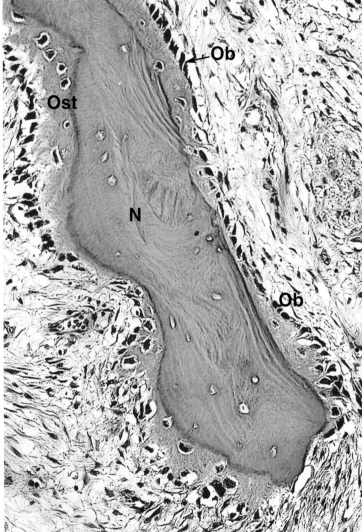

(b)

Fig. 22.1 Osteomyelitis
(a) (HP)
(b) Necrotic bone (HP)

Micrograph (a) shows a high power view of acute purulent osteomyelitis in the amputated toe of a diabetic patient. There is an acute inflammatory reaction in the marrow space **M** at the lower left of the field which is infiltrated by plentiful neutrophils in a fibrin meshwork. The bony trabecula is necrotic with no viable osteocytes in the lacunae **L**. In the upper right, the marrow is fibrotic indicating ongoing repair.

In micrograph (b), the process has progressed to a chronic phase with necrotic bone undergoing remodelling. The trabecula of necrotic bone **N** in the centre is surrounded by active osteoblasts **Ob** which are laying down new matrix or osteoid **Ost** on the outer surface of the dead trabecular bone.

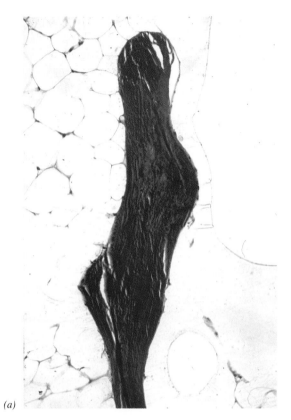

(a)

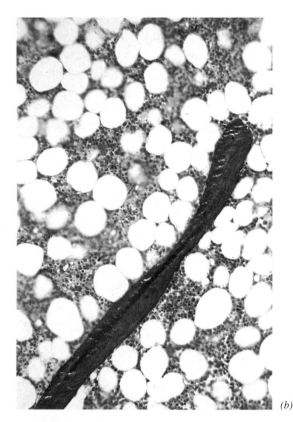

(b)

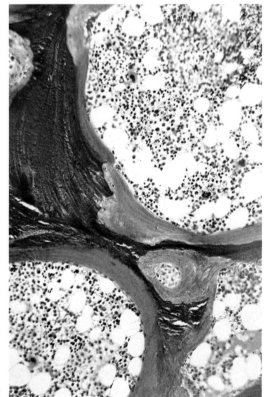

(c)

Fig. 22.2 Osteoporosis and osteomalacia (undecalcified resin sections, Goldner's trichrome) (MP)
**(a) Normal bone   (b) Osteoporosis
(c) Osteomalacia**

In *normal trabecular bone*, the entire trabecula is fully calcified (stained green by the Goldner trichrome method).

In *osteoporosis*, the bone appears qualitatively normal but its mass is diminished with the trabeculae being reduced in both number and size. Osteoporosis is extremely common in the elderly, especially in post-menopausal women, and is exacerbated by immobility. It may also occur in an isolated limb if immobilised for any reason and probably represents disuse atrophy. Osteoporosis is also caused by some endocrine disorders and is particularly seen with corticosteroid excess.

In *osteomalacia*, the trabeculae are of normal or increased thickness, but there is deficient mineralisation so that each trabecula has a central core of calcified bone (stained green) coated by an outer shell of unmineralised osteoid (stained orange-red). Osteomalacia is usually the result of vitamin D deficiency. Vitamin D deficiency in the growing child (rickets) is identical to osteomalacia pathologically; it results in gross skeletal deformity by disruption of bone mineralisation at growth plates.

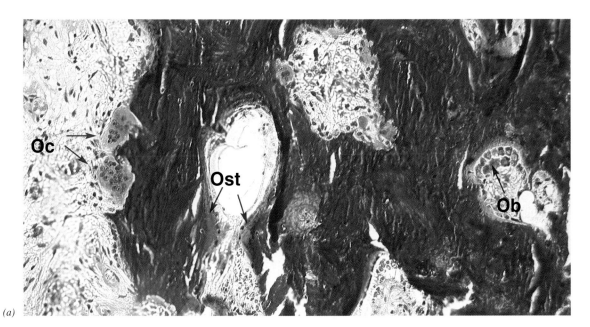

(a)

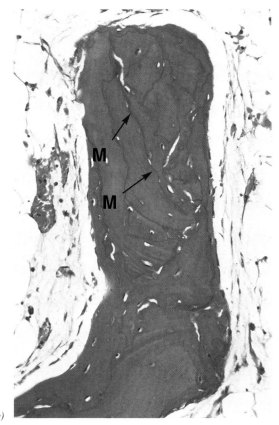

(b)

Fig. 22.3 Paget's disease of bone (MP)

(a) **Active osteolytic lesion (undecalcified resin
section, Goldner's trichrome)**

(b) **Inactive sclerotic lesion (decalcified paraffin
section, H&E)**

In *Paget's disease of bone*, there is indiscriminate and
uncontrolled osteoclastic erosion of bone followed by
excessive osteoblastic activity producing excess osteoid
which subsequently becomes mineralised, leading to
irregular trabecular thickening. Micrograph (a) shows
abnormally large multinucleate osteoclasts **Oc** actively
eroding a bone surface. Another trabecular surface shows
a layer of newly deposited red-staining osteoid **Ost**
underlying rows of large active cuboidal osteoblasts **Ob**.
This progressive haphazard remodelling results in gross
distortion of bone, often with marked thickening; the
condition tends to be confined to a relatively small number
of long bones, vertebrae or cranial bones which may
become inadequate to withstand functional stresses
leading to severe skeletal deformity (e.g. bowing of long
bones) or even pathological fracture.

With time, disease activity slowly diminishes, the
initially highly cellular bone becoming progressively
sclerotic; usually the bone is left thicker than before but
paradoxically weaker, as much of the former strong
lamellar bone is replaced by weaker woven bone. The
disruption of the optimum lamellar pattern can be readily
viewed by polarising microscopy, and in old lesions as in
micrograph (b), the limits of separate episodes of previous
bone destruction and irregular new bone formation are
marked by thin dark *mosaic lines* **M**.

BASIC SYSTEMS PATHOLOGY

Bone tumours

Primary tumours of bone may arise from all the cell types found in bone; the essential features of the more important of these tumours are tabulated in Figure 22.4.

Osteoid osteoma is a benign but painful tumour of bone and is illustrated in Figure 22.5. The most common malignant primary tumour of bone is the *osteogenic sarcoma* (Fig. 22.6); it mainly occurs in children and adolescents.

Chondromas (Fig. 22.7) are benign tumours of hyaline cartilage and may arise either on the surface of bone or within the medullary cavity where they are known as *enchondromas*; they rarely undergo malignant transformation. *Chondrosarcomas* are malignant tumours mainly arising in middle-aged and elderly individuals. Malignant tumours may also arise from lymphoid cells of the bone marrow, for example myeloma, lymphoma, leukaemia etc. (Ch. 16).

In addition to true bony neoplasms, there is a miscellaneous group of *tumour-like lesions* also found in bone, the main features of which are presented in Figure 22.9. The cartilage-capped *exostosis (osteochondroma)* is the most common of these and is illustrated in Figure 22.10.

Bone is a frequent and important site of haematogenous metastatic spread of malignant epithelial tumours, particularly carcinomas of bronchus, breast, kidney, thyroid and prostate (see Fig. 16.5). Metastatic tumour deposits usually destroy bone trabeculae, although carcinoma of the prostate (Fig. 19.11) sometimes stimulates excessive new bone formation, resulting in osteosclerotic rather than the more usual osteolytic deposits.

Fig. 22.4 Important primary tumours of bone

Name	Presumed cell of origin	Age and sex incidence	Common sites	Behaviour
Osteoid osteoma	Osteoblast	Adolescents M>F	Lower limb	Benign, osteosclerotic; painful
Osteogenic sarcoma (osteosarcoma)	Primitive osteoblast	(i) 10–25 years (ii) Over 65 years M>F	(i) Around knee (ii) At site of Paget's disease	Highly malignant; early metastasis to lungs
Chondroma (enchondroma)	Chondrocyte	Young adults M>F	Bones of hands	Usually benign and expansile
Chondrosarcoma	Chondrocyte	30–60 years M>F	Spine and pelvis	Malignant; local spread and distant metastasis
Non-ossifying fibroma	Uncertain	Child/adol M>F	Long bones of lower limb	Benign, osteolytic; occasionally multiple
Chondromyxoid fibroma	Uncertain	Adol/young adult M>F	Long bones, especially tibia	Benign osteolytic
Giant cell tumour	Osteoclast	20–40 years M>F	Around knee	Mostly benign, may recur; rarely malignant
Chordoma	Notochord tissue	40+ years M>F	Sacrum	Local bone destruction and invasion
Ewing's tumour	Uncertain	Child/adol M>F	Midshaft of long bones	Malignant; early and extensive metastasis

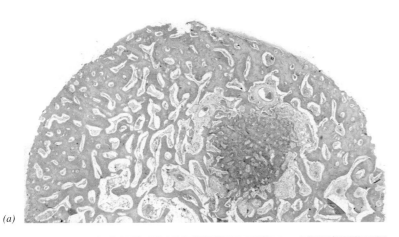

(a)

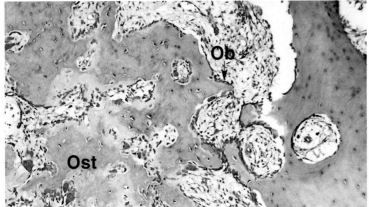

(b)

Fig. 22.5 Osteoid osteoma
(a) **Osteoid osteoma in medullary cavity (LP)**
(b) **Histology of edge of lesion (MP)**

Osteoid osteoma is a benign tumour of osteoblasts which usually arises in the medullary cavity of the shaft of long bones, commonly the tibia or femur. Micrograph (a) shows the typical low power appearance of this benign tumour. Micrograph (b) shows the edge of the lesion. There is a central 'nidus' composed of partially mineralised osteoid **Ost** in irregular masses surrounded by a rim of actively proliferating osteoblasts **Ob**.

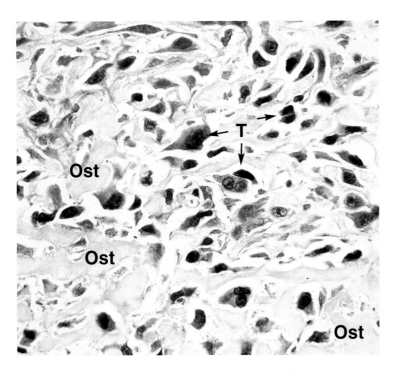

Fig. 22.6 Osteogenic sarcoma (osteosarcoma) (HP)

This relatively uncommon tumour is nevertheless the most frequently occurring primary malignant tumour of bone. Most cases occur in children and adolescents (usually around the knee), but it may occasionally occur in elderly patients with longstanding Paget's disease. Histologically, the tumour has a very variable appearance, but islands of delicately pink-stained osteoid **Ost** are usually present. The tumour cells **T**, which are derived from osteoblasts, are usually poorly differentiated and pleomorphic with much mitotic activity. These tumours are generally highly vascular and early bloodstream metastasis to the lungs is common.

BASIC SYSTEMS PATHOLOGY

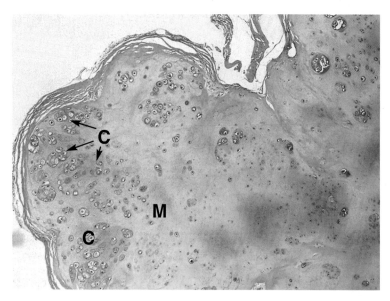

Fig. 22.7 Chondroma (LP)

Chondromas are made up of well-circumscribed nodules of benign cartilage. The gross appearance is characteristic with a semi-translucent, grey-blue appearance which is due to the hyaline matrix **M**. The neoplastic chondrocytes **C** seen within the lacunae are benign, with no dysplastic features, and are embedded in well-formed cartilage matrix.

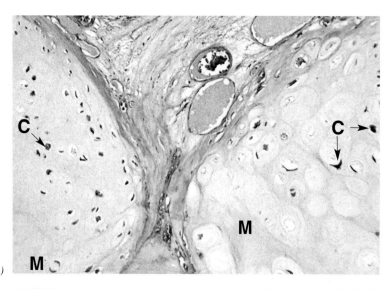

(a)

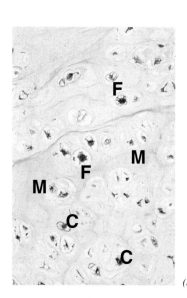

(b)

Fig. 22.8 Chondrosarcoma
(a) MP   (b) HP

This malignant cartilaginous tumour arises usually in the axial skeleton at middle age and later. The tumours vary in their behaviour from indolent low grade malignancy to very poorly differentiated aggressive neoplasms with little obvious cartilage formation.

The tumour shown here is a well-differentiated chondrosarcoma consisting of nodules of pale hyaline matrix **M**. Embedded within the matrix are malignant chondrocytes **C** which differ from normal chondrocytes in that they are enlarged atypical cells which may be binucleate or show crowding of two or more cells in a single lacuna. Mitotic figures **F** may be seen. A well-differentiated chondrosarcoma such as this may be difficult to differentiate from a benign chondroma.

Fig. 22.9 Tumour-like lesions in bone

Name	Age and sex incidence	Common sites	Behaviour
Osteochondroma	Child/adol M>F	Upper tibia, lower fibula	Benign (hamartomatous?) cartilage and bone outgrowth from bone surface; rare potential for malignant transformation
Aneurysmal bone cyst	Adol/young adult M>F	Shaft of long bones, spine	Osteolytic, predispose to fracture
Fibrous dysplasia	Child/adol M>F	Femur, tibia, fibula, facial bones	Osteolytic, predispose to fracture
'Brown tumour' of hyperparathyroidism	Adults M>F	Anywhere	Osteolytic lesions, often multiple

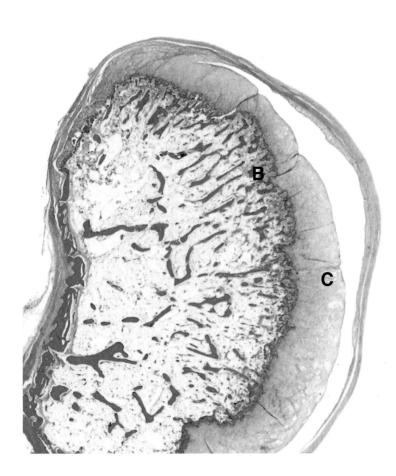

Fig. 22.10 Osteochondroma (LP)

Osteochondromas or *exostoses* are mushroom-shaped bony protuberances with a cartilage cap **C**, arising in the region of the epiphysis.

Endochondral ossification takes place at the deep surface of the cartilage to form cortical bone **B**. The stalk consists of medullary bone. Very occasionally a chondrosarcoma may arise in an osteochondroma and this is much more common in individuals with the hereditary syndrome *multiple hereditary exostosis*.

In this photomicrograph there has been artefactual separation of the perichondrium.

Diseases of the joints

The three most important disorders of joints are osteoarthritis, gout and rheumatoid arthritis. *Osteoarthritis* (Fig. 22.11) is the name given to the wear and tear degenerative changes which occur in some joints with increasing age. *Gout* is an inflammatory arthropathy caused by the deposition of urate crystals within the joints; this is illustrated in Figure 22.12. *Rheumatoid arthritis* (Fig. 22.13) is a chronic inflammatory synovitis and arthritis of probable autoimmune origin.

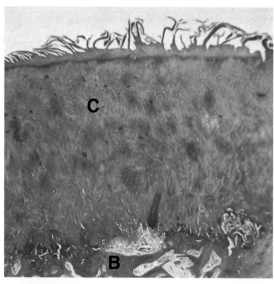

(a)

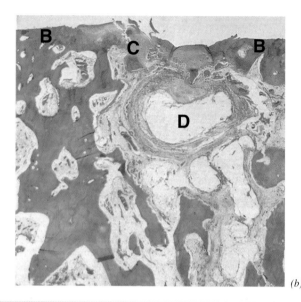

(b)

Fig. 22.11 Osteoarthritis
(a) Early changes (MP)   (b) Established lesion (LP)

Osteoarthritis is a degenerative disorder of articular cartilage as a result of excessive wear and tear, with secondary inflammatory changes in the soft tissue components of the joint. In the earliest stages, the articular cartilage **C** loses its smooth appearance and develops surface fibrillations and flaking as shown in micrograph (a). The damaged cartilage is progressively eroded until the underlying cortical bone **B** is exposed. After prolonged articulation of naked bone with the opposing surface, the bone becomes slightly thickened, hard, dense and highly polished, a process known as

eburnation. At the same time, there is irregular outgrowth of new bone (*osteophytes*) at the articular margins.

In the established case shown in micrograph (b), only a small amount of cartilage **C** remains and the exposed bone **B** has undergone eburnation. The bone underlying the traumatised eburnated surface may undergo cystic degeneration **D**.

All of these changes lead to joint pain and progressive limitation of movement at the joint. The hips, knees and finger joints are most commonly and severely affected.

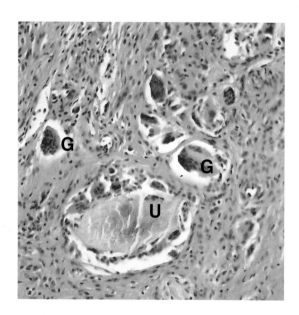

Fig. 22.12 Gout (MP)

Gout is an acute relapsing form of arthritis found in individuals with hyperuricaemia. Gout is most often 'primary', i.e. of unknown cause; however, a small proportion of cases arises owing to increased nucleic acid turnover as in leukaemia or in patients with chronic renal disease who cannot excrete urate.

Acute attacks of gout are precipitated by crystallisation of urate within joints causing an acute inflammatory reaction. Over time, chronic arthritis may develop with the formation of a chronic granulomatous response with giant cells **G**. The giant cells are seen aggregated around the residual material of the urate crystals **U**. The synovium is inflamed and fibrotic, and this inflammatory mass or *pannus* may erode the underlying cartilage.

Gouty tophi in the soft tissues have a similar histological appearance.

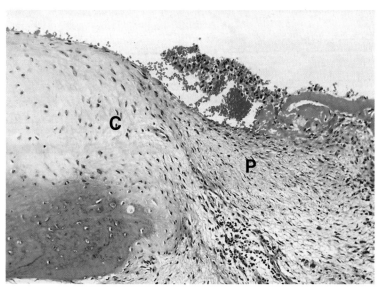

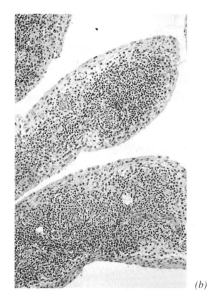

(a) *(b)*

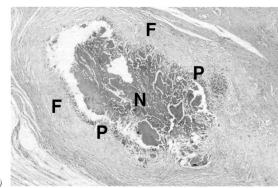

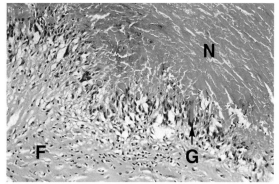

(c) *(d)*

Fig. 22.13 Rheumatoid arthritis
(a) Articular cartilage (MP)   (b) Synovium (MP)
(c) Rheumatoid skin nodule (LP) (d) Rheumatoid skin nodule (HP)

Rheumatoid arthritis is a systemic disorder, the predominant feature of which is chronic relapsing inflammation of articular joints, particularly in the hands and knees. The disease affects both the synovium lining the joint capsule and the cartilage on the articular surfaces.

The earliest changes occur in the synovium which becomes thickened, excessively vascular and thrown up into papillary folds as a result of oedema and heavy lymphoplasmacytic infiltration; this is seen in micrograph (b). This is accompanied by exudation of excess fluid into the joint space with precipitation of fibrin on the synovial surface.

The articular cartilage changes shown in micrograph (a) follow later and involve localised destruction of cartilage **C** and its replacement by fibrovascular granulation tissue known as *pannus* **P**. Initially, joint mobility is limited by pain and swelling, then later by gross cartilage and bone destruction and fibrous ankylosis across the joint space owing to fusion of transjacent granulation tissue pannus.

Rheumatoid nodules are found in the subcutaneous tissue most commonly in individuals with *seropositive rheumatoid arthritis*, i.e. those who have *rheumatoid factor* in their serum. The nodules are usually found on the extensor surfaces of the limbs and clinically are firm, non-tender and mobile. Rheumatoid nodules may also occur rarely in almost any other tissue, for example lung, spleen.

The rheumatoid nodule, shown at low power in micrograph (c), consists of a central core of *necrosis* **N** rimmed by a palisade of histiocytes and fibroblasts **P** which is in turn surrounded by fibrosis **F** containing lymphocytes and plasma cells.

The palisading or lining up of histiocytes and fibroblasts is better appreciated at high magnification in micrograph (d). An occasional giant cell **G** can be identified. The rheumatoid nodule in fact represents a large granuloma.

23. Nervous system

Diseases of the nervous system

There is nothing special about the nervous system and its diseases. It is prone to infection, trauma and the processes of infarction, inflammation, and neoplasia in the same way as other tissues.

Diseases affecting the nervous system may be divided into two types:

- **General pathological phenomena** which affect all cellular constituents – for example, processes such as cerebral infarction and acute inflammation affect neurones, specialised support cells (glia), blood vessels and associated supporting (connective) tissues including the meninges. The nervous system is particularly vulnerable to relatively transient metabolic insults such as hypoxia or hypoglycaemia causing death of neurones and their axons; other tissue elements are less immediately affected.
- **Specific disease processes** affecting particular cell types – for example in *Alzheimer's disease* (a form of dementia), neurones alone are affected causing generalised brain atrophy; in *Parkinson's disease*, there is focal loss of neurones from the substantia nigra; in *multiple sclerosis*, damage is specific to myelin sheaths and in this case lesions are distributed in a patchy manner throughout the central nervous system (CNS).

Tissues of the CNS

- **Neurones** are the functional units of the nervous system. A typical neurone is composed of a cell body rich in rough endoplasmic reticulum (*Nissl substance*), short afferent cell processes termed *dendrites*, and a main efferent cell process termed the *axon*. Except in development, neurones are not capable of replication and hence, once a neuronal cell body dies, regeneration is not possible. Damage to the axon with preservation of the nerve cell body can, however, be repaired by regeneration of the axon.
- **Specialised support cells (glial cells)** are of four types: astrocytes, oligodendrocytes, microglia and ependymal cells. *Astrocytes*, with their delicate cytoplasmic processes, form a 'fibrillary' supporting framework for the neurones and other cells of the CNS, and proliferate following damage. *Oligodendrocytes* are responsible for myelin formation around axons in the CNS; their counterparts in the peripheral nervous system are the *Schwann cells*. *Microglia* are cells with small processes and are the CNS equivalent of quiescent macrophages elsewhere. *Ependymal cells* provide a lining to the ventricles and central canal of the spinal cord.
- **Blood vessels** in the brain have a specialised structure for maintenance of the *blood–brain barrier*; this limits transport and diffusion from the vascular compartment into the CNS. Connective tissues in the CNS are limited to the meninges, choroid plexuses and around blood vessels. The relative paucity of fibroblastic cells means that healing in the CNS is generally not marked by fibrous scarring. In the peripheral nervous system, connective tissue and associated blood vessels are found in association with individual axons (endoneurium), bundles of axons (perineurium) and peripheral nerves (epineurium).

Response of CNS tissues to injury

Neurones have a limited ability to survive significant changes in their metabolic or physical environment and are said to be *selectively vulnerable* when compared to the more robust astrocytes or microglial cells. Neurones may undergo reversible cell damage which is recognisable histologically by swelling of the cell body associated with loss of Nissl substance, a process termed *chromatolysis*. This process is particularly seen in the cell body of a neurone after damage to the axonal process. As discussed in Chapter 1, necrosis of brain tissue usually results in liquefaction, leaving a fluid-filled space.

Following injury or necrosis, healing through granulation tissue and fibrous scarring does not generally occur owing to a relative lack of fibroblasts in the CNS. Initially, there is an exudative response with activation of local microglia and recruitment of phagocytic monocytes to phagocytose dead tissue. This is followed by proliferation of astrocytes to form an *astrocytic scar*. This process is generally termed *gliosis* and is a common end product of damage to the specialised structures of the CNS. If there is extensive tissue necrosis, for example following infarction, the gliotic response is insufficient to repair the whole defect and a fluid-filled space lined by gliosis remains.

Healing through granulation tissue and collagenous fibrosis occurs in relation to healing of bacterial inflammatory processes such as around a cerebral abscess; it also occurs in disease involving the meninges, such as acute meningitis (Fig. 2.6) and tuberculous meningitis (Fig. 4.9).

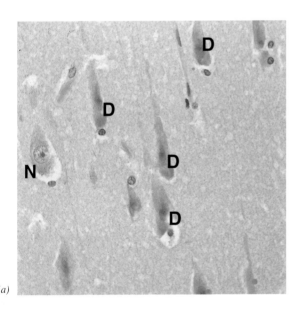

(a)

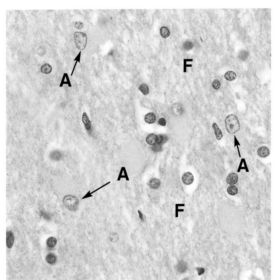

(b)

Fig. 23.1 Neuronal death and astrocytic response
(a) **Early response (HP)** (b) **Later response (HP)**

Neurones are especially vulnerable to hypoxia such as may occur following cardiac or respiratory arrest. At an early stage, dead neurones become shrunken and eosinophilic with pyknosis of the nuclei. This change particularly affects large pyramidal neurones and is shown in micrograph (a) where recently dead neurones **D** in the hippocampus contrast with normal surviving cells **N**. Note that surrounding cells such as oligodendrocytes and astrocytes are unaffected.

Following such damage, dead neurones will be removed by phagocytic cells, and there is associated proliferation of astrocytic cells in the damaged area. This is seen in micrograph (b) which is a similar area of the hippocampus to that shown in micrograph (a), but subject to an episode of hypoxia several weeks earlier. No neurones are seen and the area is replaced by large pink-stained astrocytic cells **A** and their fibres **F**. This process, termed gliosis, is a common end result of damage to neurones in the central nervous system.

Vascular disorders of the CNS

Cerebral arteries are prone to all of the diseases affecting vessels described in Chapter 11, particularly atheroma, arteriosclerosis, thrombosis, aneurysm formation and vasculitis.

The main consequence of disease of cerebral blood vessels is *stroke*, a term used to describe the sudden onset of a persistent focal neurological deficit such as paralysis, disturbance of speech, coordination or sensation. The majority of strokes are owing to *cerebral infarction* as a result of atheroma, thrombosis or embolism. *Cerebral haemorrhage* is also an important cause of stroke and is the consequence of rupture of small intracerebral vessels. A generalised term used clinically to describe these sudden vascular events is *cerebrovascular accident* (commonly abbreviated to *CVA*).

Cerebral infarction may follow thrombosis of a cerebral artery, commonly superimposed on atheroma of cerebral vessels. This is commonly seen in the vertebro-basilar territory resulting in brain stem infarction. Cerebral infarction may also result from occlusion of a vessel by embolus; such emboli most commonly arise from complicated atheroma of the carotid arteries (usually at the bifurcation), from the left side of the heart (frequently from mural thrombus after myocardial infarction), from atrial thrombosis in atrial fibrillation, or from thrombotic vegetations on the aortic or mitral valves. More insidious disease results from progressive arteriosclerosis of small vessels in the brain causing degeneration of white matter with small areas of micro-infarction in the cerebral cortex. This is a common cause of dementia (progressive intellectual deterioration) in the elderly and is termed *multi-infarct dementia*.

Intracerebral haemorrhage is usually a complication of hypertension. The muscular walls of small vessels in the brain are replaced by collagenous tissue and the vessels are then prone to rupture. The three most common sites for intracerebral haemorrhage are in the basal ganglia, the pons and the cerebellum.

Intracranial haemorrhage may also occur from vessels outside the brain. *Subarachnoid haemorrhage* is due to rupture of vessels in the subarachnoid space; the most common reason is rupture of a small aneurysm arising on one of the main cerebral arteries, descriptively termed a *berry aneurysm* (Fig. 11.12). Intracerebral or subarachnoid haemorrhage may also be owing to congenital abnormalities of cerebral vessels forming *arteriovenous malformations*. *Subdural haemorrhage* results from bleeding from fragile veins which traverse the subdural space. This most commonly occurs in the elderly as a result of trauma which may be relatively trivial. *Extradural haemorrhage* is a result of bleeding from arterial vessels outside the dura. This is a common complication of trauma to the head, especially with skull fracture; the middle meningeal artery is most vulnerable.

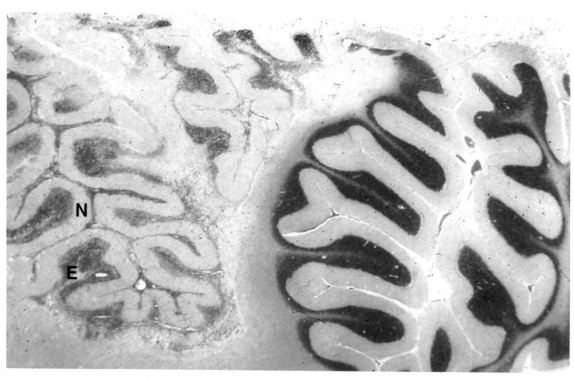

(a)

Fig. 23.2a Cerebral infarction *(caption opposite)*

Fig. 23.2 Cerebral infarction
(a) Early infarct (LP) *(illustration opposite)*
(b) Later infarct (MP)   (c) Old (cystic) infarct (LP)

These three micrographs illustrate important histological features of cerebral infarction.

The earliest histological manifestations involve the neurones which become shrunken, eosinophilic and exhibit nuclear pyknosis. These changes are seen between 6 and 12 hours after infarction and are accompanied by microscopic disruption of small capillary vessels with extravasation of red cells. Unlike other tissues, in cerebral infarction a neutrophilic response is only transient and macrophage infiltration dominates the cellular reaction in necrotic tissue from about 2 days post-infarction. This is accompanied by proliferation of small vessels at the margin of the infarcted territory.

Macroscopically, cerebral infarcts can be either haemorrhagic or 'anaemic' (pale). The haemorrhagic pattern is thought to be caused by blood flowing back into capillaries damaged by the initial ischaemic episode.

Micrograph (a) illustrates an area of infarction in the cerebellum of a patient dying 2 days after infarction. The infarcted area on the left exhibits loss of basophilia because of necrosis **N** of the small neurones of the granular layer and extravasation of erythrocytes **E**.

Following the infarct, organisation and repair take place. The dead tissue becomes infiltrated by macrophages recruited from blood monocytes which phagocytose lipid-rich myelin and take on a foamy appearance. By about 7 to 10 days post-infarction, the infarct has become liquefied and partly cystic. Micrograph (b) shows this phase in a cortical cerebral infarct; the infarcted area **Inf** consists of a homogeneous mass of necrotic tissue with remnants of karyorrhectic nuclei. Surrounding this area is a zone of lipid-containing macrophages **M** and beyond this is a peripheral zone of proliferating astrocytic glial cells and blood vessels **G**. Glial proliferation (*gliosis*) is the equivalent of granulation tissue in infarcts elsewhere in the body and is intended to fill the infarcted territory. The resulting glial scar is formed not of fibrous tissue but of the cell bodies and processes of astrocytes. This phase lasts up to 2 months post-infarction.

When an infarct is large, the process of gliosis does not completely fill the defect and a cyst-like cavity remains lined by dense astrocytic tissue. Micrograph (c) shows an old cystic infarct in the internal capsule with the central cavity **C** surrounded by glial tissue **G**. There is no neuronal regeneration following a cerebral infarct. Some of the early clinical manifestations of cerebral infarction may be due to oedema occurring in the relatively undamaged tissue at the margins of the infarcted territory. This oedema resolves and explains some of the clinical improvement which a patient may experience with time.

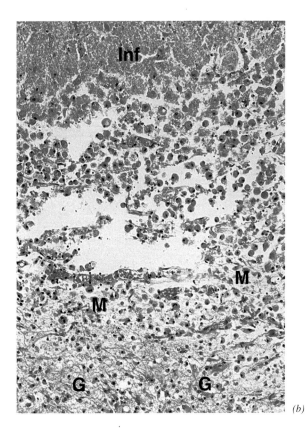

(b)

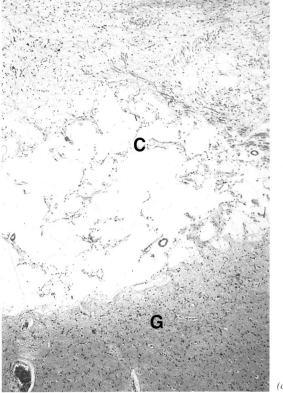

(c)

Degenerative diseases of the CNS

Certain disease of the CNS are characterised by progressive degeneration of neurones, and/or white matter:

- **Alzheimer's disease** causes dementia mainly in the elderly. The disease is of unknown aetiology but there are distinct histological abnormalities (Fig. 23.3) which distinguish the condition from multi-infarct dementia and dementia with Lewy bodies (see below).
- **Parkinson's disease** (Fig. 23.4) causes clinical features of tremor, slow movement and rigidity and is a result of degeneration of nerve cells in the substantia nigra. The cause is unknown.
- **Dementia with Lewy bodies** is clinically similar to Alzheimer's disease and causes dementia. It has brain stem pathology identical to that seen in Parkinson's disease but, in addition, the same type of neuronal pathology destroys cortical neurones and causes dementia.
- **Motor neurone disease** is the result of specific degeneration of motor neurones in the cerebral cortex, brain stem and spinal cord. Cells degenerate over a period of a few years and this results in progressive denervation of muscle with insidious paralysis and death. The cause of this disease is unknown.
- **Creutzfeldt–Jakob disease** (**CJD**) is a cause of rapid dementia resulting from extensive death of neurones in the cerebral cortex (Fig. 23.8). The disease is unique amongst degenerative disease in that a transmissible cause has been demonstrated (**variant CJD**) although poorly characterised. The infective agent, known as *prion protein*, is closely related to that which causes scrapie in sheep and bovine spongiform encephalopathy in cattle.
- **Leukodystrophies** are a group of degenerative diseases of white matter, usually resulting from an inborn error of metabolism; they usually cause progressive neurological impairment in childhood.

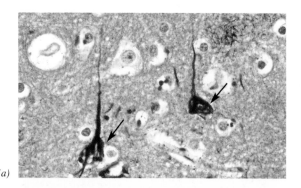

(a)

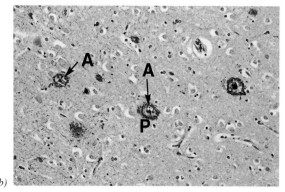

(b)

Fig. 23.3 Alzheimer's disease
(a) Silver stain (HP) (b) Silver stain (MP)

Alzheimer's disease is a cause of dementia usually occurring after the age of 70 years but in some cases at an earlier age. The cause of the disease is unknown; however, there are distinctive changes in the brain which allow the diagnosis to be made histologically.

Macroscopically, there is thinning of gyri (cerebral atrophy), particularly of the frontal and temporal lobes.

As seen in micrograph (a), neurones accumulate abnormal filaments forming flame-shaped skeins termed *neurofibrillary tangles* (arrows). These are composed of tau protein, a microtubule-associated protein.

In addition, there is extracellular deposition of amyloid (see Fig. 5.2) in association with distorted dendrites which form structures termed *senile plaques*. The plaques **P** are deposits of amyloid protein which are associated with distorted nerve cell processes. A peripheral zone of amyloid and neurites **A** is separated from a compact core of amyloid in the mature form of lesion. The amyloid is composed of a fragment of a normal neuronal protein termed β**APP** (beta amyloid precursor protein).

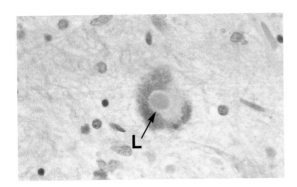

Fig. 23.4 Parkinson's disease (HP)

Parkinson's disease is caused by idiopathic destruction of neurones in the substantia nigra resulting in loss of the neurotransmitter dopamine. Histologically, distinctive inclusions are seen in the remaining neurones.

This specimen, from the substantia nigra of a patient with Parkinson's disease, shows a typical melanin-containing neurone containing a rounded pink-staining inclusion known as a *Lewy body* **L**. These bodies are composed of aggregates of the protein alpha synuclein with other proteins. Similar inclusions occur in neurones of the cerebral cortex in *dementia with Lewy bodies*, which has recently become recognised as a common cause of dementia.

Inflammatory and related conditions of the CNS

Inflammatory processes involving the CNS are divided into those involving the meninges (termed *meningitis*) or the CNS proper (termed *encephalitis* in the brain, *myelitis* in the spinal cord).

Encephalomyelitis and *meningo-encephalitis* describe conditions where a mixed pattern of involvement occurs. Inflammatory diseases are due to bacterial, viral or immunological causes.

Meningitis

Viral meningitis is commonly due to an *enterovirus* and is rarely fatal; it results in a transient lymphocytic response in the meninges.

In contrast, *bacterial meningitis* is a severe life-threatening disease; survivors are commonly left with severe brain damage. The common infective agents are the meningococcus (*Neisseria meningitidis*), the pneumococcus (*Streptococcus pneumoniae*) and *Haemophilus influenzae*.

Histologically, there is an acute purulent neutrophilic response in the meninges with secondary thrombosis of many of the blood vessels supplying the CNS. Treatment with antibiotics may allow recovery; however, healing may be complicated by fibrosis in the meninges.

Tuberculosis may also cause meningitis, which is characterised by a lymphocytic response in the cerebrospinal fluid (CSF) and the formation of caseating granulomas in the meninges (Fig. 4.9). *Fungal meningitis* may be caused by *Cryptococcus* (Fig. 4.22), and is increasingly seen in immunosuppressed patients, for example AIDS. Tertiary syphilis may cause chronic meningitis, the resultant meningeal fibrosis resulting in cranial nerve entrapment.

Encephalitis and myelitis

Encephalitis and myelitis are usually caused by viral infections, some having a particular propensity to affect specific types of neurones. In viral encephalitis or myelitis, there are three main histological features:

- focal neuronal loss and phagocytosis as a direct result of viral infection
- lymphocytic 'cuffing' of vessels with increase in microglial cells; this is because of a local immune response
- astrocytic reaction with increase in number and size of astrocytes in response to loss of neurones.

Herpes viruses cause a severe form of generalised encephalitis with extensive necrosis of brain tissue; this is illustrated in Figure 23.5. In contrast, the *polio virus* tends to attack motor cells of the anterior horn of the spinal cord causing *poliomyelitis* (Fig. 23.6) and for this reason is termed a *neurotropic virus*. *Rabies virus* is also neurotropic and results in a meningo-encephalitis with virus inclusions visible in neuronal cells. *Papovavirus* infection of the CNS occurs in immunosuppressed patients and particularly affects oligodendroglial cells resulting in loss of myelin in white matter; the disease is termed *progressive multifocal leucoencephalopathy*. The *human immunodeficiency virus* (*HIV-1*), which causes AIDS, also affects the CNS and can result in *HIV encephalitis* (Fig. 23.7). Persistent viral infection of the brain occurs in some cases with *measles virus* and results in a chronic degeneration of nerve cells in a disease termed *subacute sclerosing panencephalitis*.

Brain abscesses

Cerebral abscesses may develop as a part of a meningitis or may be the result of direct spread of infection from the middle ear (into the temporal lobe) or of blood-borne spread from an infection elsewhere in the body such as the lung. In cerebral abscesses, there is commonly a mixed infection including anaerobic organisms. Histologically, there is a pus-filled cavity walled off by fibrosis generated through granulation tissue derived from local blood vessels. Around this fibrous cavity wall, there is a reactive astrocytic response.

Fungal infections of the CNS proper are mainly confined to immunosuppressed patients and are most commonly due to *Aspergillus, Zygomycoses* and *Cryptococcus* species; lesions usually take the form of a brain abscess.

Other CNS inflammatory disorders

The CNS is also affected by parasitic infections, particularly *toxoplasmosis*, a disease which affects neonates and increasingly those who are immunosuppressed.

Damage to the CNS may be mediated by immunological mechanisms. The most common pattern is lymphocytic infiltration around blood vessels and immune-mediated destruction and phagocytosis of myelin. One type of disease in which this process is seen is *post-infectious encephalomyelitis*, where the trigger to such an immune reaction is a recent viral infection or vaccination. *Multiple sclerosis* is a much more common disease which is also thought to be mediated by an abnormal immune response causing myelin destruction (Fig. 23.9), although the triggering factor in this disease is as yet unknown.

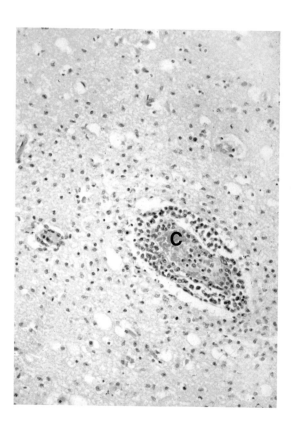

Fig. 23.5 Herpes simplex encephalitis (MP)

Viral encephalitis may be caused by *herpes simplex type 1*, the same virus which causes 'cold sores'. The virus spreads to involve the frontal lobes, limbic system and temporal lobes of the brain. The typical histological features of an encephalitis are seen, namely neuronal death, lymphocytic cuffing of vessels and astrocyte proliferation. There is, however, severe necrosis of the affected areas of brain, which become semi-liquid as macrophages phagocytose dead tissue.

This micrograph shows an area of cortex replaced by a mixture of macrophages and astrocytes (the cytological detail is not discernible at this magnification), with a small vessel cuffed by lymphoid cells **C**. Careful examination of tissue may reveal eosinophilic viral inclusion bodies in nuclei of remaining neurones. Immunofluorescence tests can detect herpes viral antigen and are used diagnostically. Electron microscopy is another method used to detect the virus. Prompt treatment with the drug *acyclovir* may halt progression of the disease; however, late presentation commonly results in death or severe neurological deficit.

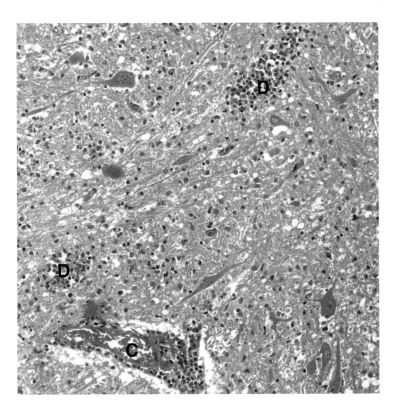

Fig. 23.6 Poliomyelitis (MP)

Although it may cause a diffuse encephalomyelitis, the polio virus most commonly attacks the anterior horn cells of the spinal cord (lower motor neurones), resulting in paralysis of associated skeletal muscle. It may also affect cranial nerve motor nuclei and result in a bulbar paralysis.

Nerve cells are invaded by viral particles and die. The dead cells excite a phagocytic response and are marked by clusters of microglial cells engulfing cellular debris **D**. As with other viral infections of the nervous system, the histological hallmark of lymphocytic vascular cuffing **C** is prominent. The spaces occupied by the destroyed cells are replaced by gliosis.

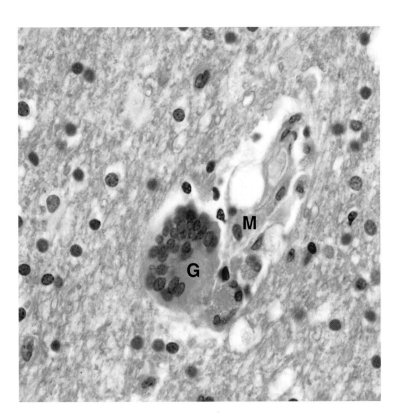

Fig. 23.7 HIV encephalitis (HP)

Neurological dysfunction is very common in AIDS, including opportunistic infections, primary central nervous system lymphoma and direct or indirect effects of the HIV virus itself. One such condition, *HIV encephalitis*, is shown here. The characteristic feature is inflammation of white matter with aggregates of mononuclear cells **M** and associated multinucleate giant cells **G**. These are found throughout the central nervous system, usually close to a small blood vessel, and may be associated with foci of necrosis and reactive gliosis. Virus can be detected within cells in these areas. The clinical features are of insidious dementia, mood disorders and motor abnormalities.

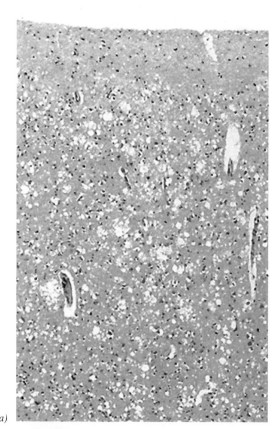

(a)

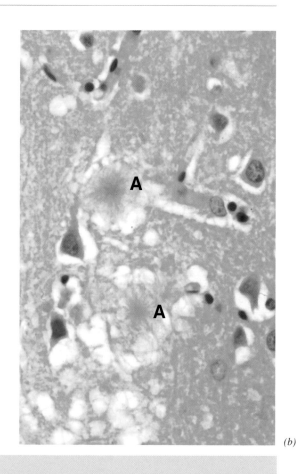

(b)

Fig. 23.8 Prion diseases
(a) Spongiform change in cerebral cortex (LP)
(b) Amyloid plaque in variant Creutzfeldt–Jakob disease (HP)

The prion diseases are also known as the ***transmissible spongiform encephalopathies*** and have a common molecular pathological basis. These include the following neurodegenerative disorders: ***Creutzfeldt–Jakob disease (CJD)*** and ***variant Creutzfeldt–Jakob disease (vCJD)***, ***Gerstmann-Sträussler-Sheinker syndrome (GSS)***, and ***fatal familial insomnia (FFI)***. Prion diseases occur in several species in addition to man, the most notable being scrapie in sheep and bovine spongiform encephalopathy (BSE) in cattle.

These diseases are biologically unique as they are believed to be transmitted by a protein-only agent. Prion protein is a normal cellular protein associated with the cell membrane. In disease it is believed that the three dimensional configuration of the protein becomes altered such that it aggregates in cells and is resistant to degradation. Importantly, it is believed that the abnormal configuration of the protein is able to bring about conversion of normal prion protein to a pathological form, such that disease can be transmitted.

The main pathological changes seen in the nervous system are neuronal loss, vacuolation (termed spongiform change) and astrocytic change and astrocytic gliosis. These features can be seen in micrograph a) where the cerebral cortex shows loss of neurons and is largely replaced by rounded vacuoles. Astrocytic gliosis is best seen if special stains are used to detect astrocyte proliferation. In some cases accumulated prion protein forms plaques of amyloid. This is particularly seen in vCJD as shown in micrograph (b) where plaques of amyloid **A** are surrounded by spongiform change. In vCJD, but not other forms, prion protein accumulates in lymphoid tissues, such as tonsil, where it can be demonstrated using immunohistochemical techniques.

Most human prion diseases occur sporadically. They can, however, be transmitted by inoculation, both to other species and also iatrogenically, from person to person, by corneal transplantation, use of cadaveric dural grafts, neurosurgery with contaminated instruments, and treatment with human growth hormone or gonadotrophins obtained from cadavers. vCJD is believed to have been transmitted to man from BSE in cattle through consumption of contaminated beef. In addition, several human prion diseases can be inherited in an autosomal dominant fashion if there are mutations in the prion gene that give rise to an abnormal protein configuration. Importantly, protein derived from a genetic cause can transmit disease by innoculation.

In a health care setting, prion diseases represent a potential biological hazard mainly from inoculation and so autopsy and histological procedures have to be carried out to appropriate health and safety standards.

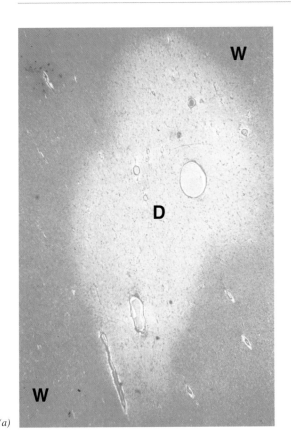

(a)

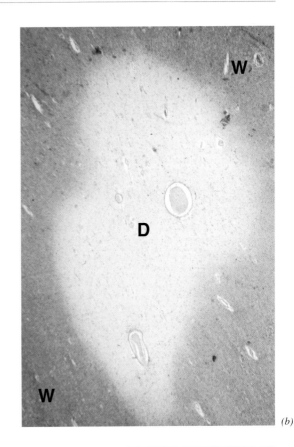

(b)

Fig. 23.9 Multiple (disseminated) sclerosis
(a) H&E stain (LP)   (b) Loyez staining method (LP)

Multiple sclerosis is a disease caused by the selective destruction of myelin in the central nervous system; hence it is termed a *demyelinating disease*. It is postulated that there is an abnormal immunological reaction in the central nervous system, possibly triggered by a viral infection, resulting in focal myelin destruction.

There are three histological stages in the demyelinating process. First, during an acute episode, myelin breakdown occurs associated with lymphocyte and macrophage infiltration of the affected area which is termed a *plaque*; at this stage there is clinical evidence of focal neurological dysfunction. Although this process is directed against myelin, secondary damage to axons also occurs. In the second phase of the process, astrocytes proliferate and gradually infiltrate the demyelinated area which exhibits continued evidence of lymphocytic infiltration. In the final phase of evolution of the plaque, cellularity is reduced, astrocytes shrink in size, and the process becomes 'burnt out'.

Macroscopically, areas of old demyelination appear as pale-grey, rubbery, sharply defined areas in the white matter.

Micrograph (a) shows the typical H&E appearance of an established focus of demyelination. The pale-staining demyelinated area **D** is easily distinguished from the normal-staining white matter **W**. Micrograph (b) illustrates the same lesion stained by a method to demonstrate myelin; the demyelinated area is unstained.

Multiple sclerosis runs a variable but usually prolonged course characterised by periods of focal demyelination which are disseminated both in location within the central nervous system and time of occurrence. During episodes of active demyelination, focal neurological signs often appear, but at times of remission there may be partial or even complete resolution of the neurological deficit, possibly as a result of resolution of inflammatory oedema surrounding the active lesions.

Tumours of the CNS

Primary tumours of the CNS arise from four main cell types: neurones and their precursors, glial cells, meningeal arachnoidal cells and lymphoreticular cells. Primary tumours of the nervous system vary greatly in behaviour from slow-growing (*low grade*) to rapidly growing (*high grade*). They exert harmful effects by growing into vital structures or by causing swelling of the brain around the tumour resulting in secondary compression of vital structures. The different types of primary brain tumour have preferred sites of origin and patterns of age incidence which are summarised in Figure 23.10.

Fig. 23.10 Primary tumours of the CNS				
Tumour	**Cell of origin**	**Site**	**Age**	**Behaviour**
Oligodendroglioma	Oligodendrocyte	Hemisphere	Adulthood	Low to high grade
Astrocytoma	Astrocyte	Hemisphere Cerebellum	Adulthood Childhood	Low to high grade Low grade
Glioblastoma multiforme	Astrocyte	Hemisphere	Adulthood	High grade
Ependymoma	Ependyma	IVth ventricle Spinal cord	Childhood Adulthood	High grade Low grade
Meningioma	Arachnoidal	Meninges	Adulthood	Low grade
Medulloblastoma	Neuroectoderm	Cerebellum	Childhood	High grade
Haemangioblastoma	Unknown	Cerebellum	All ages	Low grade
Lymphoma	Lymphocyte	Hemisphere	Adulthood	High grade

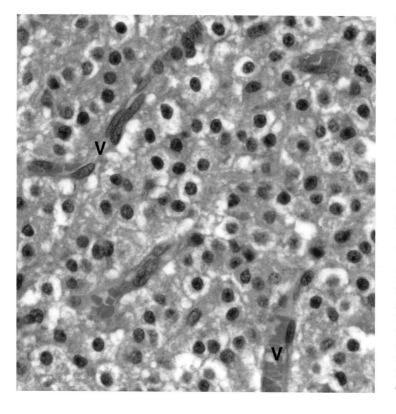

Fig. 23.11 Oligodendroglioma (HP)

These tumours are most commonly seen in the cerebral hemispheres; they are believed to derive from oligodendrocytes on the basis of cytological similarity and recent evidence of expression of lineage-specific markers. The tumour is composed of homogeneous sheets of cells with uniform rounded nuclei, a vacuolated cytoplasm forming a 'halo' around each nucleus and a network of finely branching small blood vessels **V**. Microscopic foci of calcification are frequently seen.

. While many oligodendrogliomas behave in a relatively low grade manner, the presence of nuclear pleomorphism, necrosis, a high mitotic count and endothelial proliferation in blood vessels is associated with rapid growth and recurrence. Tumours exhibiting such features are termed *anaplastic oligodendrogliomas*.

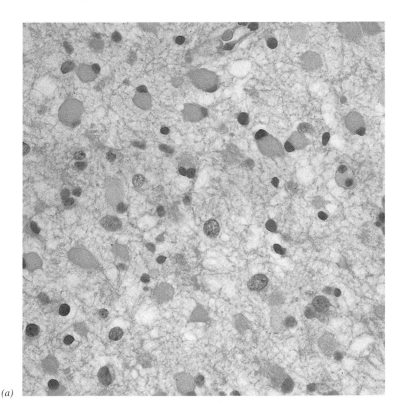

(a)

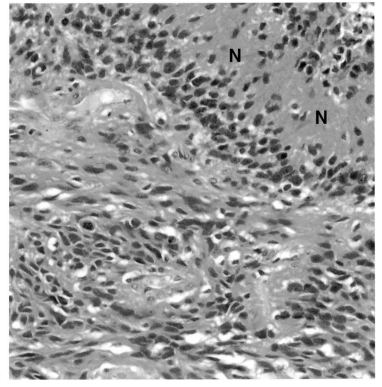

(b)

BASIC SYSTEMS PATHOLOGY

Fig. 23.12 Tumours of astroglial origin
(a) Low grade astrocytoma (HP)
(b) Glioblastoma multiforme (MP)

There is a spectrum of differentiation in tumours of astroglial origin from low grade (benign) to high grade (malignant).

A *low grade astrocytoma* in the cerebral hemispheres is illustrated in micrograph (a). Tumour cells have pink cytoplasm and cellular processes characteristic of astrocytic cells. Low grade astrocytomas do not exhibit great cellularity and show no necrosis or endothelial proliferation in blood vessels.

Glioblastoma multiforme is a tumour composed of pleomorphic glial cells of varying sizes. As seen in micrograph (b), these vary from small cells which exhibit little tendency to differentiation, to cells exhibiting astrocytic morphology, through to large bizarre giant tumour cells. Necrosis **N** is a typical feature of this type of tumour, together with a high cellularity and proliferation of endothelial cells in blood vessels. These tumours have a very poor prognosis even when treated by surgery and radiotherapy.

In between these two extremes are astrocytomas which exhibit high cellularity, mitotic activity and endothelial proliferation in blood vessels. These are termed *anaplastic astrocytomas* and have an intermediate rate of growth and recurrence.

Astrocytic tumours can be graded according to histological criteria. The St. Anne/Mayo scheme evaluates cellular pleomorphism, mitoses, vascular proliferation and necrosis, and is used to establish tumour grade for astroglial tumours in the cerebral hemispheres. Using these criteria, the tumour in micrograph (a) is Grade II, and that in micrograph (b) is Grade IV.

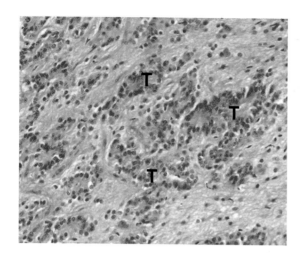

Fig. 23.13 Ependymoma (HP)

These tumours are derived from the ependymal cells which normally line the ventricular system. Histologically, the tumour cells are uniform and arranged around blood vessels leaving a perivascular 'nuclear free zone'. In addition, areas of tumour form epithelial tubules **T** which recapitulate the structure of the central canal of the spinal cord.

Ependymomas are most commonly seen in the region of the fourth ventricle and are also the commonest intrinsic tumour of the spinal cord in childhood. Tumours range from low grade lesions to high grade (anaplastic) ependymomas. There is a propensity for tumour to spread via the leptomeninges, seeding via the CSF pathways.

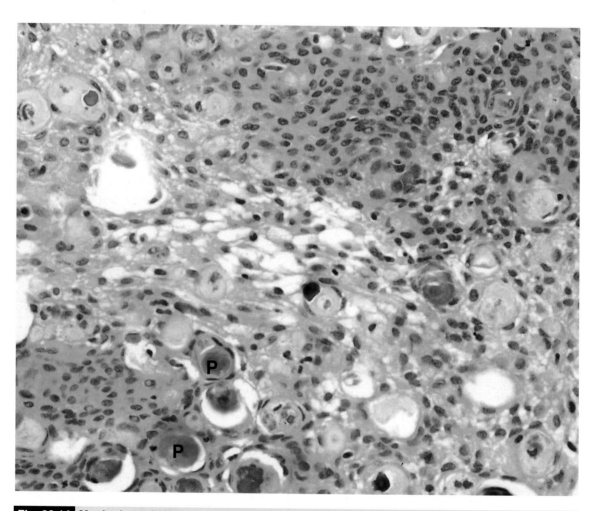

Fig. 23.14 Meningioma (HP)

Meningiomas are thought to arise from arachnoidal epithelial cells of the meninges and are common tumours in adults. The tumours are nearly always benign and produce symptoms by slow compression of underlying brain or spinal cord. There are several histological patterns of meningioma varying from epithelial-type lesions to spindle-cell lesions.

This micrograph illustrates a meningioma composed of a mixture of spindle cells and epithelial cells arranged in whorls. At the centre of the whorls there may be areas of calcification termed *psammoma bodies* **P**. Mitotic figures are not common in meningiomas. While most are benign, some meningiomas show mitotic activity and areas of necrosis, and are then termed *atypical meningiomas*. Such tumours are prone to regrowth as local recurrences.

Disorders of peripheral nerves

Diseases of the peripheral nerves, *peripheral neuropathies*, result in abnormal motor or sensory function in the territory of the nerve affected. There are two main patterns of disease. *Axonal neuropathies* are due to primary damage to axons, while *demyelinating neuropathies* are because of primary damage to Schwann cells and myelin.

Generalised peripheral neuropathies may be found in association with a variety of diseases such as diabetes mellitus, lead poisoning, alcoholism, uraemia and some malignancies. Several specific peripheral neuropathy syndromes are associated with segmental loss of myelin; these include *post-infectious polyneuropathy (Guillain-Barré syndrome)*, and a large group of *hereditary sensory-motor neuropathies*. Axonal degeneration underlies other causes of peripheral neuropathy, for example those due to toxins, trauma or ischaemia. As a world problem, an important cause of peripheral nerve disease is leprosy (Fig. 4.12) in which nerve trunks are infiltrated by large numbers of macrophages filled with *Mycobacterium leprae* with resulting loss of nerve fibres.

Tumours of peripheral nerve are common and are derived from Schwann cells (the cells forming peripheral myelin sheaths) and perineurial cells; examples are shown in Figures 23.15 and 23.16.

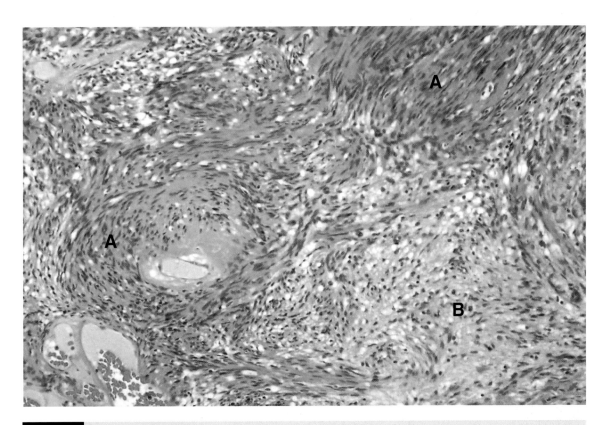

Fig. 23.15 Schwannoma (MP)

These tumours, derived from Schwann cells, typically arise in peripheral nerves; they are commonly seen arising from the eighth cranial nerve when they are termed *acoustic neuromas*.

There are two patterns of growth seen histologically. Compact areas of spindle cells with pink cytoplasm forming palisades and whorls are termed *Antoni A tissue* **A**, while degeneration in the tumour results in loosely arranged vacuolated tumour areas termed *Antoni B tissue* **B**.

Schwannomas are usually solitary, rounded tumours found in relation to nerve trunks. They are benign and usually slow growing. Schwannomas arising from the acoustic nerve (acoustic neuromas) can be part of the syndrome of neurofibromatosis type 2.

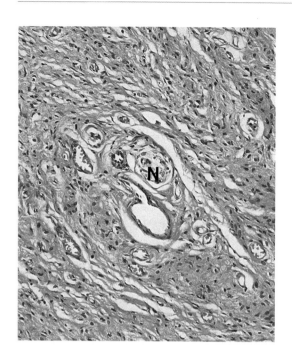

Fig. 23.16 Neurofibroma (HP)

The *neurofibroma* is a tumour of peripheral nerves derived from perineurial cells. Tumours may be solitary but are frequently multiple, especially in the genetically determined disease *neurofibromatosis type 1* (Von Recklinghausen's disease). Lesions on peripheral nerves are visible as subcutaneous nodules; lesions on spinal nerve roots within the spinal canal may cause spinal cord compression.

Histologically, the tumour is composed of loosely arranged spindle cells with varying amounts of intervening collagen. A frequent feature is accumulation of connective tissue mucopolysaccharides resulting in a gelatinous or myxoid tumour. In contrast to the schwannoma, neurofibromas expand the nerve trunks in a diffuse manner; as in this micrograph, it is possible to identify axons and nerve fibres of the underlying nerve **N**. Neurofibromas are benign tumours; however, malignant tumours may also arise from perineurial cells when they are termed *neurofibrosarcomas*.

Disorders of skeletal muscle

Diseases of skeletal muscle present clinically with weakness, wasting of muscle, or pain on exercise. These symptoms and signs can be either due to primary disease of muscle (*myopathy*) or may be secondary to degeneration in the innervation of the muscle (*denervation*); for this latter reason, muscle diseases are commonly considered together with diseases of the nervous system. Histology often provides the only satisfactory method for distinguishing between myopathies and certain neuropathies.

Myopathies can be classified according to aetiology into three main groups:

- **muscular dystrophies** – genetically determined skeletal muscle disorders
- **myositis** – inflammatory diseases
- **myopathies secondary to systemic diseases**.

The muscular dystrophies are characterised by degeneration of muscle fibres resulting in muscle wasting and weakness. There are several syndromes differing in age and sex incidence, time of onset and clinical course. It is now recognised that many are due to mutations in genes coding for structural proteins in muscle: *Duchenne muscular dystrophy* is shown in Figure 23.17. Histologically, there are abnormalities of size and internal structure of muscle fibres, often associated with fibrous replacement of damaged muscle.

Myositis is most commonly due to immunologically mediated muscle damage in a disease termed *polymyositis* (Fig. 23.18). Cushing's disease, thyrotoxicosis and carcinomatosis may be associated with muscle weakness and wasting secondary to the systemic disease process. An example of *neurogenic muscular atrophy* (Fig. 23.19) completes the chapter.

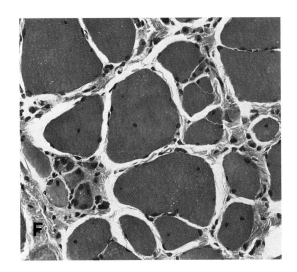

Fig. 23.17 Duchenne muscular dystrophy (HP)

This form of dystrophy is an X-linked recessive trait and thus almost exclusively manifest in boys. Symptoms of proximal muscular weakness develop early in childhood causing difficulty in standing up.

Histologically, there is destruction of muscle fibres with replacement of the muscle by fibrous tissue **F**. Residual muscle fibres exhibit a markedly abnormal variation in fibre size because of atrophy of some and hypertrophy of others. As the disease progresses, the muscle becomes virtually replaced by fibrosis and later adipose tissue. This gives rise to apparent swelling of the affected muscles and accounts for the *pseudohypertrophy* of the calf muscles seen in affected children.

Duchenne dystrophy has a relentless course and results in death in early adult life. Other forms of muscular dystrophy may have a more benign clinical course.

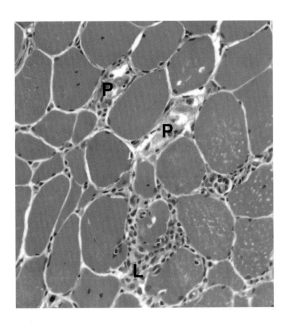

Fig. 23.18 Polymyositis (HP)

As seen in this muscle biopsy, *polymyositis* is characterised by necrosis of individual muscle fibres, associated with lymphoid infiltration **L** and phagocytosis **P** of muscle fibre debris. The disease is believed to be autoimmune in origin and can be treated by immunosuppression. Clinically, patients develop muscle weakness and have an elevated serum creatine kinase level, reflecting active muscle necrosis.

Dermatomyositis is another form of inflammatory myopathy associated with characteristic skin rashes.

Inclusion body myositis is a further common form of inflammatory muscle disease, typically seen in the elderly, with pathological features of muscle fibre necrosis and inflammation. The affected muscle fibres also show characteristic intracellular inclusion bodies. In contrast to polymyositis and dermatomyositis, this form of disease is generally not responsive to immunosuppressive therapy.

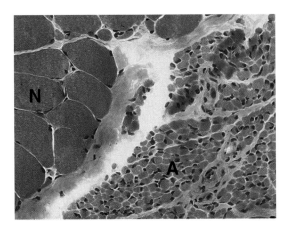

Fig. 23.19 Neurogenic muscular atrophy (HP)

Weakness and wasting of skeletal muscle may occur as a result of lower motor neurone damage rather than primary muscle disease. Histologically, *neurogenic muscle atrophy* affects groups of muscle fibres supplied by damaged motor neurones in contrast to the haphazard pattern of atrophy seen in the muscular dystrophies.

In this micrograph, normal sized fibres **N** contrast sharply with a large group of atrophic fibres **A** from a denervated motor unit. This is an example of *spinal muscular atrophy* in which there is loss of spinal anterior horn cells. Similar changes are seen in a variety of peripheral nerve diseases.

Notes on commonly used staining methods

● Haematoxylin and eosin (H&E)

This is the most commonly used stain in animal histology and routine pathology. Haematoxylin is a dye which stains acidic structures a purplish blue, and eosin a dye which stains basic structures pinkish-red. In the animal cell, most of the acidic structures reside in the nucleus due to nuclear DNA, whereas most of the cytoplasmic structures are basic. Thus nuclei stain purplish-blue, and cytoplasm is pinkish-red unless the cell contains abundant RNA, in which case there may be a purplish tint to the cytoplasmic staining (e.g., plasma cells – see Fig. 3.2).

The intensity of cell staining by H&E depends on many factors, including the particular formulation of the H&E stain (there are many recipes), but the thickness of the tissue section is most important; you will note that the staining intensity is greater when we have used thick sections (e.g. Fig. 13.21c) for low power pictures than when we have used very thin sections for very high power pictures (e.g. Fig. 13.21d).

● PAS and DPAS (periodic acid–Schiff and diastase periodic acid–Schiff)

The periodic acid–Schiff (PAS) reaction essentially demonstrates complex carbohydrates by staining them an attractive magenta colour. Not only does it stain pure complex carbohydrates such as glycogen, it also stains carbohydrates which are complexed with proteins and lipids. Many of these complexes are present in animal tissues as structural proteins, for example in basement membranes (see Fig. 15.9e), fungal cell walls (see Fig. 4.19), and mucins secreted by some epithelial cells. Staining due to glycogen can be eradicated by pretreatment of the tissue section by the specific enzyme, diastase (amylase).

● Ziehl–Neelson and Wade–Fite stains

These two stains are used to demonstrate bacteria belonging to the Mycobacterium group, which all possess a protective capsule containing lipids which affect the rate at which dyes move into and out of the bacterium during staining. Two dyes are used, basic fuchsin mixed with phenol, and methylene blue. The first dye (which is red) is forced into all the tissues in the section (including any Mycobacteria) by heating. The section is then exposed to acid and alcohol which wash the red dye out of everything except the Mycobacteria, which hold onto it because of the lipid capsule. All the other tissues are then free to take up the contrasting blue dye, but the Mycobacteria remain red against a blue background (see Fig. 4.11).

● Giemsa stain

Although this stain is mainly used in a slightly modified form to stain red and white blood cells in blood and bone marrow smears, it can also be used to demonstrate some microorganisms (see Fig. 13.7b).

● Gram stain

This method is mainly used in smears of bacteria in diagnostic microbiology, but can also be used in histological sections to show whether any bacteria present are Gram-positive or Gram-negative (see Fig. 11.8b).

● Congo Red and Sirius Red

These two dyes have a special affinity for proteins with a β-pleated sheet pattern, for example, amyloid. Amyloid stains red with both methods (see Fig. 5.3b), and shows an apple green birefringence when examined by polarizing microscopy.

● Van Gieson

This is a method which uses two coloured solutions, picric acid (yellow) and acid fuchsin (red) as a mixture. The acid fuchsin stains collagen orangey-red, and all other tissues yellow (see Fig. 14.9c). Now rarely used on its own, it is more frequently combined with a stain for elastin (***Elastic-van Gieson***). This method is particularly useful for the staining of arteries because it clearly distinguishes between the elastic lamina (black), the smooth muscle of the tunica media (yellow) and collagen (red) (see Fig. 11.12). It is also used to demonstrate the mixture of collagen and elastic fibres in the dermis of the skin.

● Perls stain

This old method is used to demonstrate the presence of ferric iron in tissues, usually at the site of old bleeding where the iron-containing pigment, haemosiderin (which is derived from local haemoglobin breakdown), accumulates. It is also used to demonstrate the excess accumulation of iron in various tissues in the primary iron-storage disease, haemochromatosis (see Fig. 14.10).

● Goldner's trichrome

This method was developed for use in resin sections of undecalcified bone in the elucidation of metabolic bone disease such as osteomalacia and Paget's disease. It uses a combination of different dyes which distinguish between calcified bone (blue green colour) and uncalcified osteoid (orange red colour). Haematoxylin stains the nuclei of osteoblasts and osteoclasts, so that the level of cellular activity can also be assessed (see Fig. 22.2).

● Silver methods

Many histological staining methods use silver salts such as silver nitrate in solution to demonstrate a wide range of structures, including fungi and cells and fibres, particularly cells and fibres in the central nervous system. In general, these methods can be temperamental, and are becoming less popular. Some examples are shown in Figs 4.20d, 23.3.

● **Loyez haematoxylin method**
Haematoxylin is a very versatile dye, and in the past was used to demonstrate a wide range of specific structures. The Loyez method is an iron haematoxylin method which demonstrates myelin (see Fig. 23.9b).

● **Immunocytochemical and immunofluorescent methods**
One of the great advances in histotechnology has been the development of these methods. The details are complicated, but basically a specific monoclonal antibody is raised against a specific chemical in the tissues. This is then applied to a tissue section and the antibody binds selectively to any of its specific antigen in the tissue. The site of this antibody binding is visualised using either a fluorescent or a coloured marker. Using techniques such as this, it is possible to localise substances such as insulin and other hormones, immunoglobulins, and a wide range of other substances within tissues (see Figs 13.17b and 15.4b).

Index